GENES, BRAIN, AND BEHAVIOR

Research Publications:
Association for Research in Nervous and Mental Disease
Volume 69

ASSOCIATION FOR RESEARCH IN NERVOUS AND MENTAL DISEASE

OFFICERS 1989

Paul R. McHugh, M.D.
President
The Johns Hopkins University
School of Medicine
Baltimore, MD

Ivan Bodis-Wollner, M.D.
Secretary-Treasurer
Mt. Sinai School of Medicine
New York, NY

Daniel Moros, M.D.
Assistant Secretary-Treasurer
Mt. Sinai School of Medicine
New York, NY

TRUSTEES

Melvin D. Yahr, M.D.
Chairman

Shervert Frazier, M.D.
Seymour Kety, M.D.
Paul R. McHugh, M.D.
Robert Michels, M.D.
Herbert Pardes, M.D.
Fred Plum, M.D.
Herman van Praag, M.D.
Dominick Purpura, M.D.
Lewis P. Rowland, M.D.
Albert J. Stunkard, M.D.
Stephen G. Waxman, M.D.

Honorary Trustee
Clarence C. Hare, M.D.

COMMISSION—1989

David Botstein, Ph.D.
San Francisco, CA

Susan Folstein, M.D.
Baltimore, MD

Uta Francke, M.D.
Stanford, CA

James F. Gusella, Ph.D.
Charlestown, MA

Kenneth K. Kidd, Ph.D.
New Haven, CT

Louis M. Kunkel, Ph.D.
Boston, MA

Paul R. McHugh, M.D.
Baltimore, MD

Victor A. McKusick, M.D.
Baltimore, MD

Robert Plomin, Ph.D.
University Park, PA

Reed E. Pyeritz, M.D., Ph.D.
Baltimore, MD

Lewis P. Rowland, M.D.
New York, NY

Douglas C. Wallace, Ph.D.
Atlanta, GA

Genes, Brain, and Behavior

Research Publications:
Association for Research in Nervous and Mental Disease
Volume 69

Editors

Paul R. McHugh, M.D.
Department of Psychiatry
The Johns Hopkins University School of Medicine
Baltimore, Maryland

Victor A. McKusick, M.D.
Department of Medical Genetics
The Johns Hopkins University School of Medicine
Baltimore, Maryland

Raven Press ◆ New York

Raven Press, Ltd., 1185 Avenue of the Americas, New York, New York 10036

© 1991 by Raven Press, Ltd. All rights reserved. This book is protected by copyright. No part of it may be reproduced, stored in a retrieval system, or transmitted, in any form or by any means, electronic, mechanical, photocopy, or recording, or otherwise, without the prior written permission of the publisher.

Made in the United States of America

Library of Congress Cataloging-in-Publication Data

Genes, brain, and behavior / editors, Paul R. McHugh, Victor A. McKusick.
    p.   cm. — (Research publications / Association for Research in Nervous and Mental Disease ; v. 69)
    Includes bibliographical references.
    Includes index.
    ISBN 0-88167-725-6
    1. Mental illness—Genetic aspects. 2. Nervous system—Diseases—Genetic aspects. I. McHugh, Paul R. (Paul Rodney), 1931– . II. McKusick, Victor A. (Victor Almon), 1921– . III. Series: Research publications (Association for Research in Nervous and Mental Disease) ; v. 69.
    [DNLM: 1. Mental Disorders—genetics. 2. Nervous System Diseases—genetics. W1 RE233P v. 69 / WM 100 G3265]
RC455.4.G4G43   1991
616.8′0442—dc20
DNLM/DLC
for Library of Congress   90-8978
                                                                                                                            CIP

    The material contained in this volume was submitted as previously unpublished material, except in the instances in which credit has been given to the source from which some of the illustrative material was derived.
    Great care has been taken to maintain the accuracy of the information contained in the volume. However, neither Raven Press nor the editors can be held responsible for errors or for any consequences arising from the use of the information contained herein.
    Materials appearing in this book prepared by individuals as part of their official duties as U.S. Government employees are not covered by the above-mentioned copyright.

9 8 7 6 5 4 3 2 1

RESEARCH PUBLICATIONS: ASSOCIATION FOR RESEARCH IN NERVOUS AND MENTAL DISEASE

I.	(1920)	*ACUTE EPIDEMIC ENCEPHALITIS (LETHARGIC ENCEPHALITIS)
II.	(1921)	*MULTIPLE SCLEROSIS (DISSEMINATED SCLEROSIS)
III.	(1923)	*HEREDITY IN NERVOUS AND MENTAL DISEASE
IV.	(1924)	THE HUMAN CEREBROSPINAL FLUID
V.	(1925)	*SCHIZOPHRENIA (DEMENTIA PRAECOX)
VI.	(1926)	*THE CEREBELLUM
VII.	(1922)	*EPILEPSY AND THE CONVULSIVE STATE (PART I)
	(1929)	*EPILEPSY AND THE CONVULSIVE STATE (PART II)
VIII.	(1927)	*THE INTRACRANIAL PRESSURE IN HEALTH AND DISEASE
IX.	(1928)	*THE VEGETATIVE NERVOUS SYSTEM
X.	(1929)	*SCHIZOPHRENIA (DEMENTIA PRAECOX) (COMMUNICATION OF VOL. V)
XI.	(1930)	*MANIC-DEPRESSIVE PSYCHOSIS
XII.	(1931)	*INFECTIONS OF THE CENTRAL NERVOUS SYSTEM
XIII.	(1932)	*LOCALIZATION OF FUNCTION IN THE CEREBRAL CORTEX
XIV.	(1933)	*THE BIOLOGY OF THE INDIVIDUAL
XV.	(1934)	*SENSATION: ITS MECHANISMS AND DISTURBANCES
XVI.	(1935)	*TUMORS OF THE NERVOUS SYSTEM
XVII.	(1936)	*THE PITUITARY GLAND
XVIII.	(1937)	*THE CIRCULATION OF THE BRAIN AND SPINAL CORD
XIX.	(1938)	*THE INTER-RELATIONSHIP OF MIND AND BODY
XX.	(1939)	*HYPOTHALAMUS AND CENTRAL LEVELS OF AUTONOMIC FUNCTION
XXI.	(1940)	*THE DISEASE OF THE BASAL GANGLIA
XXII.	(1941)	*THE ROLE OF NUTRITIONAL DEFICIENCY IN NERVOUS AND MENTAL DISEASE
XXIII.	(1942)	*PAIN
XXIV.	(1943)	*TRAUMA OF THE CENTRAL NERVOUS SYSTEM
XXV.	(1944)	*MILITARY NEUROPSYCHIATRY
XXVI.	(1946)	*EPILEPSY
XXVII.	(1947)	*THE FRONTAL LOBES
XXVIII.	(1948)	*MULTIPLE SCLEROSIS AND THE DEMYELINATING DISEASES
XXIX.	(1948)	*LIFE STRESS AND BODILY DISEASE
XXX.	(1950)	*PATTERNS OF ORGANIZATION IN THE CENTRAL NERVOUS SYSTEM
XXXI.	(1951)	*PSYCHIATRIC TREATMENT
XXXII.	(1952)	*METABOLIC AND TOXIC DISEASE OF THE NERVOUS SYSTEM
XXXIII.	(1953)	*GENETICS AND THE INHERITANCE OF INTEGRATED NEUROLOGICAL PSYCHIATRIC PATTERNS
XXXIV.	(1954)	*NEUROLOGY AND PSYCHIATRY IN CHILDHOOD
XXXV.	(1955)	*NEUROLOGIC AND PSYCHIATRIC ASPECTS OF DISORDERS OF AGING
XXXVI.	(1956)	*THE BRAIN AND HUMAN BEHAVIOR
XXXVII.	(1957)	*THE EFFECT OF PHARMACOLOGIC AGENTS ON THE NERVOUS SYSTEM
XXXVIII.	(1958)	*NEUROMUSCULAR DISORDERS
XXXIX.	(1959)	*MENTAL RETARDATION
XL.	(1960)	*ULTRASTRUCTURE AND METABOLISM OF THE NERVOUS SYSTEM
XLI.	(1961)	*CEREBROVASCULAR DISEASE
XLII.	(1962)	*DISORDERS OF COMMUNICATION
XLIII.	(1963)	*ENDOCRINES AND THE CENTRAL NERVOUS SYSTEM
XLIV.	(1964)	*INFECTIONS OF THE NERVOUS SYSTEM

XLV.	(1965)	*SLEEP AND ALTERED STATES OF CONSCIOUSNESS
XLVI.	(1968)	*ADDICTIVE STATES
XLVII.	(1969)	SOCIAL PSYCHIATRY
XLVIII.	(1970)	*PERCEPTION AND ITS DISORDERS
XLIX.	(1971)	*IMMUNOLOGICAL DISORDERS OF THE NERVOUS SYSTEM
50.	(1972)	NEUROTRANSMITTERS
51.	(1973)	BIOLOGICAL AND ENVIRONMENTAL DETERMINANTS OF EARLY DEVELOPMENT
52.	(1974)	AGGRESSION
53.	(1974)	BRAIN DYSFUNCTION IN METABOLIC DISORDERS
54.	(1975)	BIOLOGY OF THE MAJOR PSYCHOSES: A COMPARATIVE ANALYSIS
55.	(1976)	THE BASAL GANGLIA
56.	(1978)	THE HYPOTHALAMUS
57.	(1979)	CONGENITAL AND ACQUIRED COGNITIVE DISORDERS
58.	(1980)	PAIN
59.	(1981)	BRAIN, BEHAVIOR, AND BODILY DISEASE
60.	(1983)	GENETICS OF NEUROLOGICAL AND PSYCHIATRIC DISORDERS
61.	(1983)	EPILEPSY
62.	(1984)	EATING AND ITS DISORDERS
63.	(1985)	BRAIN IMAGING AND BRAIN FUNCTION
64.	(1986)	NEUROPEPTIDES IN NEUROLOGIC AND PSYCHIATRIC DISORDERS
65.	(1987)	MOLECULAR NEUROBIOLOGY IN NEUROLOGY AND PSYCHIATRY
66.	(1988)	LANGUAGE, COMMUNICATION, AND THE BRAIN
67.	(1990)	VISION AND THE BRAIN: THE ORGANIZATION OF THE CENTRAL VISUAL SYSTEM
68.	(1990)	IMMUNOLOGIC MECHANISMS IN NEUROLOGIC AND PSYCHIATRIC DISEASE
69.	(1991)	GENES, BRAIN, AND BEHAVIOR

Titles marked with an (*) are out of print.

Preface

This volume has both the characteristics of a course of instruction and a forum for presentation of recent findings. The overall goal is to provide a general understanding of the current status of medical genetics and show how concepts and methods emerging in that discipline can be applied to the study of particular neurological and psychiatric disorders. It, therefore, emphasizes recent conceptual and technical advances in basic science, relates them to a background of knowledge in both biology and general medicine, and displays contemporary achievements in genetics that have rendered neurological and psychiatric problems comprehensible and accessible to better diagnosis, prognosis, and treatment.

In this volume are individuals who are contributing to the contemporary advances in the field and are committed teachers of the subject whose views have shaped the discourse of the discipline of medical genetics. The authors, as well as the readers, will find the means to follow the reasoning and logic of genetics applied to clinical matters and come to appreciate the excitement of the current discoveries in neurology and psychiatry.

With these overall goals and their significance in mind, there are a number of important practical issues that shaped this volume. For example, there are at least two areas of basic science in which clinicians are particularly uncertain. The first is a simple matter of information on the basic issues of the anatomy of chromosomes and their characteristic actions during cell division and gamete formation. This is crucial information in comprehending disorders emerging in individuals and within family groups. These issues are addressed in the first three chapters. They are followed by the chapter by Dr. Pyeritz that emphasizes the importance of clinical assessments in understanding the phenotypes of disorders, indicating that heterogeneity of expression is the rule among human genetic disorders. A clear concept of how psychiatric and neurological genetics is a branch of medical genetics and how that field has emerged with progressive specificity of some fundamental principles over the past 25 years should encourage clinicians by identifying the crucial value of clinical skills in this time when advances in technology seem the only characteristic of genetic research.

The second area of uncertainty is the genetic technology itself. Clinicians are uncertain about a whole variety of issues such as the difference between the human gene map, in which the location of genes on specific chromosomes is defined by several different methods, and the human genome project, in which a complete nucleotide sequencing of the human genome is the goal. Several contributors are employing these technical methods in the direct study of psychiatric and neurological disorders.

In considering the clinical issues that would provide the best examples of the advances in contemporary genetics and the applications of its technology, we thought it was important to cast the net widely in the domains of neurology and psychiatry. Although the title is *Genes, Brain, and Behavior*, and this obviously encompasses clinical conditions such as Alzheimer's disease, Huntington's disease, manic depression, and schizophrenia, the enormous importance of the achievements in the definition of the genetic abnormality in muscular dystrophy also is presented in this volume. The discoveries by Dr. Kunkel in this condition are exciting both as a model of how an abnormal gene is identified and followed through to a comprehension of the molecular pathogenesis of the disorder, and as a crucial issue in contemporary neurological practice.

A major emphasis in this book is on mendelizing conditions because these provide the best illumination of how classical genetic concepts are applied to medical disorders. This emphasis focuses attention on a number of issues such as the importance of pedigrees, LOD scores, the "founder" effect within apparent genetic isolates, phenotypic heterogeneity, genetic heterogeneity, and "reverse" genetics as an approach to pathogenesis.

A variety of other issues are also discussed in this volume. Specifically, Dr. Coyle presents a contemporary study of a chromosome disorder (Down syndrome). Dr. Wallace identifies the place of mitochondrial genetics and the disorders that relate to the mitochondria that give us intriguing insights into pathogenesis from that site that can be compared to the pathogenetic mechanisms tied to nuclear genes. Finally, we focus on behavioral issues both in a general sense of behavioral genetics as an emerging field and in such specific conditions as obesity and alcoholism, where the genetic contributions are becoming more confidently established.

All in all, our attempt in this volume as in other ARNMD volumes, is to emphasize again the importance of the collaboration of basic scientists and clinicians in producing understanding of the nature of neurological and psychiatric diseases and thus providing a rational approach to their treatment and prevention. We believe that the "new genetics" provides our disciplines with analytic tools comparable to those brought to general medicine by bacteriology and microbiology in the past century. The genetic techniques offer a future set of opportunities for the control of these impairing disorders similar to those experienced in the field of infectious disease.

Paul R. McHugh, M.D.
Victor A. McKusick, M.D.

Contents

Basic Genetics

1   Advances in Medical Genetics in the Past 30 Years
    Victor A. McKusick

19   The Chromosome, Its Anatomy, and Its Aberrations
    Teresa L. Yang-Feng

39   Genetic Variation and the Meiotic Process
    Renee Z. Dintzis

47   Formal Genetics in Humans: Mendelian and Nonmendelian Inheritance
    Reed E. Pyeritz

Application of the Basic Genetic Science to Specific Conditions

75   The Search for the Genetic Defects in Huntington's Disease and Familial Alzheimer's Disease
    James F. Gusella

85   Down Syndrome and the Trisomy 16 Mouse: Impact of Gene Imbalance on Brain Development and Aging
    Joseph T. Coyle, Mary Lou Oster-Granite, Roger Reeves, Christine Hohmann, Patrizia Corsi, and John Gearhart

101   Mitochondrial Genes and Neuromuscular Disease
    Douglas C. Wallace

121   Muscular Dystrophy Research: What Have We Learned and Where Do We Go from Here?
    Frederick M. Boyce, Alan H. Beggs, and Louis M. Kunkel

129   Genetics of Alzheimer's Disease
    Marshal F. Folstein and Andrew Warren

137   The Current Status of Linkage Studies in Schizophrenia
    Joel Gelernter and Kenneth Kidd

153   Genetics of Manic Depressive Illness: Current Status and Evolving Concepts
    Miron Baron

Behavioral Expression of Genetic Disorder

165 Behavioral Genetics
Robert Plomin

181 The Psychopathology of Huntington's Disease
Susan E. Folstein

193 Molecular Genetic Analysis of Phenylketonuria and Mental Retardation
Savio L. C. Woo

205 Genetic Contributions to Human Obesity
Albert J. Stunkard

219 The Genetics of Alcoholism
Donald W. Goodwin

227 Subject Index

Contributors

Miron Baron
Department of Psychiatry
Columbia University College of
 Physicians and Surgeons
New York State Psychiatric Institute
722 W. 168th Street
New York, New York 10032

Alan H. Beggs
Division of Genetics and
 Mental Retardation Center
The Children's Hospital
300 Longwood Avenue
Boston, Massachusetts 02115
Department of Pediatrics
Harvard Medical School
Howard Hughes Medical Institute
Boston, Massachusetts 02115

Frederick M. Boyce
Division of Genetics and
 Mental Retardation Center
The Children's Hospital
300 Longwood Avenue
Boston, Massachusetts 02115

Patrizia Corsi
Department of Psychiatry
The Johns Hopkins University
 School of Medicine
Meyer Building 4-163
6700 N. Wolfe Street
Baltimore, Maryland 21205

Joseph T. Coyle
Departments of Psychiatry, Neuroscience,
 Pharmacology, and Pediatrics
The Johns Hopkins University
 School of Medicine
Meyer Building 4-163
6700 N. Wolfe Street
Baltimore, Maryland 21205

Renee Z. Dintzis
Departments of Cell Biology and
 Anatomy, and Biophysics
The Johns Hopkins University
 School of Medicine
Wood Basic Science Building 606A
725 N. Wolfe Street
Baltimore, Maryland 21205

Marshal F. Folstein
Department of Psychiatry
The Johns Hopkins Hospital
Osler 320
600 N. Wolfe Street
Baltimore, Maryland 21205

Susan E. Folstein
Department of Psychiatry
Division of Psychiatric Genetics
The Johns Hopkins University
 School of Medicine
Meyer Building 2-181
600 N. Wolfe Street
Baltimore, Maryland 21205

John Gearhart
The Developmental Genetics Laboratory
 of the Department of Physiology
The Johns Hopkins University
 School of Medicine
700 N. Wolfe Street, Phys. 202
Baltimore, Maryland 21205

Joel Gelernter
Department of Psychiatry
Yale University School of Medicine
333 Cedar Street
New Haven, Connecticut 06510

Donald W. Goodwin
Department of Psychiatry
Kansas University Medical Center
39th and Rainbow Boulevard
Kansas City, Kansas 66103

James F. Gusella
Molecular Neurogenetics Laboratory
Massachusetts General Hospital
Department of Genetics
Harvard University
Boston, Massachusetts 02114

Christine Hohmann
Department of Psychiatry
The Johns Hopkins University
  School of Medicine
Meyer Building 4-163
6700 N. Wolfe Street
Baltimore, Maryland 21205

Kenneth K. Kidd
Departments of Psychiatry
  and Human Genetics
Yale University School of Medicine
333 Cedar Street
New Haven, Connecticut 06510

Louis M. Kunkel
Division of Genetics and Mental
  Retardation Center
The Children's Hospital
300 Longwood Avenue
Boston, Massachusetts 02115
Department of Pediatrics
Harvard Medical School
Howard Hughes Medical Institute
Boston, Massachusetts 02115

Victor A. McKusick
Department of Medical Genetics
The Johns Hopkins University
  School of Medicine
Blalock 1007
600 N. Wolfe Street
Baltimore, Maryland 21205

Mary Lou Oster-Granite
Department of Neuroscience
The Developmental Genetics Laboratory
  of the Department of Physiology
The Johns Hopkins University
  School of Medicine
700 N. Wolfe Street, Phys. 202
Baltimore, Maryland 21205

Robert Plomin
Center for Developmental
  and Health Genetics
College of Health and Human
  Development
The Pennsylvania State University
S211 Henderson Building South
University Park, Pennsylvania 16802

Reed E. Pyeritz
Department of Medicine and Pediatrics
Center for Medical Genetics
The Johns Hopkins University
  School of Medicine
Blalock 1012
600 N. Wolfe Street
Baltimore, Maryland 21205

Roger Reeves
The Developmental Genetics Laboratory
  of the Department of Physiology
The Johns Hopkins University
  School of Medicine
700 N. Wolfe Street, Phys. 202
Baltimore, Maryland 21205

Albert J. Stunkard
Department of Psychiatry
University of Pennsylvania
133 South 36th Street
Suite 507
Philadelphia, Pennsylvania 19104-3246

Douglas C. Wallace
Departments of Biochemistry, Pediatrics,
  and Neurology
Emory University School of Medicine
109 Woodruff Memorial Building
Atlanta, Georgia 30322

Andrew Warren
Department of Psychiatry
The Johns Hopkins Hospital
Osler 320
600 N. Wolfe Street
Baltimore, Maryland 21205

Savio L. C. Woo
Howard Hughes Medical Institute
Department of Cell Biology and Institute
 for Molecular Genetics
Baylor College of Medicine
One Baylor Plaza
Houston, Texas 77030

Teresa L. Yang-Feng
Department of Human Genetics
Yale University School of Medicine
333 Cedar Street
New Haven, Connecticut 06510

Genes, Brain, and Behavior, edited by
P. R. McHugh and V. A. McKusick.
Raven Press, Ltd., New York © 1991.

Advances in Medical Genetics in the Past 30 Years

Victor A. McKusick

Department of Medical Genetics, The Johns Hopkins University School of Medicine, Baltimore, Maryland 21205

Dr. McHugh suggested I write on "Advances in Medical Genetics in the past *25* years." I increased it to 30 because a major change took place in 1959; it was then that clinical cytogenetics had its birth. In that year Lejeune announced the finding of trisomy 21 in Down syndrome (or mongoloid idiocy as it was then called). In rapid succession in those exciting early months of 1959, the chromosome abnormalities of the Turner and Klinefelter syndromes were also described. (These findings demonstrated the role of the Y chromosome in testis determination in the human, i.e., the existence of a testis-determining factor (TDF) coded by the Y—a phenomenon that to this day still awaits elucidation in full detail.)

Actually even 30 years is a bit artificial because it is now 31 years since the Lejeune publication. Furthermore, Lejeune had the information in December 1958, when he visited Baltimore. He was on his way home from Pasadena where, on the invitation of George Beadle, he had given a course on human genetics at Cal Tech in the fall semester. (Speaking little English, he wrote out his lectures verbatim and in the process learned to speak the language.) I remember Lejeune telling a group of us in my living room that he felt certain he knew the nature of the abnormality in mongoloid idiocy. I confess that the significance of the finding escaped me at the time, just as I did not fully appreciate, I fear, the presentation by Tjio and Levan of the correct chromosome number, with exhibition of metaphase spreads, at the first World Congress of Human Genetics in Copenhagen in August 1956.

Before the dawn of clinical cytogenetics, biochemical genetics in humans—both the inborn errors of metabolism conceived by Garrod (1908) and molecular diseases conceived by Pauling (1948)—had added significant dimensions to medical genetics that previously had little more methodology than the construction of pedigrees and little more theoretical basis than the laws of Mendel bolstered by methods of segregation analysis. But the capability to study the chromosomes with some ease gave medical geneticists their organ, just as cardiologists had the heart and neurologists the nervous system. Studies of the chromosomes and especially the mapping of genes to specific chromosomal sites—these are really anatomic approaches—have provided a neo-Vesalian basis for clinical genetics; indeed, as I shall attempt to show, for all of medicine. In 1543, the anatomy text of Vesalius was a turning point for medicine. It turned the profession from useless theorizing to a rugged empiricism. It gave the profession a body of knowledge uniquely its own. It formed the basis for subsequent scientific advances, e.g., the physiology of Harvey (1628) and the morbid anatomy of Morgagni (1761). On a smaller scale, in the past 30 years the development of knowledge about the human genetic anatomy has done the same for clinical genetics and for medicine in general. A leading paradigm for the elucidation of disorders in all areas of medicine is that of "reverse genetics," which starts with determination of the anatomic arrangement of genes on chromosomes.

SOME DEFINITIONS

Medical genetics might be defined as "all of medicine that is genetic and all of genetics that is medical." That may be too inclusive a definition; one may find more useful the following "nested" set of definitions:

Genetics = the science of biologic variation
Human genetics = the science of biologic variation in humans
Medical genetics = the science of human biologic variation as it relates to health and disease
Clinical genetics = that part of medical genetics concerned with the health of individual humans and their families
(Clinical genetics = the science and practice ("art") of diagnosis, prevention, and management of genetic disorders)

It can be argued that medical genetics is a more extensive discipline than human genetics because it is impossible to think of any aspect of human genetics that is not relevant to medical genetics but the converse is not true. I wish, however, to avoid definitions that suggest the existence of a highly categorized specialty, either scientific or clinical. It is true that clinical genetics has become a specialty with "boards" (first given in 1980) and all the other appurtenances of a clinical specialty (1). This is a device for maintaining standards of training and practice and for regulating the use of the increasing diagnostic and therapeutic armamentarium that is at the disposal of clinical genetics. But the medical genetics whose progress in the past 30 years I trace here belongs to all of medicine and, more than a specialty, it is an aggregate of concepts, methods, principles, and fundamental knowledge.

Since the definition of medical genetics should not suggest a narrow specialization, perhaps my first definition is best after all: *Medical genetics is all of medicine that is genetic and all of genetics that is medical.*

I have been in medical genetics for over 40 years (2)—although in the early years I did not realize medical genetics was my field. Indeed, I have been a published medical geneticist for 40 years because my first works on the syndrome of polyps and spots appeared in two successive issues of the *New England Journal of Medicine* in December 1949 (3). Claiming the privilege of seniority, allow me to trace progress in medical genetics in the past 30 years by reviewing the progressive growth during that time of my catalogs of mendelian traits and the two derivative compendia: the human gene map (chromosome-by-chromosome gene lists) and the tabulation of molecular defects in mendelian disorders.

MENDELIAN INHERITANCE IN MAN, AN ENCYCLOPEDIA OF GENE LOCI

I have recounted elsewhere (4) how the catalogs began about 1960 with the listing of X-linked traits (designed to define the genetic constitution of the X chromosome) (5), continued with the autosomal recessive catalog (initially designed as an aid to studies of inbred Amish populations) (6), were completed with the autosomal dominant catalog and were computerized in 1964. Now in its 9th print edition (7), the published book has been computer-based from the beginning. The first three editions (1966, 1968, 1971) were produced by photo-offset of the output of the printer—all uppercase. Beginning with the 4th edition, computer tapes have been used to drive an automatic phototypesetter, which produces conventional typography, thereby resulting in improved legibility and economy of page space. Between editions, the computer files have been continually updated. Since 1985 an "online" version has been maintained and used in connection with a search method that is very useful to the "authoring" process and to the application of the database in the clinic and laboratory. Since August 1987, the online version, OMIM, has been available worldwide from the Welch Medical Library of the Johns Hopkins University via Telenet. This alternative type of "publication" complements, but will not in the near future replace, the "hard copy" edition. OMIM has two advantages over the print version: timeliness and capacity for rapid and exhaustive search of a scope impossible with print indices. MIM has the advantage of portability. The computer-based publication narrows to 4 months the gap between closure of the file for publication and delivery of the finished book. We are now on an every-other-year publication schedule with closure of the file March 1 and availability of books July 1 in even numbered years. The 9th edition became available, on schedule, July 1, 1990.

The entries in *Mendelian Inheritance in Man* have grown from about 1,500 to almost 5,000 over the period of almost 25 years of publication (Fig. 1). The intent is to create only one entry per gene locus. Thus, the numbers give some indication of the portion of the 50,000 to 100,000 genes for which we have some information. In the early days of the catalogs, indeed until relatively recently, the only method we had for identifying genes was by mendelizing phenotypes. In the past few years, an increasing number of entries have been created, when genes were cloned, sequenced, and mapped, even though no mendelizing phenotype had been related to that gene. Some of the genes uncovered by cell biology and molecular genetics are ones we had no inkling of 30 years ago; for example, oncogenes, the genes that normally have important functions in development and differentiation but which when mutated cause cancer.

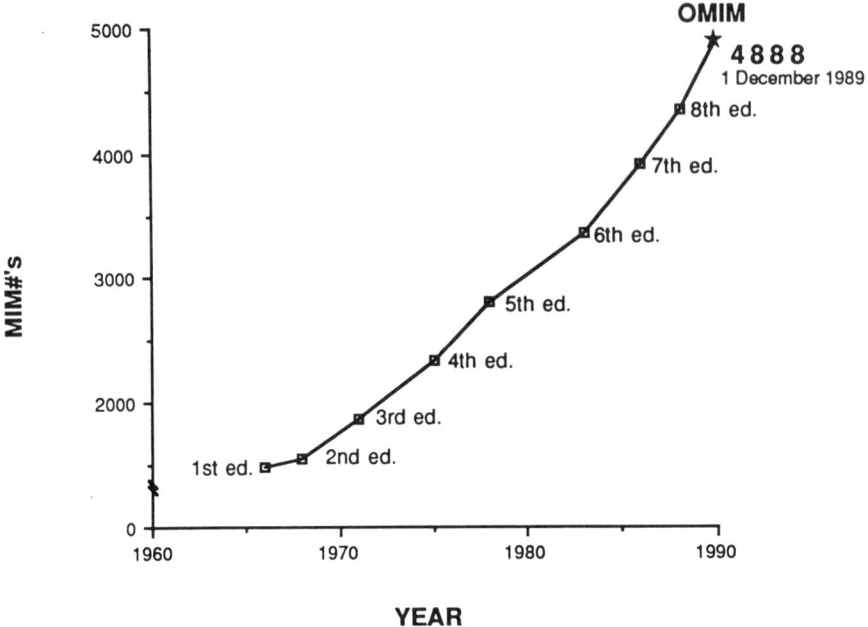

FIG. 1. The growth of *Mendelian Inheritance in Man* through eight print editions and the continuously updated online version (OMIM). Total number of entries graphically illustrated.

In the earlier stages when gene delineation depended on mendelizing phenotypes, the increase in number of entries represented not so much the identification of new major phenotypes, but rather identification of different genetic "causes" of the same phenotype, i.e., the recognition of genetic heterogeneity (Table 1). We had clinical, biochemical, and genetic methods for recognizing heterogeneity within categories such as muscular dystrophy, mental retardation, congenital deafness, and other categories. The mucopolysaccharidoses illustrate the point. In the edition of 1966 (MIM1) I listed 6 types of mucopolysaccharidosis. Types I and II had been distinguished 10 years earlier, in the 1st edition of my *Heritable Disorders of Connective Tissue* (8), on the basis of clinical and genetic differences. The Sanfilippo, Morquio, and Maroteaux-Lamy syndromes had been added later, on the basis of biochemical and clinical differences. A separate entry had been added for Scheie syndrome, or MPS V, but later fibroblast-mixing experiments proved this disorder to be allelic with the Hurler syndrome; the two disorders did not show cross-correction. By the 4th edition the asterisk was removed from MPS V and by the 5th edition (1978) the write-up was "folded into" that for MPS I. This illustrates the counterforces in genetic nosology: splitting and lumping. The principles of genetics force one to think of mutation as a specific etiologic mechanism that results in specific disease entities. In 1930, in his *Nosography*, Knut Faber, professor of medicine in Copenhagen, traced the development of understanding of the classifica-

TABLE 1. *Methods for identifying genetic heterogeneity*

I. Genetic methods
   A. Mode of inheritance. For example, spastic paraplegia and Charcot-Marie-Tooth disease occur in all three major modes: autosomal dominant, autosomal recessive, and X-linked.
   B. Nonallelism of recessive. For example, all children of parents with phenotypically identical recessive congenital deafness may have normal hearing indicating that the parents are homozygous at different loci.
   C. Linkage relationships. For example, one form of Charcot-Marie-Tooth disease linked to chromosome-17 markers, one form to chromosome-1 markers, and yet a third autosomal dominant form is linked to neither.
II. Analysis of phenotype. For example, mucopolysaccharidoses I and II (Hurler and Hunter syndromes, respectively) are distinguishable by the presence or absence of corneal clouding and the severity of the disorder including age at death.
III. Biochemical analysis. For example, hereditary nonspherocytic hemolytic anemia has many different forms, each involving deficiency of a different enzyme.
IV. Physiologic studies. For example, the X-linked hemophilias can be distinguished by mutual cross-correction of the clotting defect *in vitro* and *in vivo*.
V. Studies of cells in culture (somatic cell genetics).
   A. For example, many of the mucopolysaccharidoses are distinguishable by cell-mixing experiments. The defect in degradation of mucopolysaccharides is mutually corrected by transfer of enzymes between cells.
   B. For example, cell hybridization studies permit recognition of distinct forms of xeroderma pigmentosum, depending on whether or not the defect in DNA repair disappears in the heterokaryon. Complementation is usually an indication that the gene defects are at different loci; however, complementation may in some circumstances (e.g., through favorable change in the tertiary structure of a polymeric molecule) occur between cells homozygous for different allelic mutations. For instance, cells from the infantile form of GM1-gangliosidosis complement those from the juvenile or adult type, despite the fact that beta-galactosidase, the enzyme that is deficient in both disorders, has a single species of polypeptide change. Another example: Conversely, lack of complementation is not incontrovertible proof of identity or allelism. The fibroblasts of mucosulfatidosis do not complement those of the Maroteaux-Lamy syndrome or those of metachromatic leukodystrophy, yet other evidence indicates that these are clearly separate entities.
VI. Molecular genetic analysis. For example, several types of familial amyloid polyneuropathy have been shown to be "caused" by allelic mutations in the transthyretin (prealbumin) gene but the Iowa or Van Allen type has been shown to be due to a mutation in the gene for apolipoprotein AI.

tion of disease. Through Gregor Mendel's principles, he assigned a leading role in directing thought along the lines of specific entities. One other factor of comparable impact was the advent of the bacteriologic era, with its focus on specific etiology and specific entities. One must only recall that it was little more than a century ago that in many circles jaundice, dropsy, anemia, fever, dysentery, etc., were thought of as entities, to realize the influence of bacteriologic and genetic discoveries on the conceptual base of medicine.

In medical genetics there is little place for expressions such as "spectrum of disease," "disease A is a mild form, or a variant, of disease B," etc. Disease A and disease B are either the same disease, if they are based on the same mutation, or different diseases. Phenotypic overlap is not necessarily grounds for considering them fundamentally the same or even closely related. The only justification I can see for use of the expression "disease A is a variant of disease B" is in relation to allelic forms; it might, with validity be said, for example, that the Scheie syndrome has been found to be a variant of the Hurler syndrome; to say that the Hurler and Scheie syndromes are allelic variants of alpha-L-iduronidase deficiency would be more precise. With the identification of at least two phenotypes due to different mutations in the alpha-L-iduronidase gene, the possibility of the existence of compound heterozygotes (genetic compounds) at this locus came to mind, and we identified patients that seemed to correspond to what one would expect for the Hurler/Scheie compound. We were guided in this by the example of SS disease, CC disease, and the SC genetic compound; SC disease is intermediate in severity between SS disease and CC disease and has some qualitatively distinctive phenotypic features. So it is also with the Hurler/Scheie compound heterozygote. This line of thinking led us to point out the importance of allelic series in determining variability in autosomal recessive disorders.

With MIM4 (1975) MPS VII (beta-galactosidase deficiency) was placed on record. With the MIM5 (1978) MPS VIII was added, with asterisk, but this did not stand the test of time and lost its asterisk in the MIM6 (1983) and thereafter was retained "for historic purposes only" after the previously reported enzyme deficiency was found to have been in error, possibly because of scientific fraud. The Sanfilippo syndrome was divided progressively into four separate entities each due to deficiency of a different enzyme involved in the degradation of heparan sulfate and each due to mutation at a separate gene locus. We knew about two of these, MPSIIIa and MPS IIIb, by the MIM4 (1975); we knew about all four by the MIM6 (1983). By the MIM5 (1978), we recognized that the Morquio syndrome could be produced not only by mutation at the gene for N-acetylglucosamine-6-sulfatase but also in beta-galactosidase, the enzyme that in another mutant form is responsible for GM1-gangliosidosis (generalized gangliosidosis).

Thus the mucopolysaccharidoses are a superb example of lumping and splitting in genetic nosology. I say that in the creation of the catalogs I am continually taking about 30 steps forward and 1 step backward, i.e., for every 30 entries I create, I eliminate an entry by "folding it in" with another entry.

Molecular genetics has been a powerful tool for genetic nosology; it has led to much splitting but it has also led to lumping. For example, several varieties of amyloid polyneuropathy, which were listed previously as separate asterisked entries in MIM, we now know are the result of different amino acid substitutions in the transthyretin (TTR; prealbumin) gene and therefore, following the philosophy of 1 entry–1 genetic locus, must be combined under one heading. (The Van Allen or Iowa form of amyloid neuropathy is an exception; the causative lesion resides in the gene for apolipoprotein AI, not TTR.)

An earlier example of lumping came with the hemolytic anemias due to specific red cell enzymopathies. Entries might be created in the dominant catalog on the basis of discovery of an electrophoretic polymorphism of a red cell enzyme in a clinically normal individual; the polymorphism was dominant (or co-dominant). Deficiency of the same enzyme might later be identified (before or after the polymorphism) as the cause of hemolytic anemia and receive a separate entry in the recessive catalog, if it were not appreciated that these were one and the same gene locus, i.e., that several phenotypes, "normal" and pathologic, resulted from alleles.

There are admittedly some problems in attempting to maintain an encyclopedia that is at the same time a catalog of phenotypes and a catalog of genes. This follows directly from the fact that some disorders can be produced by two or more separate gene loci and conversely that two or more very disparate disorders may be caused by different mutations at the same locus. In the cases of hemoglobin (Fig. 2) and type-I collagen, one sees evidence of these two principles. The alpha and beta loci encoding the two kinds of subunits of adult hemoglobin are located on chromosome 16 and 11, respectively; the alpha-1 and alpha-2 loci encoding subunits of type-I collagen are located on chromosomes 17 and 7, respectively. Mutations at either of the two collagen loci may cause any one of several types of osteogenesis imperfecta or of the Ehlers-Danlos syndrome and different mutations at either of the two beta-globin loci can cause thalassemia, Heinz body anemia, polycythemia, or methemoglobinemia. In order to maintain the integrity of the "one gene locus–one MIM entry" rule, it is necessary to make the gene locus, not the disorder, the primary designation. In some cases, where there is considerable phenotypic and genetic information about a particular form of osteogenesis imperfecta or Ehlers-Danlos syndrome, for example, a separate entry (without an asterisk) may be retained, even though we recognize that mutations at any one of two or more loci may cause the particular disorder. We must depend on the indices (print and computerized search) to find the phenotypes desired. In clinical medicine it is, of course, the phenotype that is of primary interest.

We have recognized for a long time that to some extent the categorization *dominant* and *recessive* are arbitrary. The closer one gets to the primary gene expression, the more the terms lose their distinction. *Dominant* and *recessive* are terms invented

	Heinz body hemolytic anemia	Thalassemia	Erythremia	Methemoglobinemia
HBA	e.g., Hb Toyama Hb King County	α - thalassemias Mainly deletion types	e.g., Hb Chesapeake	HbM (several types) e.g., HbM (Boston) HbM (Kankakee)
HBB	e.g., Hb Köln Hb Hammersmith Hb Bristol	β - thalassemias Deletion and non-deletion types	e.g., Hb Osler	HbM (several types) e.g., HbM (Saskatoon)

FIG. 2. An example from the hemoglobinopathies: A matrix showing the occurrence of the same phenotype resulting from mutations at different loci and strikingly different phenotypes resulting from mutations in a single locus.

by Mendel himself and used by him to refer to what he called the *character* and what we would call the *phenotype*. Strictly speaking, it is not correct to refer to a gene as dominant or recessive, although this is a useful shorthand. New entries created on the basis of cloned genes for which no mendelizing phenotype has yet been identified have been placed in the dominant catalog arbitrarily. The continuation of the system of putting allelic mutations at a given locus in the same entry, regardless of whether the phenotype is dominant or recessive, may create trouble for those who do not read the information carefully. I recall some people who were confused by the fact that sickle cell anemia was discussed in the dominant catalog (in the entry for beta-globin) rather than in the recessive catalog. In the fullness of time, the print version of MIM can be expected to fill many volumes, at least as many as there are chromosomes, and organization by chromosome will probably be the logical system used in the ultimate gene encyclopedia.

MOLECULAR DEFECTS IN MENDELIAN DISORDERS

Beginning with MIM 3 (1971), I have maintained a list called at first "Enzymopathies," more recently "Protein defects in inherited disorders," and most recently "Molecular defects in mendelian disorder." The intellectual ancestry (Fig. 3) of these lists goes back on one side to Garrod with his inborn errors of metabolism and the principles that were elaborated genetically and biochemically in *Neurospora* by Beadle and Tatum; and on the other side to Pauling's concept of molecular disease with sickle cell anemia as a prime example—substantiated at the level of protein amino acid sequence by Ingram. These two intellectual/scientific streams converged in the "holy trinity" of DNA-RNA-protein, revealed between 1953, when Watson and Crick proposed the structure of DNA, and 1966 when the genetic code was finally worked out.

The list of enzymopathies given in 1971 numbered 103. The present list, which

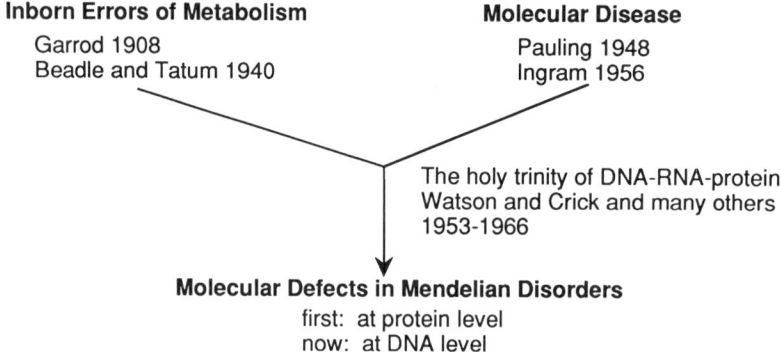

FIG. 3. The intellectual/scientific ancestry of the list of molecular defects in mendelian disorders.

includes any defect identified at least at the protein level, has 443 entries. The methods for identifying molecular defects are listed in Table 2. The level of proof varies from the most secure ("confirmed"), #1, a change in DNA itself, to #15, the least definitive ("tentative"), homology with an animal model.

Intragenic Lesions

The mutational changes *within* the gene have been cataloged in recent editions. All the variant hemoglobins have been cataloged from the beginning, i.e., MIM 1 (1966); the amino acid change indicated the nature of the intragenic lesion. In recent

TABLE 2. *Methods of defining the molecular defect in mendelian disorders*

C = confirmed
1. Change in the cloned gene that is not a polymorphism, e.g., C → T in codon 39 of HBB (nonsense mutation leading to beta-thalassemia); T → A in codon 6 of HBB (missense mutation leading to sickle cell anemia).
2. Absent, reduced, or abnormal mRNA, e.g., absent or abnormal mRNA for alpha-1, 4-glucosidase in type-II glycogen storage disease.
3. Correction of the defect in cultured cells by transfection of the normal gene. (Negative results do not exclude the possibility that the gene is the basis of the abnormality.) Example: HPRT.
4. "Reverse genetics": demonstration of change in a DNA segment where the disease maps and determination of the normal function of the DNA segment. Example: cystic fibrosis.
5. Altered primary structure of the protein, i.e., altered amino acid sequence that is not a polymorphism. Example: sickle cell anemia.

P = provisional
6. Failure of complementation in cell fusion studies with cells of known defect. (Complementation is useful negative information, indicating that a different defect may be involved.)
7. Physical abnormality of a protein, as indicated, e.g., by electrophoretic difference or immunologic change.
8. Absolute linkage (no recombination) of a disease phenotype to an RFLP related to the gene for the molecule (a "candidate gene" approach). Example: COL1A2 and osteogenesis imperfecta tarda.
9. Deficiency of enzymatic or other functional activity, e.g., deficiency of glucose-6-phosphatase in type-I glycogen storage disease or quantitative deficiency of nonenzymic protein.
10. An intermediate level of enzyme activity (or other basic function) in heterozygotes for a recessive disorder. Many examples known.

T = tentative
11. The disease phenotype maps to the same area of the genome as the gene for a given molecule (another "candidate gene" approach). Example: elliptocytosis and protein 4.1; amelogenesis imperfecta and amelogenin.
12. Inference of enzyme deficiency from accumulation of substrate and/or deficiency of product(s); inference of deficiency of nonenzymic protein from a functional defect, e.g., blue cone pigment in tritan colorblindness.
13. Correction by providing substance not synthesized, e.g., biotin in biotinidase deficiency and growth hormone releasing factor in some cases of isolated growth hormone deficiency.
14. Morphologic abnormality, e.g., of tonofibrils, in "harlequin fetus."
15. Argument from homology: identification of molecular defect in phenotypically and genetically homologous disease in other species, most often the mouse. Example: *jimpy* in mouse and Pelizaeus-Merzbacher disease in human.

times lesions in the DNA, the gene itself, have been demonstrated by methods of molecular genetics. Remarkable is the variety of intragenic lesions that can lead to the same phenotype. Specific diagnostic tests based on specific changes have been devised for use in prenatal, presymptomatic, and carrier diagnosis. Use of the information for DNA diagnosis is a main reason I consider it important to keep track of the many allelic mutations that are being discovered at an accelerating pace in many mendelian disorders. The information also has considerable theoretical interest to students of mutation and to population geneticists.

Intragenic lesions can be classified according to the part of the gene that they involve, e.g., coding region, splice sites, initiator codon, terminator codon, promoter, etc. Alternatively, mutation can be divided into two large classes, point mutations and length mutations; each of these has several members, as follows:

Point Mutation (PM)

1. Point mutation in initiator codon (PMi). An example is the demonstration of change of the initiator methionine codon in the abnormal Gs-alpha protein in pseudohypoparathyroidism.
2. Point mutation, missense type (PMm). There are many examples in which change in a single nucleotide leads to substitution of one amino acid for another. The first and most famous example is that of sickle cell anemia in which valine is substituted for glutamic acid as residue 6 of the beta-globin chain.
3. Point mutation, nonsense type (PMn). A single nucleotide change in codon 39 of the beta-globin gene converts the code from that for glutamine to a stop codon. This is the cause of a frequent form of beta-0-thalassemia in the Mediterranean area.
4. Point mutation in promotor (PMp). Examples are known among the beta-thalassemias and hereditary persistence of fetal hemoglobin.
5. Point mutation affected RNA processing (other than splicing) (PMp). Examples are mutation in the AATAAA signal sequence at the 3' end of the gene. Transcription normally proceeds well beyond the 3' end of the gene and cleavage of the RNA transcript occurs 10 to 15 nucleotides downstream of the signal sequence. Mutation in the signal sequence causes failure of RNA cleavage.
6. Point mutation affecting splicing of RNA (PMs). Mutation in the donor or receptor splice site can interfere with splicing. This occurs in forms of beta-thalassemia; in the PAH gene in the form of PKU most frequent in Caucasians; and in one of the HexA mutations that is frequent in Ashkenazi Jews.
7. Point mutation in a terminator codon (PMt). Mutation in the terminator codon of the alpha-globin gene leads to an abnormally long gene product called hemoglobin Constant Spring. The Hb Tak and Hb Cranston have extra long beta-globin chains, but the change appears to have been a frame-shift resulting from deletion or insertion proximal to the end, such that transcription "reads through" the terminator codon.

Length Mutations (LM)

1. Deletion (LMd). A majority of cases of Duchenne muscular dystrophy and Becker muscular dystrophy are due to deletion in the dystrophin gene.
2. Insertion (LMi). Type-I hyperlipidemia in a large portion of cases is due to insertion in the gene coding lipoprotein lipase. Insertion of a LINE sequence (L1) in the factor VIII gene has been found as a "cause" of hemophilia A. Hemophilia B El Salvador is due to an insertion. The most frequent form of Tay-Sachs disease in Ashkenazi Jews is due to an insertion. Hemoglobin Grady is due to an insertion of three amino acids between normal amino acids numbers 18 and 19 of the alpha chain; the insert is a repeat of normal residues 116, 117, and 118. Thus, this is, in fact, a duplication. (This illustrates that, like most classifications, the categorization of mutation is somewhat arbitrary. The point mutation in the terminator codon in Hb Constant Spring results in an abnormally long gene product and could be called a length mutation; however, the genetic material itself is not longer and it is the gene, not the gene product, on which the classification is based.)
3. Rearrangement (LMr). Complex rearrangements of the LDLR gene in familial hypercholesterolemia and of the GPIIIa gene in Glanzmann thrombasthenia have been described.
4. Duplication (LMdu). There are reports of duplications within the dystrophin gene in cases of DMD, in the factor VIII gene in hemophilia A, in the LDLR gene in familial hypercholesterolemia, and in the CollAI gene in osteogenesis imperfecta congenita.

THE HUMAN GENE MAP

I would now like to review the history of the development of our information on the human gene map during the past 20 years (9).

Almost all of the 1,900 genes (Fig. 4) for which we know the chromosomal location were mapped since 1968, when the first specific gene (that for Duffy blood group) was mapped to chromosome number 1 by our group in Baltimore (10). At that time, about 68 genes were known to be on the X chromosome although their regional location was not known; furthermore, a few pairs and triplets of gene loci were known to be linked to each other, but the chromosome that carried them was not known.

The growth of information in this field has been exponential. In the early 1970s somatic cell hybridization came into the picture. About 1980 molecular genetics entered the scene, contributing to family studies by providing DNA markers (RFLPs and VNTRs); to somatic cell hybridization by providing probes that could be applied to somatic cell hybrid DNAs, thus obviating the necessity of having expression of the gene at the cellular level; and to mapping by chromosomal *in situ* hybridization. The latter method was made to work reliably for single-copy genes

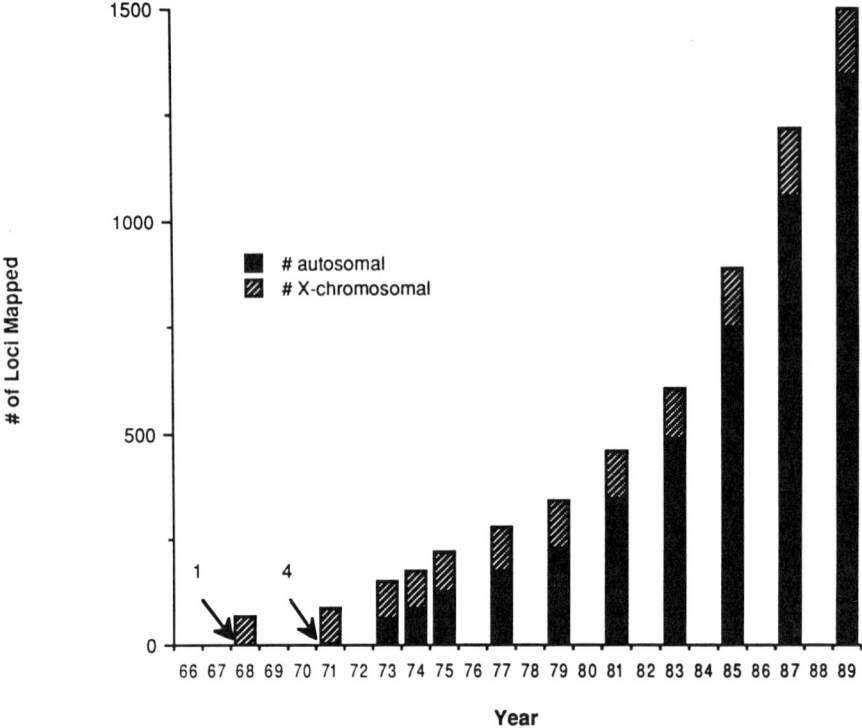

FIG. 4. Growth of information on the specific chromosomal location of expressed genes (to June 1989).

for the first time in 1981 and since that time has rapidly become, in its several improved forms, a leading method of mapping.

Up until about 1970, mapping was done entirely by genetic means, i.e., studies of meiotic segregation in families. This gave information about the distance between any two gene loci; assigning genes or groups of genes ("linkage groups") to specific chromosomes and chromosome regions required correlation with a chromosome heteromorphism such as that of chromosome 1 ("the Donahue chromosome") found to be linked to Duffy blood group or with a balance translocation such as those involving chromosome 16 used for mapping the haptoglobin locus. Because of the limited number of proteins ("gene product") available to use as markers and because of the genetically disadvantageous characteristics of human families, mapping was a slow process until the development of surrogate methods, particularly somatic cell hybridization, and before the development of the more direct methods for getting at the gene provided by molecular genetics.

The 1,900 genes that have been mapped code for a great variety of protein products: blood groups, enzymes, hormones, clotting factors, growth factors, receptors (e.g., for hormones, growth factors), oncogenes, structural proteins (e.g., collagens, elastins), etc. Also, some code for various RNAs such as tRNA, ribosomal RNA, and so on.

The Human Genome Project, the undertaking to map and sequence completely the human genome (11), has a great advantage over some other projects that must wait for results until a major instrument or resource has been constructed: the spin-off begins immediately. The spin-off from human gene mapping just outlined has represented a main justification for undertaking the complete job—the insight the map gives into human genetic disease. In this connection, the "morbid map" is of interest. Of the 1,900 genes that have been mapped to specific sites, disease-producing mutations are known at more than 400. Indeed, many of the gene loci have been identified only on the basis of mapping of the disease phenotype itself. For example, Huntington disease mapped to chromosome 4 by linkage to a DNA marker was the first of these; Duchenne muscular dystrophy and cystic fibrosis are outstanding later examples. Some of the diseases that are listed on the morbid map are positioned there by virtue of the fact that the "wild-type" gene that underwent mutation to result in the disorder has been mapped to that location. In other cases, e.g., one form of elliptocytosis located on the short arm of chromosome 1, the gene was mapped by both approaches: eliptocytosis had been linked to Rh blood group, which was later assigned to that location, and protein 4.1, which is defective in that form of elliptocytosis, was mapped to the same site. Figures 5, 6, and 7 give three examples of mapped chromosomes. Part A in each case gives the location of selected anchor genes; Part B is the "morbid map."

As stated earlier, the human is estimated to have 50,000 to 100,000 genes. How do we arrive at this estimate of the gene number, "soft" as it is? A number of this order of magnitude was suggested in the past on indirect grounds. We have more direct basis for estimation now because some short segments have been mapped in a fairly saturated manner. One of these is the segment of llp that contains five expressed globin genes in 50 kb of DNA—genes coding for epsilon-, 2 gamma-, delta-, and beta-globins. Given a uniform distribution of genes, this would mean 300,000 genes in all. But there is reason to think that the correct number is much smaller, partly because the beta-globin cluster is separated from neighboring genes by a significant amount of DNA and especially because the globin genes are themselves atypically small—the alpha globin gene is the smallest gene I know.

Genes, like jeans, come in many sizes. There are small genes with genomic sizes less then 10 kb, there are medium-sized genes with genomic sizes less than 50 kb, such as albumin (25 kb) and LDL receptor (45 kb); there are large genes with genomic sizes less than 100 kb, such as the gene for phenylalanine hydroxylase, which is mutant in PKU (90 kb); there are giant genes such as those for factor VIII (186 kb), cystic fibrosis (~250 kb) and thyroglobulin (>300 kb); and there are mammoth genes such as that for dystrophin, which is mutant in Duchenne muscular dystrophy (>2 million kb). Thus, the estimate of 50,000 to 100,000 genes seems reasonable.

The genes that have been mapped also include an ever-increasing number of mendelian genetic disorders in which the basic biochemical defect is not known or

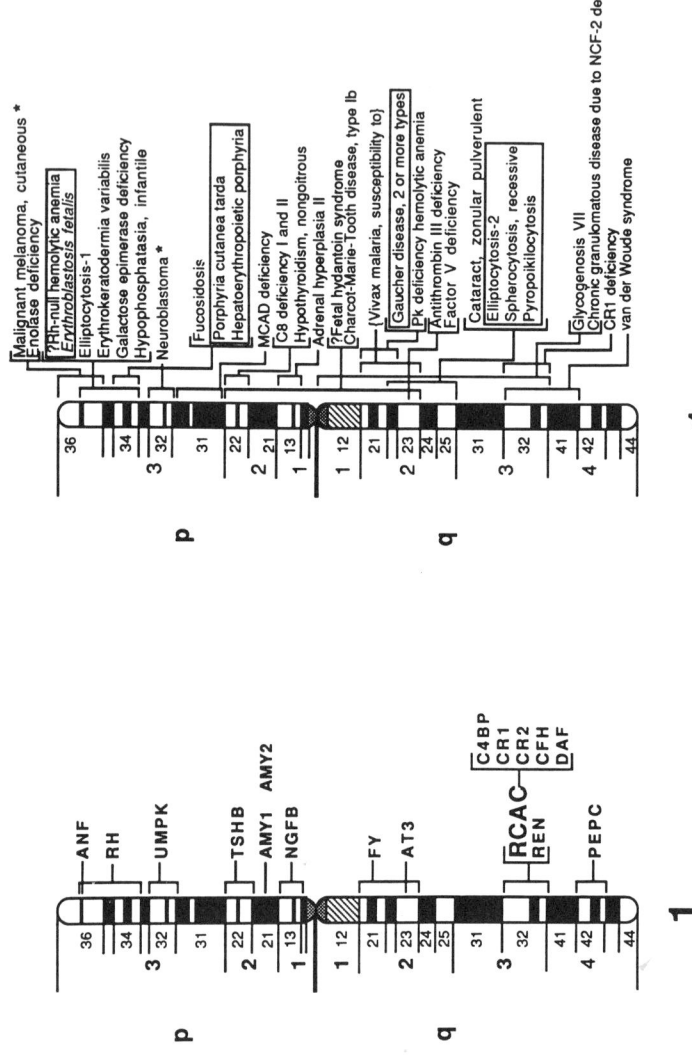

FIG. 5. Gene maps of chromosome 1. **Left:** Selected "anchor" loci; e.g., RH, Rh blood group locus; AMY, amylase; FY, Duffy blood group locus; REN, renin, etc. **Right:** The "morbid map." Boxes indicate that the enclosed disorders are allelic, i.e., mutations caused by different mutations at the same locus. *, neoplasm. Braces indicate specific susceptibility/resistance with monogenic basis. See ref. 9.

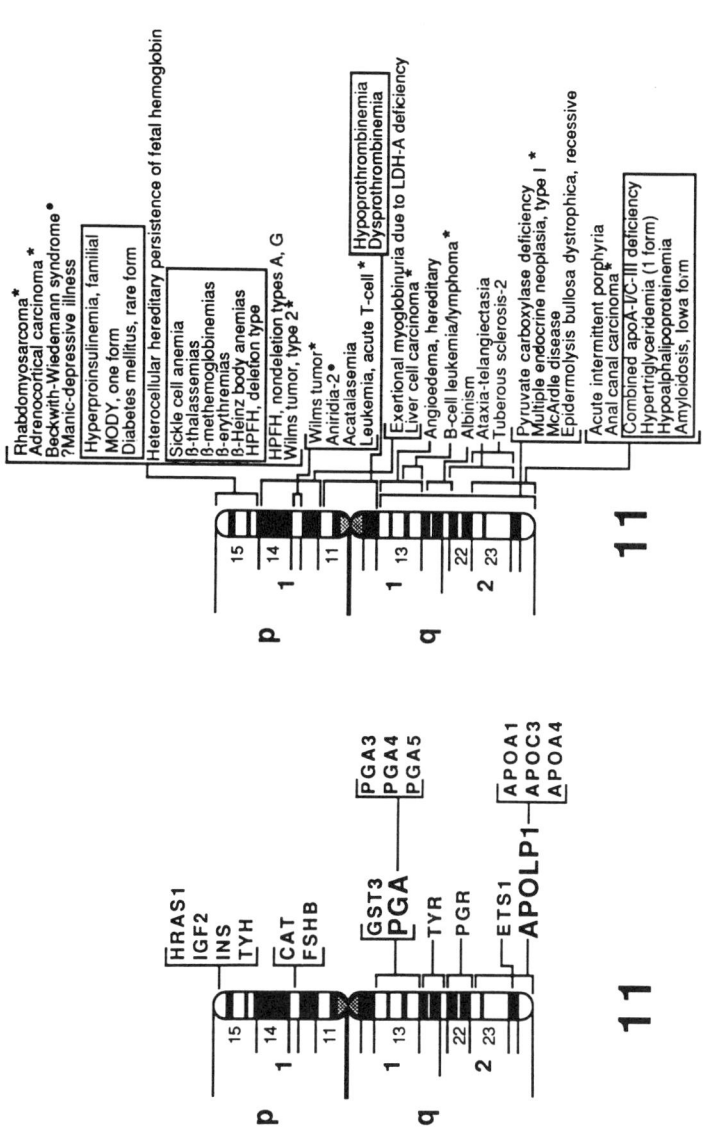

FIG. 6. Gene maps of chromosome 11. **Left:** Selected "anchor" loci. INS, insulin; TYH, tyrosine hydroxylase; TYR, tyrosinase; APOLP1, apolipoprotein cluster I; etc. **Right:** The "morbid map." Symbols as in Fig. 5 right, plus the following: ●, malformation with restricted chromosomal change.

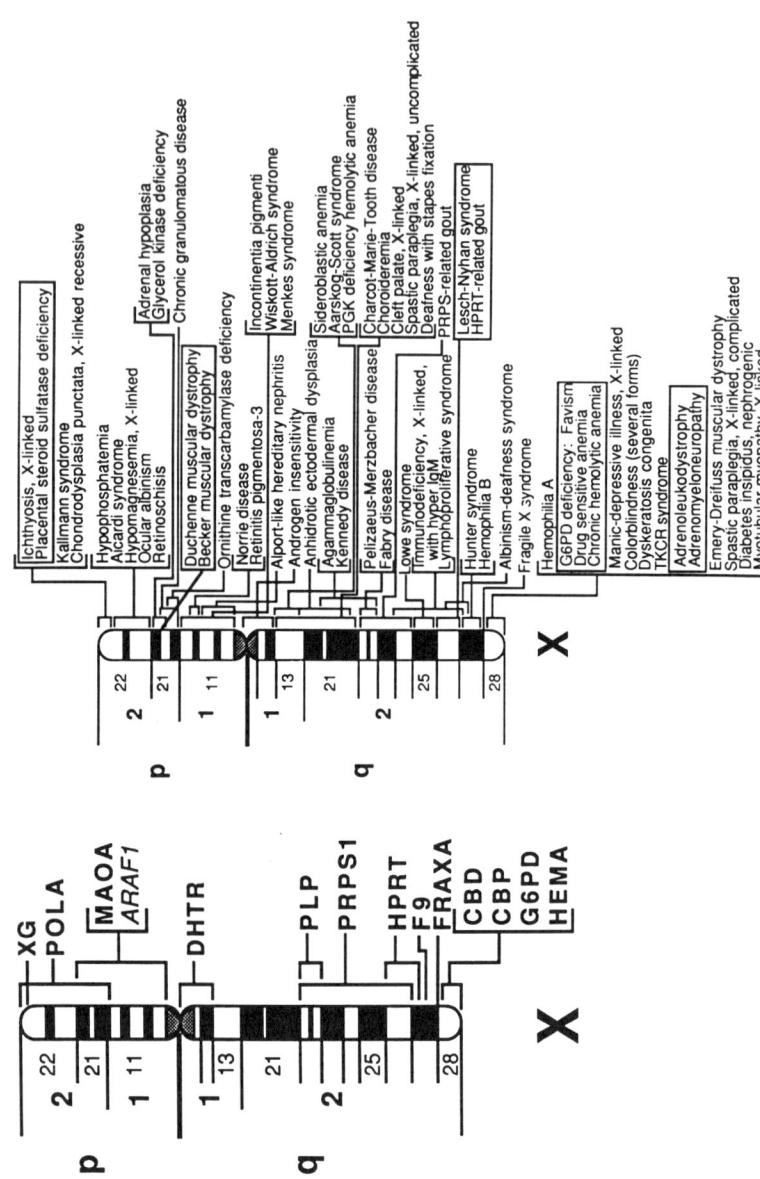

FIG. 7. Gene maps of the X chromosome. **Left:** Selected "anchor" loci; e.g., XG, Xg blood group; MAOA, monoamine oxidase A; CBC,CBP, deutan and protan colorblindness; etc. **Right:** The "morbid map."

was not known at the time of the original mapping. Immediate usefulness of gene mapping has been particularly in relation to these disorders. Because the basic biochemical defect was not known, it was impossible to design an "iron-clad" test for the disorder and for carriers of the gene. Furthermore, a basic understanding of the "cause" of the disease was lacking so that rational therapy could not be designed.

As indicated by the schema shown in Fig. 8, once the gene for disease is mapped it then is possible to do diagnosis (prenatal, presymptomatic, and clinical) by the linkage principle. Even more important in the long run is the ability it provides to "go for the gene," i.e., to determine what normal gene is defective in the given disorder and the nature of the defect. Given this information one can design gene-specific diagnosis and working back from the gene, one can elucidate the pathogenetic chain that connects gene and phene.

Someone introduced the term *reverse genetics* for the process of "going for the gene" and then working back to the phenotype. It is the reverse of how we usually work in medical genetics going from the phenotype to a defective or deficient protein and then to the gene. As pointed out by David Botstein and others, however, it is not the reverse of the process that has been standard for classic genetics, in *Drosophila*, for example. For this and other reasons, the suggestion of Ed Southern seems legitimate: In medical genetics we have traditionally worked from outside in; reverse genetics might better be called the inside-out approach.

Besides the value of genomics (mapping, sequencing, and otherwise analyzing complex genomes) to the understanding of diagnosis and management of mendelian disorders, usefulness in the category of somatic-cell genetic disease represented by

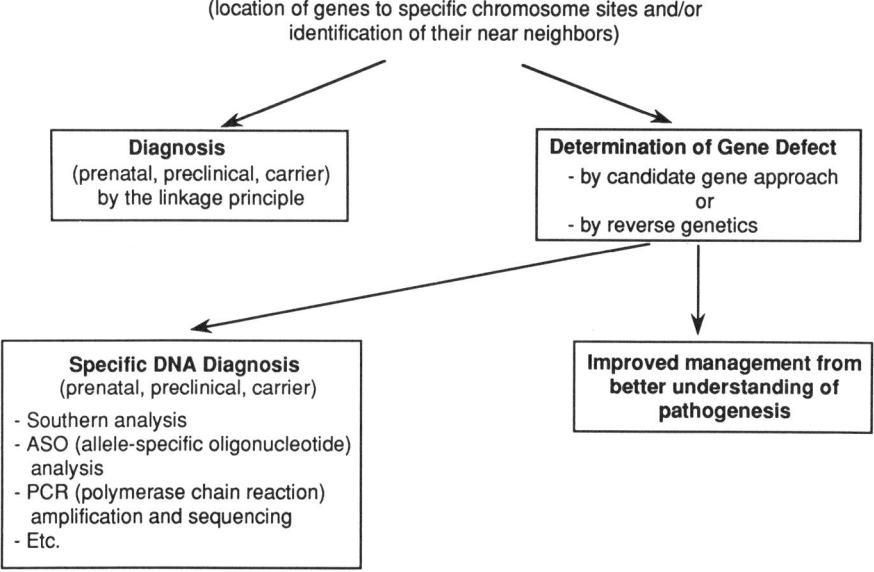

FIG. 8. The clinical applications of gene mapping.

cancer (12) is becoming ever more evident. Mapping and sequencing studies have provided extensive support for Theodor Boveri's chromosome theory of cancer and indicate the relationship between specific changes in the genome and specific types and stages of cancer. Even in carcinogen-induced cancers such as small-cell cancer of the lung, specific genomic changes are being identified as the fundamental cause or mechanism of abnormal growth. Increasingly, such specific changes in the DNA of tumors will be the basis of tumor diagnosis, staging, prognosis, and therapy. Dulbecoo was right.

A fifth category of genetic disease comprises those disorders resulting from mutations in the mitochondrial genome. The mitochondrial chromosome has been completely sequenced and mapped and therefore is a paradigm for what might be achieved for the 25 nuclear chromosomes. Mitochondrial mutations causing neurologic, muscle, hematologic, and even oncologic disorders are being described.

In summary, it might be said that genetic nosology, defining molecular defects in genetic disorders, and mapping genes to specific chromosomal sites are all interrelated processes arrived at the delineation of genes. And it can be said that although the human is a notoriously unsuitable subject for genetic study because of his (and her) long generation time, small number of progeny, and refusal to breed according to experimental protocols, the development of surrogate methods such as study of the genetics of cultured somatic cells and the analysis of the gene itself or the gene product have made man (and woman) one of the genetically best studied organisms.

REFERENCES

1. McKusick, V. A. (1975): Presidential address: the growth and development of human genetics as a clinical discipline. *Am. J. Hum. Genet.*, 27:261–273.
2. McKusick, V. A. (1989): In retrospect: forty years of medical genetics. *JAMA*, 261:3155–3158.
3. Jeghers, H., McKusick, V. A., Katz, K. H. (1949): Generalized intestinal polyposis and melanin spots of the oral mucosa, lips and digits. *N. Engl. J. Med.*, 241:993–1005, 1031–1036.
4. McKusick, V. A. (1989): Historical perspectives: the understanding and management of genetic disorders. *Md. Med. J.*, 38:901–910.
5. McKusick, V. A. (1962): On the X chromosome of man. *Q. Rev. Biol.*, 37:69–175.
6. McKusick, V. A., ed. *Medical Genetic Studies of the Amish. Selected Papers.* Baltimore: The Johns Hopkins University Press, 1978.
7. McKusick, V. A. (1990): *Mendelian Inheritance in Man. Catalogs of Autosomal Dominant, Autosomal, Recessive, and X-linked Phenotypes*, 9th ed. The Johns Hopkins University Press, Baltimore.
8. McKusick, V. A. (1956/1972): *Heritable Disorders of Connective Tissue*, 1st, 4th eds. St. Louis, CV Mosby.
9. McKusick, V. A. (1986–1988): The morbid anatomy of the human genome: a review of gene mapping and clinical medicine. *Medicine*, 65:1–33, 66:11–63, 237–296, 67:1–19.
10. Donahue, R. P., Bias, W. B., Renwick, J. H., McKusick, V. A. (1968): Probable assignment of the Duffy blood group locus to chromosome 1 in man. *Proc. Natl. Acad. Sci. USA*, 61949–61955.
11. McKusick, V. A. (1989): Mapping and sequencing the human genome. *N. Engl. J. Med.*, 320:910–915.
12. McKusick, V. A. (1985): Marcella O'Grady Boveri (1865–1950) and the chromosome theory of cancer. *J. Med. Genet.*, 22:431–440.

Genes, Brain, and Behavior, edited by
P. R. McHugh and V. A. McKusick.
Raven Press, Ltd., New York © 1991.

The Chromosome, Its Anatomy, and Its Aberrations

Teresa L. Yang-Feng

Department of Human Genetics, Yale University School of Medicine, New Haven, Connecticut 06510

Chromatin is the basic unit of chromosome structure and is composed of DNA and proteins. The uniform supercoil model of chromatin structure has just recently been established. The long strand of DNA is packaged, together with histone and non-histone proteins, into a chromosome through a stepwise process. Higher orders of coiling finally lead to the condensed mitotic chromosomes, which are the basic subjects for human cytogenetics.

In 1956, it was determined that the correct number of human chromosomes is 46, thus providing the basic principles for the studies of human chromosomes and chromosomal disorders. Subsequently, several numerical abnormalities and some structural aberrations were discovered. In 1970, however, the introduction of chromosome banding techniques revolutionized cytogenetic analysis. Each chromosome could now be precisely identified on the basis of its unique banding pattern. Previously obscure structural abnormalities and new deletion or duplication syndromes were uncovered. The addition of high-resolution banding techniques made it possible to study the chromosomes in greater detail and allowed for the detection of previously undetectable aberrations, hence identifying the contiguous gene syndromes that are associated with very subtle and specific abnormalities.

Aside from the constitutional chromosome abnormalities, acquired nonrandom chromosomal defects are important in the diagnosis and evaluation of human hematologic disorders. Also, site-specific chromosomal changes have identified the chromosomal regions containing genes crucial to the malignant development.

The combination of molecular and cytogenetic methods has aided in the detection of submicroscopic structural changes, the characterization of marker chromosomes and has advanced our understanding of cytogenetic defects in chromosomal disorders as well as cancers. Most recently, the observations of genomic imprinting effects on the phenotypic expressions of some genetic diseases, including chromosomal disorders, have added a new perspective to the evaluation of the consequences of chromosome abnormalities.

CHROMOSOME STRUCTURE

The amount of DNA in the human genome is about 7.1×10^9 base pairs, which are organized into 23 pairs of chromosomes. Each chromosome is composed of a single continuous DNA molecule, histone, and nonhistone proteins. The chromosomal DNA associated with protein is packed and folded in an orderly fashion in a nucleus at a packing ratio of about 1:10,000 (40,72). A 140-base pair length of DNA is wound in two left-handed turns around a histone core of two identical tetrameres (H2A, H2B, H3, H4) to form each disc-shaped core particle; this structure is known as a nucleosome. Nucleosomes are connected by linker DNA of 20 to 100 bp per subunit associated with histone H1 to form the 100-Å chromatin fiber with the "beads-on-a-string" appearance. The nucleosome-free short regions of the 100-Å chromatin fiber are the DNase I hypersensitive sites because of the relative sensitivity of the DNA in chromatin to the cleavage by DNase I and other reagents. These sites are often found at or near the 5′ end of genes suggesting a role in gene activation. Histone H1 interacts with the linker DNA and leads to establish the next unit of structural organization, the 300-Å fiber. The chromatin fibers with various nonhistone proteins are further folded or coiled into a metaphase chromosome or within the confines of an interphase nucleus.

CHROMOSOME ORGANIZATION

Euchromatin

Chromatin, the basic unit of chromosome organization, is divided into two types: euchromatin and heterochromatin (9). Euchromatin regions are specific portions of chromosomes with certain patterns of condensation and staining properties and are found mainly on the arms of chromosomes. Most known genes are located in the euchromatin regions of chromosomes.

Heterochromatin

Heterochromatin represents specific regions that remain condensed throughout interphase and are genetically inactive. *Constitutive heterochromatin* forms a permanent structural characteristic of a given chromosome pair. It consists of highly repetitive DNA sequences that are not transcribed and are replicated late in the S phase. Constitutive heterochromatin is usually located in regions of the centromeres, the short arms of the acrocentric chromosomes, the distal end of the Y chromosome and the secondary constrictions of chromosomes 1, 9, and 16. It may vary in amount from chromosome to chromosome, and between homologous chromosomes without known phenotypic effects, and thus is considered a type of heteromorphism, a normal variation (34,36). *Facultative heterochromatin* contains euchromatin, which behaves as genetically inert and shows no transcription during certain stages of development. It is the type found in the inactive X chromosome in females that acts as a mechanism to produce gene dosage compensation.

Centromere. A centromere is a prominent constriction region of the chromosome at which the sister chromatids are joined and the spindle is attached during cell division. It controls chromosome segregation in both mitosis and meiosis. The centromeres are associated with blocks of heterochromatin containing several families of repetitive sequences (6,12). Some of these are made up of a few short sequences such as TTCCA. Others have a long repeat: an example is the alphoid family composed of repeating monomers approximately 170 base pairs in length. Evolutionary divergence has occurred in the sequences, so that the organization and nucleotide sequence of a multimeric higher order alphoid repeat unit present at the centromeres is specific for each particular chromosome pair (78).

Telomere. A telomere is the terminal structure of a linear chromosome and is required for the replication and stability of that chromosome. The telomere region consists of mini satellite-like DNA sequences of tandem repeat arrays of 6-nucleotide units (6,74). Recent evidence suggests that the telomere sequence and structure seem to be evolutionarily conserved, implicating its functional importance.

Nucleolus organizing region (NOR). A specialized structure on acrocentric chromosomes (human 13, 14, 15, 21, and 22) is the site of the 18S and 28S ribosomal RNA genes (rDNA) (50). NORs appear to be stalks at the end of which is a distinctive structure known as a satellite.

THE HUMAN KARYOTYPE

Chromosome Morphology

A chromosome consists of two sister chromatids and is divided into short (p) and long (q) arms by its centromere. The centromere position in a chromosome defines the chromosome as being either telocentric, acrocentric, metacentric, or submetacentric (Fig. 1). The arm ratio (q/p) for a metacentric chromosome is about 1. Prior to the introduction of banding techniques, human chromosomes were classified into seven groups (A–G) according to their sizes. Within each group, some chromosomes could be distinguished from each other based on their morphological differences.

Chromosome Banding

A variety of staining methods are available; the most useful methods are those that give chromosomes a banded appearance. In 1970, Caspersson and colleagues first demonstrated that a distinctive longitudinal differential banding pattern of each chromosome could be produced by a quinacrine derivative that binds directly to DNA (as other fluorescent dyes) and allowed identification of all human chromosomes (11,32). Soon after this, it was found that bands on chromosomes can also be

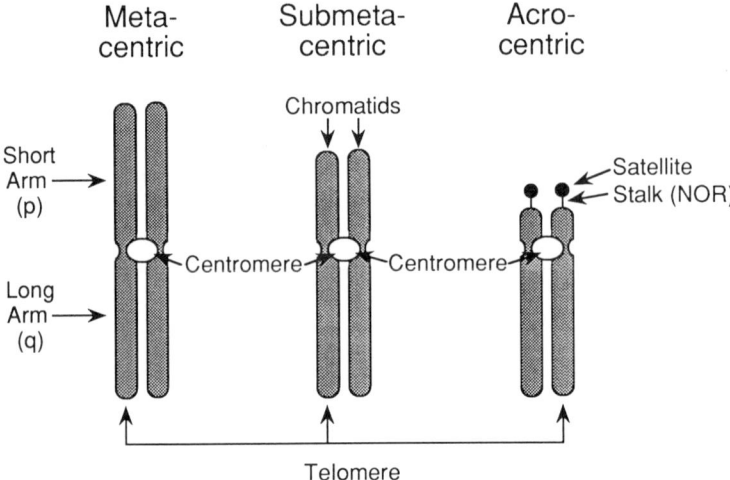

FIG. 1. Metaphase chromosome morphology.

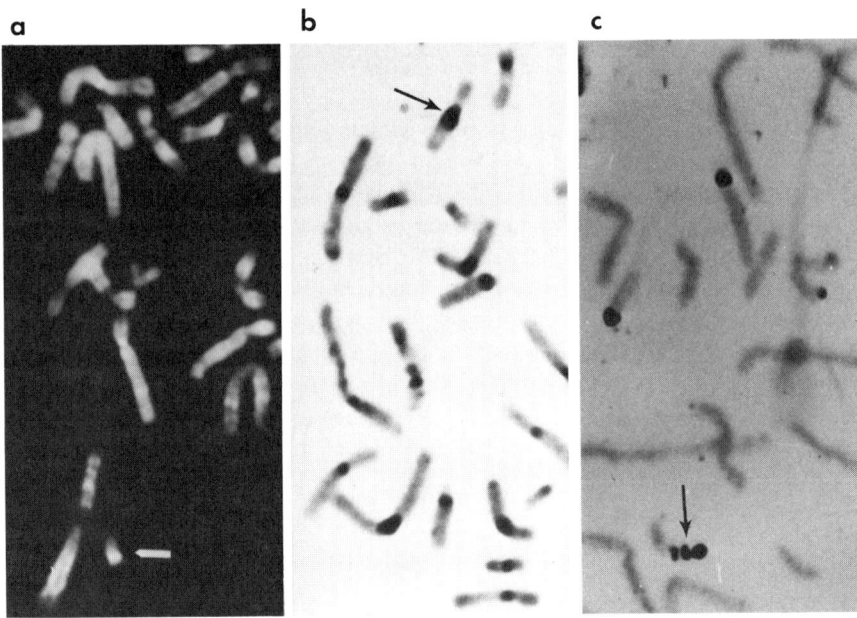

FIG. 2. Metaphase spreads after various staining procedures. *Arrows* indicate bright (**a**) fluorescence at the heterochromatic region on Yq after Q-banding; (**b**) centromeric and secondary constriction heterochromatin stained with C-banding; (**c**) three sets of stalks on an acrocentric chromosome from a normal individual by NOR-staining.

produced by other stains after pretreatments (e.g., protease, salt, alkali), which remove some protein or DNA from the chromosomes (18,63,66).

Q-banding, G-banding, and R-banding are commonly used procedures for the standard karyotyping. The patterns of Q-(quinacrine) and G-(trypsin-Giemsa) banding are almost identical except for heterochromatic regions (Fig. 2A). Some of these regions may show very bright fluorescence with Q-banding but are not noticeable by G-banding. R-banding refers to the patterns generated by techniques that give the reverse of the G- and Q-bands so the telomeric regions of most chromosomes are positively stained (20,73). Therefore, it may aid in detecting the abnormalities or defining the breakpoints involving the chromosome ends that are faintly stained by Q- and R-banding. The mechanism of these chromosome banding techniques is not clearly understood. It is known that positive Q-bands contain DNA rich in adenine and thymine residues and positive R-bands are rich in guanine-cystosine base pairs (71,75). The positive G- and Q-bands are usually later replicating than negative bands, and are generally believed to contain more heterochromatin.

There are quite a few banding techniques that stain only specific regions of some chromosomes and cannot be used to identify all chromosomes as would be necessary for the standard karyotype. Some of these are often employed in clinical applications and are discussed here. C-banding procedures stain the centromeres and other constitutive heterochromatic regions and are often used to determine if material of unknown origin is heterochromatin or euchromatin (3,67) (Fig. 2B). The G-11 banding technique, a variant of C-banding, stains the centromeric heterochromatin of chromosome 9q (7). This method can be used to distinguish human from rodent chromosomes in somatic cell hybrids because it stains human chromosomes bluish and rodent chromosomes magenta. NOR staining procedures include a precipitation of silver granules at the NOR (stalk) regions (25,49). Only the rDNA in the NORs that were actively transcribing at the last interphase are positively stained. NOR staining may be used to demonstrate that a particular rearranged chromosome contains NOR regions, and thus derived from the short arm of an acrocentric chromosome (Fig. 2C). Distamycin-DAPI-staining is specific for the distal end of the Y chromosome and the short arm of chromosome 15 (17,47).

The resolution of a chromosome is the number of bands visible on that chromosome under light microscopy. High-resolution banding is usually performed on chromosomes of cells in late prophase or early metaphase, at a time when they are less contracted, which shows larger numbers of bands per chromosome than do metaphase chromosomes (23,80). The standard metaphase banding patterns show about 400 bands per haploid set, whereas the band number of the more extended chromosomes may be up to 1,000 or more. To increase the likelihood of finding cells in early metaphase, cell synchronization is employed, using an agent such as methotrexate, which blocks and accumulates the cells in the S phase. After release from the block, many cells, at a given point, will be in approximately the same stage of mitosis, early metaphase. To further increase the yield of more extended chromosomes, agents that decrease chromosome condensation, such as actinomycin D or 5'-bromo-deoxyuridine, can be added to cultures for the last 2 to 3 hr before harvest (81). Analysis of high-resolution chromosomes allows detection of previously undetectable structural abnormalities and more precise delineation of readily identifiable ones. As shown in Fig. 3, a subtle translocation between chromosomes 5 and 20 was missed by routine chromosome studies and later identified by high-resolution banding. This translocation carrier, in fact, gave birth to a child with 5p-syndrome through whom this abnormality was first suspected.

In situ hybridization is a method combining molecular and cytogenetic techniques by hybridizing the chemically or radioactively labeled cloned DNA sequences to their complementary DNA within fixed chromosome preparations on glass slides (28). At 1,000 high-resolution chromosome band stage, each band comprises about 3,000 kb of DNA. Genetic aberrations involving less than 3,000 kb of DNA are probably not visible at the cytological level. *In situ* hybridization is very useful in the detection of submicroscopic changes in patients with clinical features typical of certain chromosomal disorders but without the specific chromosome abnormalities observed, e.g., in cases of 4p- syndrome. This procedure is also employed to characterize some chromosomal abnormalities whose nature cannot be elucidated by the currently available cytogenetic methods. As illustrated in Fig. 4, the marker chromosome found in a female Turner's patient was proven to be an isodicentric chromosome composed of two copies of the short arm of the Y chromosome by *in situ* hybridization using the hYfin probe that encodes the putative testis determining

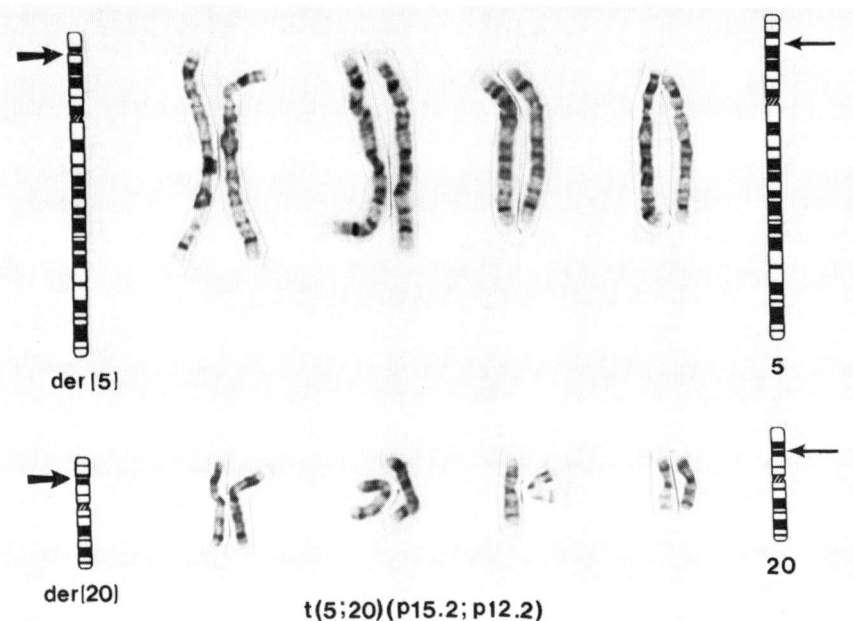

FIG. 3. Four pairs of high-resolution G-banded chromosomes 5 and 20, illustrating the subtlety of this t(5;20) translocation. *Arrows* indicate the break and rejoin points. The translocated chromosomes are the ones at the left within each pair.

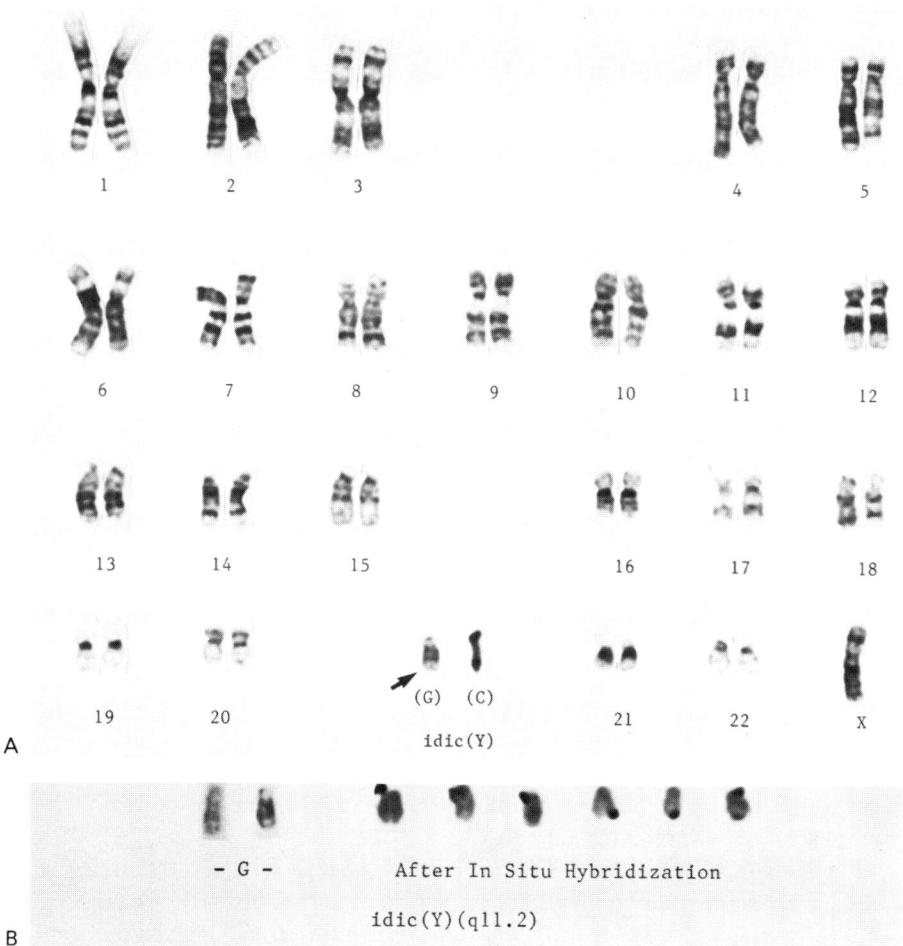

FIG. 4. A: A G-banded karyotype of 46,X,idic(Y)(q11.2) from a female Turner's patient who is mosaic for 45,X/46,X,idic(Y). **B:** *Arrow* indicates the G-banded idic (Y), which was proven to have two centromeres by C-banding. The origin of this idic (Y) was actually determined by *in situ* hybridization using a Yp-specific probe (see text). Positive singles were observed at either or both ends of the idic (Y).

factor and is located at Yp. *In situ* hybridization is a direct approach to the localization of cloned sequences and is widely used in gene mapping studies.

Heteromorphisms

As mentioned above, heterochromatin regions may vary in size, staining properties, and/or location in the chromosomes of normal individuals and are characteristic of a given chromosome in different cells in the same individual. They are almost always inherited as a dominant trait and are common enough that any two individuals are likely to differ in one or more regions. Therefore, they have been proved useful as genetic markers in determining the parental origin in cases of trisomy, triploidy, and *de novo* rearrangements or for twin zygosity and paternity testing (36). They can be readily identified by one or more specialized banding techniques.

CHROMOSOME ABNORMALITIES

As mentioned previously, the correct number of 46 human chromosomes was first determined in 1956. All cells of normal individuals have 22 pairs of autosomes and one pair of sex chromosomes, XX in the case of females and XY in the case of males.

Changes in Chromosome Numbers

Chromosome abnormalities can be classified as numerical or structural. Changes in chromosome numbers are those in which there is an increased number of sets of the basic or haploid number (polyploidy) and those with any chromosome number that is not a true multiple of a haploid set of chromosomes resulting in aneuploidy with the loss of a single chromosome and gain of one or more.

Triploidy consisting of three copies of each chromosome is very rare in live births but is one of the major abnormalities found in spontaneous abortions (15%–20%) (1,31,76). Most of these cases arise from fertilization of an ovum by two sperms (dispermy) and others arise from a diploid ovum or sperm. The karyotypes of triploidies are 69,XXX, 69,XXY, or 69XYY.

Tetraploidy (92,XXXX or 92,XXYY) is usually a lethal condition and occurs in about 2% of spontaneous abortions (24,31,55). It appears to be due to suppression of cytokinesis in the zygote (first mitotic division) with failure of the cell to divide although the chromosomes have duplicated.

Aneuploidy results from either meiotic or mitotic nondisjunction or anaphase lagging in mitosis. Nondisjunction results in two different types of aneuploid cells, trisomy and monosomy of the involved chromosome pair. Monosomy, other than the sex chromosome, is almost never observed in humans. It presumably is lethal at a very early stage of embryonic life since it is even rarely found in spontaneous abortions. Monosomy 21, which is the only autosomal monosomy, occurs in about 0.1% of spontaneous abortions (29,31).

Trisomy of the human chromosome is a rather common condition and occurs in about 4% of clinically recognized pregnancies. Most cases of trisomy are associated with the addition of a single chromosome. Trisomy for all human chromosomes except number 1 has been found in abortuses, but only trisomy 8, 9, 13, 18, and 21 have been described in liveborn individuals (27,31,33,35). Trisomy 21, known as Down's syndrome, is the most common (0.13% of live births) and the first described human chromosome disorder (46). We have now learned that the Down's syndrome phenotype can be produced by duplication of only a portion of chromosome 21 instead of a whole 21 (79). The critical region is at bands 21q22.1→q22.2. Trisomy 13 and trisomy 18 syndromes occur in 0.005% and 0.01% of livebirths, respectively, and are more frequently lethal, therefore much less common in newborn infants than trisomy 21. Trisomy for 8 and 9 is almost always found with the presence of a normal cell line (mosaicism) (10,58). Trisomy 16 is most common, about 8%, in spontaneous abortions but has never been found in newborns (8,21,31).

Sex chromosome abnormalities, in contrast to abnormalities of autosomes, are generally associated with less severe phenotype results. The common sex chromosome aneuploids include 45,X and 47,XXX in females and 47,XXY and 47,XYY in males (16,59). Individuals with sex chromosome complements of XYY, XXX, or XXY constitute the majority of sex chromosome aneuploids (27,33,35). An extra Y in males (47,XYY) and an extra X in females (47,XXX) have no obvious effects on physical development. Most Klinefelter (47,XXY) patients, in contrast to 47,XXX females, are sterile and have dull or below normal intelligence (59,64). Polysomy (multiple extra chromosomes of the same type) is almost never found in human autosomes but is not as rare in the X chromosome as that in males (49,XXXXY), and in females (49,XXXXX) up to three additional Xs have been reported (19,51,82). Individuals with additional Xs are more physically and mentally affected since there is a correlation between the number of extra Xs and the severity of developmental abnormalities.

A missing X chromosome in females (45,X) produces a distinctive phenotype with gonadal dysgenesis, short stature, and certain somatic anomalies often referred to as "Turner's stigmata" (15,16). A single Y (45,Y) or lack of any X chromosome has never been found in clinically recognized conceptions. Similar to autosomes, the loss of a sex chromosome may also have significant effects. The incidence of 45,X females, which is about 1 in 5,000, is very low in full-term births because 92% of 45,X embryos are spontaneously aborted and comprise 10% of spontaneous abortions (31,33).

The causes of nondisjunction or anaphase lag are unknown. A positive association between maternal age and the trisomies for most autosomes has been demonstrated (30). For sex chromosomes XXY and XXX trisomies, the conditions are also related to increased maternal age. The XYY condition, which is an abnormality consistent with paternal origin, therefore is not associated with advanced maternal age. The frequency of trisomies for most chromosomes rises slowly until approximately age 34, when it begins to rise exponentially with age.

Changes in Chromosome Structure

Structural abnormalities of chromosomes are the consequences of chromosome breakage. The type and nature of the abnormalities are closely related to the number of breaks and chromosomes and to the specific chromosomes involved in the rearrangements. Correlations between patients' phenotypes and chromosome rearrangements observed have identified the locations of some disease loci and led to the subsequent isolation of the implicated genes, e.g., dystrophin gene (26,39,83). Studies of abnormal X and Y chromosomes have provided some information on the critical regions for gonadal development (69,84).

Deletion of a portion of a chromosome can arise after one break forming terminal deletion or after two or more breaks and loss of the intercalary material. An apparent terminal deletion may really be an interstitial one with a telomere retained. Deletions of either the short or long arms of the X chromosome or the Y chromosome have been observed in patients with Turner stigmata or gonadal dysgenesis (69). Deletion of the short arms of chromosomes 4 (Wolf-Hirschhorn syndrome) and 5 (cri du chat syndrome) is the cause of these two well-known chromosomal disorders (41,77).

A ring chromosome is formed when a break occurs in each arm, with subsequent fusion of broken ends and is a special type of chromosome deletion with a variable amount of material lost from both arms. It is unstable and subject to various numerical or structural changes because it presents problems in the separation of chromatids at anaphase (37). Ring chromosomes of human sex chromosomes as well as autosomes have been documented.

A duplication chromosome contains an additional copy of a portion of a chromosome in a direct or inverted orientation. Duplications and deletions of all autosomes have been identified in live births with various phenotypic abnormalities, and new ones are being reported continuously.

An inversion contains a segment of a chromosome inverted through 180° relative to the remaining chromosome. Pericentric inversion, where two breaks occur in different arms, involves the centromere; while paracentric inversion does not include the centromere because the two breaks occur in the same arm. Pericentric inversion, which involves only the centromeric heterochromatin, usually has no phenotypic effects and is considered a normal variation. The most common one, pericentric inversion of chromosome 9, is found in 1% to 2% of the general population (14). At meiosis I in inversion heterozygotes, the inverted segment forms a characteristic loop in order for homologous loci to pair. An uneven number of crossovers within the loop results in chromosomally unbalanced gametes with both duplication and deletion.

An isochromosome consists of two copies of one arm and none of the other. Both arms are therefore of identical size and identical genetic composition but in a reversed sequence. Isochromosomes can result from the misdivision (transverse) of the centromere during cell division or breaks in sister chromatids near the centromere with subsequent fusion of these chromatids. The isochromosome of the long arm of the X, seen in patients with Turner's syndrome, is the most common type of isochromosome found in humans.

Translocation arises from breaks in two or more chromosomes with the subsequent transfer of a segment of one chromosome to the other chromosomes. Most translocations are found segregated within families and some are the result of new events *(de novo)*. Translocations involving the exchange of chromosome segments between two chromosomes, usually nonhomologous, are reciprocal. In this case, two rearranged chromosomes are produced. A balanced reciprocal translocation carrier, depending on the segregation patterns of the two rearranged chromosomes during meiosis, may have offspring with unbalanced chromosome complements with duplication and/or deletion (65). Therefore, parental chromosome studies are indicated when duplication or deletion is found. Reciprocal translocation is randomly found between any two chromosomes. Only the translocation between chromosomes 11 and 22 seems to occur with significant frequency (22).

Robertsonian translocation is a special type of reciprocal translocation in which the two breakpoints are at or near the centromeres. It usually occurs between two acrocentric chromosomes, which results in the fusion of the two chromosome arms to form a metacentric or submetacentric chromosome, the loss of the small chromosome consisting of short arm material and the consequent reduction of the chromosome number by one in a balanced carrier. Such a translocation between homologous chromosomes, e.g., t(21q;21q), will produce gametes of which all are unbalanced. The risk of having a Down's syndrome offspring for females carrying a Robertsonian translocation involving chromosome 21 is about 10% to 15% but for male carriers it is almost insignificant (65). The Robertsonian translocation carriers have an increased frequency of spontaneous abortions since all conceptions with trisomies of 14, 15, and 22, most with trisomy 13 and some with trisomy 21, will end in fetal wastage (8,31).

Mosaicism

Mosaicism is the presence of two or more types of cells in the same individual. In mosaicism, one of the cell lines is often normal while the other(s) involve either a numerical or structural abnormality. The ratio of normal to abnormal cells may vary from tissue to tissue. Mosaicism of numerical abnormalities is commonly seen in both autosomes and sex chromosomes; structural abnormalities are predominantly found in sex chromosomes, e.g., patients with Turner's syndrome. Phenotypic effects of an abnormal cell line in a mosaic individual are frequently ameliorated due to the presence of a normal cell line and occasionally are completely abolished.

Acquired Chromosomal Changes in Cancers

The first specific chromosome abnormality in malignant diseases, Philadelphia (Ph') chromosome, resulting from a translocation between chromosomes 9 and 22, was found in leukemic cells from patients with chronic myelogenous leukemia (CML) in 1960 (52). Since then, acquired nonrandom chromosomal changes have been found in malignant cells in various neoplasms and may serve as diagnostic and/or prognostic parameters in many hematologic disorders (42,60). Chromosomal sites involved in specific abnormalities are often found to coincide with the locations of some cellular oncogenes (61). The mechanisms of site-specific chromosome rearrangements and the involvement of oncogenes, as well as their links to cancer, have been extensively studied in Burkitt's lymphoma and certain types of leukemia (4,5,13). Three characteristic translocations between chromosomes 8 and 14, or 2 or 22 are observed in Burkitt's lymphoma (42). The oncogene, c-myc, is located at the breakpoint on chromosome 8 of these three translocations. The activation of c-myc in Burkitt's lymphoma perhaps is due to chromosome translocation that places c-myc under the control of promoters of various immunoglobulin genes (depending on the reciprocal chromosome involved in the translocation) and thereby leads to malignant transformation (4,44). Therefore, specific chromosomal changes are valuable in identifying the chromosomal sites containing genes that may be crucial to the malignant development.

Fragile X Syndrome

The fragile sites are nonstaining gaps present on specific regions on chromosomes occurring consistently in a proportion of cells of an individual and are inherited in a mendelian codominant fashion. They are only expressed under appropriate culture medium conditions. There are no known autosomal fragile sites that appear to have phenotypic effects. The fragile X syndrome is an X-linked mental retardation disorder that affects approximately 1 in 2,000 males and is associated with a folate-sensitive fragile site on the long arm of the X chromosome (Xq27) (53). Clinical features in affected males include mental retardation, speech problems, and enlarged testes.

Frequency in Population

In newborns, the chromosome abnormalities found were approximately one in every 200 (27,33,35). About 1 in 500 had a sex chromosome abnormality and another 1 in 500 had a structural abnormality, with the majority of the abnormalities being balanced. Approximately 1 in 700 had an autosomal trisomy.

The studies in spontaneous abortions revealed that 50% to 60% of the first trimester abortions had a chromosome abnormality (8,29,31). The most common abnormalities were autosomal trisomy, monosomy X, and polyploidy. In most studies, trisomy accounted for 50% to 60% of the abnormalities, monosomy X for 15% to 25%, and polyploid for 15% to 20% with two-thirds of them being triploidy. Monosomy X was the single most common abnormality found among abortuses. Of all trisomies, trisomy 16 was the most common, followed by trisomy 22, then by trisomy 21.

In stillbirths (delivery after 28th week of gestation), about 5% of them had chromosome abnormalities (2,68). Most of the abnormalities were trisomy 13, 18, and 21, sex chromosome aneuploidies and unbalanced structural aberrations.

CONTIGUOUS GENE SYNDROMES

Syndromes with recognizable patterns of malformation are caused by contiguous genes on chromosomes (21,62). These syndromes are often associated with mental retardation and growth retardation. Most of them are sporadic, but occasionally some are familial. The clinical entities of these syndromes were usually defined before their specific chromosome abnormalities were known. The specific chromosomal defects are only present in some patients and are always very subtle and can sometimes only be detected by high-resolution banding. However, submicroscopic deletions of DNA sequences within the specific chromosomal regions involved in particular syndromes have been observed in some patients without cytogenetically visible deletions (70). The syndromes and the chromosome abnormalities included in this group are deletions of 8q24 in Langer-Giedion syndrome, deletions of 11p13 in association with Wilm's tumor, deletions of 13q14 in association with retinoblastoma, deletions of 15q11-13 in both Prader-Willi (PWS) and Angelman (AS) (happy puppet) syndromes, deletions of 17p13 in Miller-Dieker syndrome, deletions of 22q11 in DiGeorge syndrome, and duplications of 11p15.5 in Beckwith-Wiedemann syndrome.

Knowledge obtained from these syndromes may allow the localization of genes important to development and growth and subsequently lead to the cloning of the implicated genes, e.g., retinoblastoma susceptibility gene was isolated by the chromosomal walking approach based on its location on 13q14 (45,54).

GENOMIC IMPRINTING AND CHROMOSOMAL DISORDERS

Recent evidence suggests that some maternal and paternal alleles in mammals can function differently due to genomic imprinting (56,57). Such an epigenetic marking process seems to influence the phenotypic expression of some genetic diseases. For example, the parental origin effects on chromosomal disorders have been well-demonstrated between PWS and AS (Fig. 5). Both contiguous gene syndromes are associated with identical cytogenetic deletions of 15 q11-13 (43,48). It seems that AS and PWS may possibly be caused by different genes because the deleted region is quite large in molecular terms. However, the deleted chromosome 15 has been shown to be of maternal origin in the cases of AS and of paternal origin in most cases of PWS suggesting the variable expressivity of gene(s) on the normal chromosome 15 due to imprinting may be responsible for the disease phenotypes (38). It is not clear if imprinting causes phenotypes consistent with AS or PWS since the molecular mechanism of the epigenetic marking process is unknown, although allele-specific differences in DNA methylation have been suggested. Nonetheless, observations of imprinting effects on phenotypes of dominant traits, recessive tumor syndromes, and chromosomal disorders certainly bring new insight to the underlying mechanism of genetic disorders.

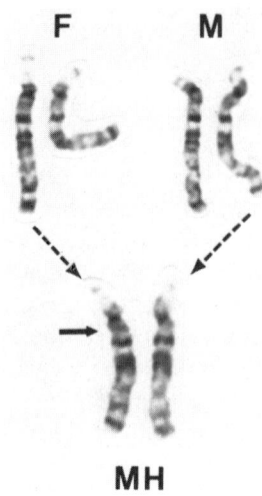

FIG. 5. Pairs of G-banded chromosome 15 from a patient, MH, with Angelman syndrome that we studied. *Arrow* (*solid line*) points to the normal chromosome 5 and indicates the region deleted on the abnormal 5 (at the right). F and M indicates the chromosome 15 pair as being from the patient's father and mother. One of the father's chromosome 15 is double satellited and was found to be the normal 15 in MH as indicated by the *arrow* (*broken line*).

ACKNOWLEDGMENT

I would like to express my appreciation to Ms. Cheryl Cyr for the preparation of this manuscript.

CYTOGENETIC TERMINOLOGY

Acrocentric   Refers to a chromosome with a nearly terminal centromere, so that one arm is very short.

Autosome   Any chromosome other than the sex chromosome.

Centromere (primary constriction)   The constricted portion of the chromosome, separating it into its two arms. It is situated in a heterochromatic region, is composed only of repetitive DNA, and is attached to the spindle fibers at mitosis and meiosis.

Chromatid   The two sister strands that make up a chromosome, held together at the centromere. Each will become a separate chromosome upon centromere division.

Chromatin   The material (DNA, RNA, and protein) of which chromosomes are composed.

Chromosome aberration   An abnormal chromosome complement resulting from the loss, duplication, or rearrangement of chromosomal (genetic) material.

   Duplication   The recurrence of a segment of chromosome resulting in an increase in the number of loci borne by the chromosome.

   Inversion   End-to-end reversal of a segment within a chromosome; pericentric if it involves the centromere and paracentric if it does not.

Deletion (in cytogenetics) Deficiency of a segment of a chromosome resulting in a reduction in the number of loci borne by the chromosome.

Translocation At least two chromosome breaks on different chromosomes, usually heterologous, followed by exchanging materials forming resultant chromosomes. If two chromosomes exchange pieces, the translocation is reciprocal.

Robertsonian translocation A translocation between two acrocentric chromosomes by fusion of the centromeres forming a large metacentric chromosome and loss of the respective short arms.

Chromosome banding Various intrachromosomal regions of varying intensities brought out by differential staining. A band is defined as part of a chromosome, clearly distinguishable from its adjacent segments by appearing darker or lighter as a result of specific staining methods. The most commonly used procedures are G-, Q-, R-, and C-banding.

Chromosomes The carriers of genetic information, consisting of long strands of DNA in a protein framework. They are constant in number in each species. The normal number in humans is 46, 22 pairs of autosomes and two sex chromosomes (XX or XY).

Contiguous gene syndromes Syndromes with recognizable patterns of malformations are caused by the involvement of contiguous genes on a chromosome through microdeletion or microduplication that is occasionally detectable at the cytological level.

Crossing over The process of exchanging genetic material between homologous chromosomes. The chiasmata seen at the diplotene of meiosis are the physical basis of a previous cross-over.

Cytogenetics The study of cell genetics, combining the methods and findings of cytology and genetics.

Cytogenetic map A map showing the locations of genes on a chromosome.

Diploid Having two complete sets of chromosomes (2n) double the number found in the gametes. In humans, the diploid chromosome number is 46. Contrast haploid, triploid.

Euchromatin Shows the staining behavior characteristic of the majority of the chromosomal material. Contrast to heterochromatin.

Fragile chromosome site A nonstaining gap that involves both chromatids and is always at exactly the same band region on a specific chromosome from an individual or kindred. Fragile sites are inherited in a mendelian codominant fashion and can be detected by specific culture and staining methods.

Haploid Having only one complete set of chromosomes, usually germ cells. Contrast, e.g., diploid. In humans, the haploid number is 23.

Heterochromatin Chromosomal material with different staining properties shows maximal condensation in interphase nuclei. It can be divided into facultative and constitutive heterochromatins. Facultative heterochromatins contain inactivated structural genes due to developmental process, e.g., one of the X chromosomes in female somatic cells. Constitutive heterochromatin is permanent and is present in all human chromosomes with quantitative differences. It is composed of repetitive DNA and transcriptional inactive, e.g., centromeres.

Homologous chromosomes   Chromosomes that pair during meiosis, have essentially the same morphology, and contain genes governing the same characteristics.

Ideogram   A diagrammatic representation of a karyotype.

In situ **hybridization (chromosomal)**   Nucleic acid sequences directly hybridized to their complementary DNA within fixed chromosome preparations on glass slides.

Interphase   The stage of the cell cycle between succeeding mitosis during which the normal metabolic processes of the cell proceed.

Isochromosome   A symmetrical chromosome with two arms of equal length and bearing the same loci in reverse sequence, formed by crosswise rather than longitudinal division of the centromere.

Karyotype   The somatic chromosomal complement of an individual. The term often refers to photomicrographs of a set of chromosomes arranged in a standard classification.

Lyonization (Lyon hypothesis)   The process by which all X chromosomes in excess of one are made genetically inactive and heterochromatic. In the female, the decision as to which X (maternal or paternal) is inactivated is taken independently for each cell, early in embryogeny, and is permanent for all descendants of that cell.

Meiosis   A process occurring in the germinal cells by which gametes, containing the haploid number of chromosomes, are produced from diploid cells.

Metacentric   Refers to chromosomes with a centrally located centromere.

Metaphase   The stage of mitosis or meiosis when the chromosomes move about within the spindle and arrange themselves on the equatorial plate.

Mitosis   Somatic cell division resulting in the formation of two cells, each with the same chromosome complement as the parent cell.

Mosaic   An individual or tissue with two or more cell lines of different genetic or chromosomal constitution, derived from the same zygote.

Nondisjunction   The failure of homologous chromosomes (in meiosis I) or sister chromatids (in meiosis II) during anaphase of cell division resulting in one daughter cell receiving both and the other daughter cell none of the chromosomes in question.

Nucleolus   An RNA-rich, round granular structure associated with specific chromosomal sites, the nucleolus organizer regions, located at the short arms of acrocentric chromosomes in humans.

Nucleosome   The repeating nucleoprotein unit of chromatin consisting of a core of eight histone molecules wrapped by a DNA segment about 146 base pairs in length.

Satellite, chromosomal   A small mass of chromatin attached to the short arm of a human acrocentric chromosome by a thin stalk (secondary constriction).

Secondary constriction Any constricted heterochromatic area in a chromosome other than the centromere, which is the primary constriction.

Sex chromosome Chromosomes responsible for sex determination. In humans, the X and Y chromosomes.

REFERENCES

1. Al Saadi, A., Juliar, J. F., Harm, J., Brough, A. J., Perrin, E. V., and Chen, H. (1976): A report on two live-born (69,XXY) and one still-born (69,XXX) infants. *Clin. Genet.*, 9:43–50.
2. Angell, R., Sandison, A., and Bain, A. (1984): Chromosome variation in perinatal mortality: a survey of 500 cases. *J. Med. Genet.*, 21:39–44.
3. Arrighi, F. E., and Hsu, T. C. (1971): Localization of heterochromatin in human chromosomes. *Cytogenetics*, 10:81–86.
4. ar-Rushdi, A., Nishikura, K., Erikson, J., Watt, R., Rovera, G., and Croce, C. M. (1983): Differential expression of the translocated and the untranslocated c-myc oncogene in Burkitt's lymphoma. *Science*, 222:390–393.
5. Ben-Neriah, Y., Daley, G. Q., Mes-Masson, A. M., Witte, O. N., and Baltimore, D. (1985): The chronic myelogenous leukemia-specific p210 protein is the product of the bcr/abl hybrid gene. *Science*, 233:212–214.
6. Blackburn, E. H., and Szostak, J. W. (1984): The molecular structure of centromeres and telomeres. *Annu. Rev. Biochem.*, 53:163–194.
7. Bobrow, M., Madan, K., and Pearson, P. L. (1972): Staining of some specific regions of human chromosomes, particularly the secondary constriction of No. 9. *Nature New Biol.*, 238:122–124.
8. Boué, J., Boué, A., and Lazar, P. (1975): Retrospective and prospective epidemiological studies of 1,500 karyotyped spontaneous human abortions. *Teratology*, 12:11–26.
9. Brown, S. W. (1966): Heterochromatin. *Science*, 151:417–425.
10. Carpenter, B. F., and Tomkins, D. J. (1982): The trisomy 9-syndrome. *Perspect. Pediatr. Pathol.*, 7:109–120.
11. Caspersson, T., Zech, L., and Johansson, C. (1970): Differential binding of alkylating fluorochromes in human chromosomes. *Exp. Cell Res.*, 60:315–319.
12. Cook, H. J., and Hindley, J. (1979): Cloning of human satellite III DNA: different components are on different chromosomes. *Nucleic Acids Res.*, 6:3177–3179.
13. Croce, C. M. (1986): Chromosome translocations and human cancer. *Cancer Res.*, 46:6019–6033.
14. de la Chapelle, A., Schröder, J., Stenstrand, K., et al. (1974): Pericentric inversions of human chromosomes 9 and 10. *Am. J. Hum. Genet.*, 26:746–766.
15. de la Chapelle, A. (1983): Sex chromosome abnormalities. In: *Emery AEH*, edited by D. L. Rimoin, pp. 193–215. Churchill Livingstone, Edinburgh.
16. DePaepe, A., and Matton, M. (1985): Turner's syndrome: updating on diagnosis and therapy. In: *Endocrine Genetics and Genetics of Growth*, edited by C. J. Papadatos and C. S. Bartsocas, pp. 283–300. Alan R. Liss, New York.
17. Donlon, T. A., and Magenis, R. E. (1983): Methyl green is a substitute for distamycin A in the formation of distamycin A/DAPI C-bands. *Hum. Genet.*, 65:144–146.
18. Drets, M. E., and Shaw, M. W. (1971): Specific banding patterns of human chromosomes. *Proc. Natl. Acad. Sci. USA*, 68:2073–2077.
19. Dryer, R. F., Patil, S. R., Zellweger, H. U., et al. (1979): Pentasomy X with multiple dislocations. *Am. J. Med. Genet.*, 4:313–321.
20. Dutrillaux, B., and Lejeune, J. (1971): Sur une nouvelle technique d'analyse du caryotype humain. *C. R. Acad. Sci.*, 272:2638–2640.
21. Emanuel, B. S. (1988): Molecular cytogenetics: toward dissection of the contiguous gene syndromes. *Am. J. Hum. Genet.*, 43:575–578.
22. Fraccaro, M., Lindsten, J., Ford, C. E., and Iselius, L. (1980): The 11q;22q translocation: a European collaboration analysis of 43 cases. *Hum. Genet.*, 56:21.
23. Francke, U., and Oliver, N. (1978): Quantitative analysis of high-resolution trypsin-Giemsa bands on human prometaphase chromosomes. *Hum. Genet.*, 45:137–165.
24. Golbus, M. S., Bachman, R., Wiltse, S., and Hall, B. D. (1976): Tetraploidy in a liveborn infant. *J. Med. Genet.*, 13:329–332.

25. Goodpasture, C., and Bloom, S. E. (1975): Visualization of nucleolar organizer regions in mammalian chromosomes using silver staining. *Chromosoma*, 53:37–50.
26. Greenstein, R. M., Reardon, M. P., and Chan, T. S. (1977): An X-autosome translocation in a girl with Duchenne muscular dystrophy, evidence for DMD gene localization. *Pediatr. Res.*, 11:475A.
27. Hamerton, J. L., Canning, N., Ray, M., and Smith, S. (1975): A cytogenetic survey of 14,069 newborn infants. I. Incidence of chromosome abnormalities. *Clin. Genet.*, 8:223–243.
28. Harper, M. E., and Saunders, G. F. (1981): Localization of single copy DNA sequences on G-banded chromosomes by in situ hybridization. *Chromosoma*, 83:431–439.
29. Hassold, T., Chen, N., Funkhouser, J., et al. (1980): A cytogenetic study of 1,000 spontaneous abortions. *Ann. Hum. Genet.*, 44:151–178.
30. Hassold, T. J., and Jacobs, P. A. (1984): Trisomy in man. *Am. Rev. Genet.*, 18:69–97.
31. Hassold, T. J. (1986): Chromosome abnormalities in human reproduction wastage. *Trends Genet.*, 2:105–110.
32. Hilwig, I., and Gropp, A. (1972): Staining of constitutive heterochromatin in mammalian chromosomes with a new fluorochrome. *Exp. Cell Res.*, 75:122–126.
33. Hook, E. B., and Hamerton, J. L. (1977): The frequency of chromosome abnormalities detected in consecutive newborn studies. In: *Population Cytogenetics, Studies in Humans*, edited by E. B. Hook and I. H. Porter, pp. 63–79. Academic Press, New York.
34. Hse, T. C. (1975): A possible function of constitutive heterochromatin: the body guard hypothesis. *Genetics*, 79:137–150.
35. Jacobs, P. A., Melville, M., Ratcliffe, S., Keay, A. J., and Syme, J. (1974): A cytogenetic survey of 11,680 newborn infants. *Ann. Hum. Genet.*, 37:359–376.
36. Jacobs, P. (1977): Human chromosome heteromorphisms. In: *Progress in Medical Genetics*, edited by A. G. Steinberg, A. G. Bearn, A. G. Motulsky, and B. Childs, pp. 251–274. Saunders, Philadelphia.
37. Kirstenmacher, M. L., and Punnett, H. H. (1970): Comparative behavior of ring chromosomes. *Am. J. Hum. Genet.*, 22:304–318.
38. Knoll, J. H. M., Nicholls, R. D., Magenis, R. E., Graham, J. M., Jr., Lalande, M., and Latt, S. A. (1989): Angelman and Prader-Will syndromes share a common chromosome 15 deletion but differ in parental origin of the deletion. *Am. J. Med. Genet.*, 32:285–290.
39. Koenig, M., Hoffman, E. P., Bertelson, C. J., Monaco, A. P., Feener, C., and Kunkel, L. M. (1987): Complete cloning of the Duchenne muscular dystrophy (DMD) cDNA and preliminary genomic organization of the DMD gene in normal and affected individuals. *Cell*, 50:509–517.
40. Kornberg, R. D., and Klug, A. (1978): The nucleosome. *Sci. Am.*, 244:52–64.
41. Lazjuk, G. L., Lurie, I. W., Ostrowkaja, T. I., et al. (1980): The Wolf-Hirschhorn syndrome. II. Pathologic anatomy. *Clin. Genet.*, 18:6–12.
42. Le Beau, M. M., and Rowley, J. D. (1986): Chromosomal abnormalities in leukemia and lymphoma: clinical and biological significance. In: *Advances in Human Genetics*, edited by H. Harris and K. Hirschhorn, pp. 1–54. Plenum Press, New York.
43. Ledbetter, D. H., Riccardi, V. M., Airhart, S. D., Strobel, R. J., Keenan, B. S., and Crawford, J. D. (1981): Deletions of chromosome 15 as a cause of the Prader-Willi syndrome. *N. Engl. J. Med.*, 304:325–329.
44. Leder, P., Bultey, J., Lenoir, G., et al. (1983): Translocations among antibody genes in human cancer. *Science*, 222:765–771.
45. Lee, W.-H., Bookstein, R., Hong, F., Young, L.-J., Shew, J.-Y., and Lee, E. Y.-H. P. (1987): Human retinoblastoma susceptibility gene: cloning, identification, and sequence. *Science*, 235:1394–1399.
46. Lejeune, J., Gautier, M., and Turpin, R. (1959): Etude des chromosomes somatiques de neuf enfants mongoliens. *C. R. Acad. Sci.*, 248:1721–1722.
47. Lin, M. S., Comings, D. E., and Alfi, O. S. (1977): Optical studies of the interaction of 4'-6-diamidino-2-phenylindole with DNA and metaphase chromosomes. *Chromosoma*, 60:15–25.
48. Magenis, R. E., Brown, M. G., Lacy, D. A., Budden, S., and LaFranchi, S. (1987): Is Angelman syndrome an alternative result of del(15)(q11q13)? *Am. J. Med. Genet.*, 28:829–838.
49. Matsui, S.-I., and Sasaki, M. (1973): Differential staining of nucleolus organizers in mammalian chromosomes. *Nature*, 246:148–150.
50. Miller, O. J. (1981): Nucleolar organizers in mammalian cells. In: *Chromosomes Today*, edited by M. D. Bennett, M. Bobrow, and G. Hewitt, pp. 64–73. Allen and Unwin, London.

51. Monheit, A., Francke, U., Saunders, B., and Jones, K. L. (1980): The penta-X syndrome. *J. Med. Genet.*, 17:392–396.
52. Nowell, P., and Hungerford, D. A. (1960): A minute chromosome in human chronic granulocyte leukemia. *Science*, 132:1197.
53. Nussbaum, R. L., and Ledbetter, D. H. (1986): Fragile X syndrome: a unique mutation in man. *Annu. Rev. Genet.*, 20:109–145.
54. Orkin, S. H. (1986): Reverse genetics and human disease: a review. *Cell*, 47:845–850.
55. Pitt, D., Leversha, M., Sinfield, C., et al. (1981): Tetraploidy in a liveborn infant with spina bifida and other anomalies. *J. Med. Genet.*, 18:309–311.
56. Reik, W. (1989): Genomic imprinting and genetic disorders in man. *Trends in Genet.*, 5(10):331–336.
57. Reik, W., and Surani, M. A. (1989): Genomic imprinting and embryonal tumors. *Nature*, 338:112–113.
58. Riccardi, V. M. (1977): Trisomy 8: an international study of 70 patients. *Birth Defects*, 13(3C):171–184.
59. Robinson, A., Lubs, A. A., Nielsen, J., and Sorensen, K. (1979): Profiles of children with 47,XXY, 47,XXX, and 47,XYY karyotypes. *Birth Defects*, 15(1):261–266.
60. Sandberg, A. A., and Turc-Carel, C. (1987): The cytogenetics of solid tumors: relation to diagnosis, classification and pathology. *Cancer*, 59:387–395.
61. Sandberg, A. A. (1988): Chromosome rearrangements, protooncogenes, and human neoplasia. In: *The Cytogenetics of Mammalian Autosomal Rearrangements*, edited by A. Daniel, pp. 835–854. Alan R. Liss, New York.
62. Schmickel, R. D. (1986): Contiguous gene syndromes: a component of recognizable syndromes. *J. Pediatr.*, 109:231–241.
63. Seabright, M. (1971): A rapid banding technique for human chromosomes. *Lancet*, 2:271–272.
64. Simspon, J. L. (1976): *Disorders of Sexual Differentiation*. Academic Press, New York.
65. Stene, J., and Stengel-Rutkowski, S. (1988): Genetic risks of familial reciprocal and Robertsonian translocation carrier. In: *The Cytogenetics of Mammalian Autosomal Rearrangements*, edited by A. Daniel, pp. 3–72. Alan R. Liss, New York.
66. Sumner, A. T., Evans, H. J., and Buckland, R. A. (1971): New technique for distinguishing between human chromosomes. *Nature New Biol.*, 232:31–32.
67. Sumner, A. T. (1972): A simple technique for demonstrating centromeric heterochromatin. *Exp. Cell Res.*, 75:304–306.
68. Sutherland, G. R., Carter, R. F., Bald, R., Smith, I. I., and Bain, A. D. (1978): Chromosomal studies at the pediatric necropsy. *Ann. Hum. Genet.*, 42:173–181.
69. Therman, E. (1983): Mechanics through which abnormal X-chromosome constitutions affect the phenotype. In: *Cytogenetics of the Mammalian X Chromosome, Part B: X Chromosome Anomalies and Their Clinical Manifestations*, edited by A. A. Sandberg, pp. 159–173. Alan R. Liss, New York.
70. van Tuinen, P. W., Dobyns, B., Rich, P. C., et al. (1988): Molecular detection of microscopic and submicroscopic deletions associated with Miller-Dieker syndrome. *Am. J. Hum. Genet.*, 43:587–596.
71. van de Sande, J. H., Lin, C. C., and Jorgenson, K. F. (1977): Reverse banding on chromosomes produced by a guanosine-cytosine specific DNA binding antibiotic: olivomycin. *Science*, 195:400–402.
72. van Holde, K. E. (1988): *Chromatin*. Springer-Verlag, New York, Berlin, Heidelberg, London, Paris, Tokyo.
73. Verma, R. S., and Lubs, H. A. (1975): A simple R banding technique. *Am. J. Hum. Genet.*, 27:110–117.
74. Weiner, A. (1988): Eukaryotic nuclear telomeres: molecular fossils of the RNP world? *Cell*, 52:155–157.
75. Weisblum, B., and de Haseth, P. L. (1972): Quinacrine, a chromosome stain specific for deoxyadenylate-deoxythymidylate-rich regions in DNA. *Proc. Natl. Acad. Sci. USA*, 69:629–632.
76. Wertelecki, W., Graham, J. M., Jr., and Sergovich, F. R. (1976): The clinical syndrome of triploidy. *Obstet. Gynecol.*, 47:69–76.
77. Wilkins, L. E., Brown, J. A., Nance, W. E., and Wolf, B. (1982): Clinical heterogeneity in 80 home-reared children with cri du chat syndrome. *J. Pediatr.*, 102:529–533.

78. Willard, H. F. (1985): Chromosome-specific organization of human minisatellite DNA. *Am. J. Hum. Genet.*, 37:524–532.
79. William, J. D., Summitt, R. L., Martens, P. R., and Kimbrell, R. A. (1975): Familial Down's syndrome due to t(10;21) translocation; evidence that the Down phenotype is related to trisomy of a specific segment of chromosome 21. *Am. J. Hum. Genet.*, 27:478–485.
80. Yunis, J. J. (1976): High resolution of human chromosomes. *Science*, 191:1268–1270.
81. Yunis, J. J. (1981): Mid-prophase human chromosomes. The attainment of 2,000 bands. *Hum. Genet.*, 56:293–298.
82. Zaleski, W. A., Houston, C. S., Prozsonyl, J., and Ying, K. L. (1966): The XXXXY syndrome anomaly: report of three new cases and review of 30 cases from the literature. *Can. Med. Assoc. J.*, 94:1143–1154.
83. Zatz, M., Vianna-Morgante, A. M., Campos, P., and Diament, A. J. (1981): Translocation (X;6) in a female with Duchenne muscular dystrophy, implications for the localization of the DMD locus. *J. Med. Genet.*, 18:442–447.
84. Zuffardi, O.(1983): Cytogenetics of X/autosome translocations. In: *Cytogenetics of the Mammalian X Chromosome, Part B: X Chromosome Anomalies and Their Clinical Manifestations*, edited by A. A. Sandberg, pp. 193–209. Alan R. Liss, New York.

Genetic Variation and the Meiotic Process

Renee Z. Dintzis

*Departments of Cell Biology and Anatomy, and Biophysics,
The Johns Hopkins University School of Medicine,
Baltimore, Maryland 21205*

All normal human somatic cells contain 46 chromosomes. These consist of 23 pairs of homologues. A homologue is one member of a pair of chromosomes, one homologue being donated by the mother, the other by the father. Homologues are related, containing the same genes in the same order in the chromosomes, but since the structure of each gene is subject to variation, the DNA molecules derived from the parents are not identical. Variant genes are called alleles. Genetic heterogeneity in a population of individuals is due to differences among the genes in their chromosomes. The 23 pairs of chromosomes are estimated to contain 50,000 to 100,000 different gene pairs, and the information carried by the DNA in these genes determines human inheritance and constitutes the human genome.

GENETIC VARIATION IS IMPORTANT FOR SPECIES SURVIVAL

During growth and repair in the body, cells divide and replace themselves by mitosis, a replication process in which DNA sequences in cells are generally maintained constant from mother cell to daughter cell. This is important for genetic stability and is crucial for the proper functioning of any particular organism. However, for a species (consisting of many organisms) to be able to adapt to a changing environment, it must be able to undergo genetic variation. Genetic heterogeneity helps to increase the chances that at least some progeny will survive unforeseeable changes in the environment.

MEIOSIS PROVIDES A NORMAL MECHANISM FOR GENETIC VARIATION

To achieve genetic variation, there must be a mechanism for reshuffling the properties of parents among their children. There must be a mechanism for DNA to undergo rearrangements that might vary the combination of genes present in an individual genome from that in another individual genome. Such a variation of chromosome content occurs during the unique type of cell division, called meiosis, which occurs only in the primordial germ cells of the body as they differentiate into gametes. The end products of meiosis are the gametes—ova in the female and spermatozoa in the male. The gametes have 23 chromosomes, the haploid number. At fertilization, two haploid gametes fuse to form a diploid zygote, which can then give rise to all the other diploid body cells. This alternation between the haploid and the diploid state is the basis of sexual reproduction.

CHROMOSOMES UNDERGO RANDOM DISTRIBUTION AND RECOMBINATION DURING MEIOSIS

During meiosis, two important mechanisms insure that the genetic constitution, or genotype, of a species will undergo variation. One mechanism involves the random distribution (independent assortment) of one member of each chromosome pair into one haploid gamete. As a result of this random distribution, each gamete receives a different mixture of maternal and paternal chromosomes. Figure 1 illustrates the eight different possible gametes resulting from the random distribution of three homologous pairs of chromosomes, ($2^3 = 8$). In humans, because we contain

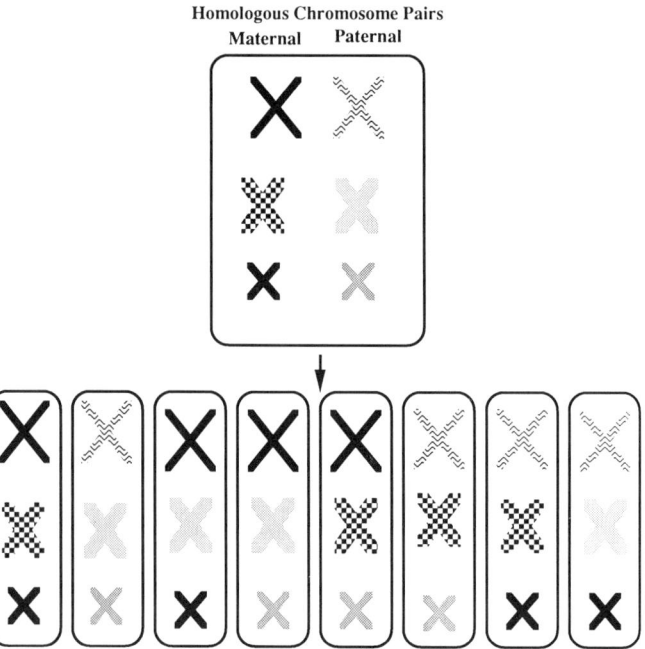

FIG. 1. The random distribution of three pairs of homologous maternal and paternal chromosomes during meiosis is illustrated. This process yields eight different possible gametes.

23 homologous pairs of chromosomes, each individual could theoretically produce at least 2^{23} (or about 8 million) genetically different gametes.

The actual number of different gametes produced is much greater than the above estimated 8 million because of the second mechanism for genetic variation taking place during meiosis. This involves a process of recombination in which genetic material is exchanged between each pair of homologous chromosomes in a unique chromosomal crossing-over that takes place during the long prophase of the first meiotic division. The crossovers recombine segments of DNA so that each gamete chromosome contains some genes derived from one parent and some from the other (Fig. 2). This type of recombination allows large sections of DNA double helix to move from one chromosome to another, but it does not normally change the arrangement of the genes in a chromosome. What it does accomplish is to permit, within the gametes from each parent, different versions (alleles) of a gene to occur in new combinations with other genes. This process leads to variations in a population that can account for differences in the resistance of individuals to challenging changes in the environment.

THE STAGES OF MEIOSIS

Meiosis is a two-staged division process. The first meiotic division (meiosis I) is a relatively long and complicated process during which DNA recombination occurs. The second meiotic division (meiosis II) is essentially a mitotic division that follows on from meiosis I without intervening duplication of the DNA.

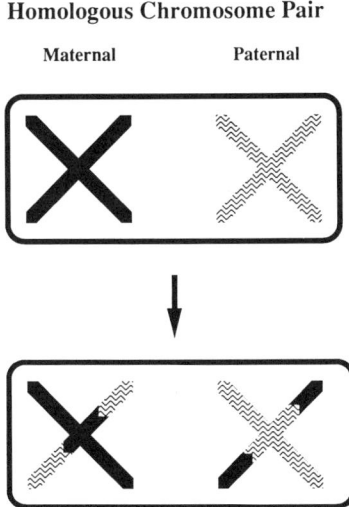

FIG. 2. Recombination involves a DNA exchange between homologous chromosomes during the crossing-over that occurs in the prophase of the first meiotic division.

MEIOTIC AND MITOTIC DIFFERENCES AND SIMILARITIES

In preparation for either mitosis or meiosis, a cell must replicate its DNA during the S (or synthesis) phase of the cell division cycle. This replication results in twin copies of each chromosome. The twin copies are called sister chromatids, and they are held together at the centromere by a structure called the kinetochore. In ordinary mitosis, the sister chromatids line up randomly on the mitotic spindle. Paternal and maternal homologues need not be near each other on the metaphase spindle. At anaphase, the kinetochores separate, the chromatids move apart, and after telophase, the resultant daughter cells again contain 48 separate chromosomes. Thus, as a result of mitosis, each diploid daughter cell contains the identical homologous pairs of chromosomes that were present in the parent cell.

In contrast, sister chromatids behave quite differently in meiosis. The homologous maternal and paternal sister chromatids recognize each other by some as yet unknown mechanism and become tightly paired during meiotic prophase. The structure containing the four paired chromatids is called a bivalent, or tetrad. It is during this tight pairing (or synapsis) that parts of homologous chromosomes are exchanged in a process called chromosomal crossing-over. Even the mostly nonhomologous X and Y sex chromosomes of the male can pair together at a short region of homology, and crossing-over can occur in this short region.

After the long prophase with its concomitant crossing-over events is completed, the tetrads line up on the metaphase spindle, and at anaphase, the homologous pairs of sister chromatids separate and move to opposite poles. This step differs from the anaphase of mitosis in that the kinetochores of sister chromatids do not separate, and therefore the sister chromatids do not separate. Instead, the sister chromatids move together, each pair going to one daughter cell. Thus, division I of meiosis results in two daughter cells that contain a diploid amount of DNA; however, they differ from normal diploid cells in that both of the two DNA copies of each chromosome have come from only one of the two homologous parental chromosomes in the original cell. Formation of the actual gamete can now proceed simply through a second cell division, meiosis II. As mentioned before, this division is similar to an ordinary mitotic division in which the sister chromatids line up on a spindle and the kinetochores separate, allowing each chromatid to segregate into a daughter cell. The progeny gametes now have a haploid DNA content. On occasion, an abnormal meiotic process may occur, in which homologues fail to separate in meiosis I or chromatids fail to separate in meiosis II. This is called nondisjunction and results in genetic abnormalities that are usually lethal.

RECOMBINATION AND CHROMOSOMAL CROSSING-OVER

In chromosomal crossing-over, actual breaks are made in single maternal and paternal DNA double helices. The two broken ends then rejoin to their opposite partners, in a reciprocal fashion. The resultant double helices each contain parts of

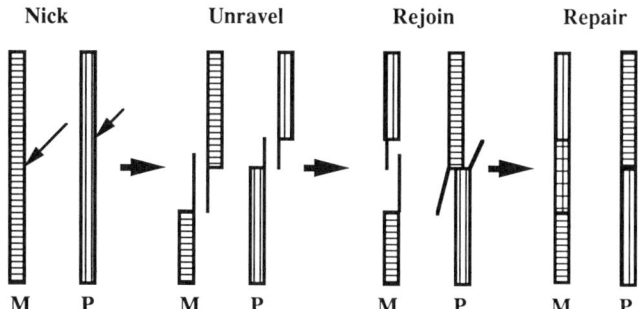

FIG. 3. In crossing-over, nicks are made in single maternal and paternal DNA double helices. The two broken ends unravel and are then rejoined in a reciprocal fashion. Repairs are then made to complete the recombined helices. M, maternal chromosome; P, paternal chromosome.

the two initial DNA molecules (Fig. 3). Among the four chromatids of the tetrad, crossovers can occur between any two of the nonsister chromatids. At the point where a crossover has taken place, the two duplicated homologues remain attached to each other. These attachment points are called chiasmata. Tetrads can contain more than one chiasma, indicating that more than one crossover can take place within a single chromosomal pair.

GENETIC RECOMBINATION OCCURS DURING THE PROPHASE OF MEIOSIS I

Chromosomes proceeding through the long prophase of meiosis I undergo dramatic shape changes as they pair and then separate. These shape changes have been classified into five stages and have been labeled: leptotene, zygotene, pachytene, diplotene, and diakinesis. For the sake of simplicity and clarity, Fig. 4 illustrates the appearance of just two homologous chromosomes (of the 23 homologues) as they undergo the shape changes of meiotic prophase I. At leptotene, the already replicated chromosomes (sister chromatids) have condensed into what appears to be a

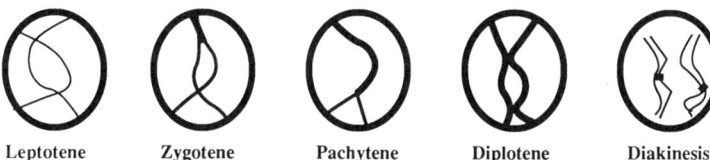

FIG. 4. The five stages of meiotic prophase I are pictured. The circles represent the nuclear envelope; inside are illustrated the shape changes undergone by a pair of homologous chromosomes. See text for more detailed description of each stage.

single thin thread. At zygotene, the homologues begin their intimate pairing, as illustrated at the upper end of the diagram of the nucleus. When pairing is complete, at pachytene, the intricate structure formed is called a synaptonemal complex. As can be seen at this stage in Fig. 4, the pairing is almost complete. Genetic recombination occurs at this stage. The tight pairing of the chromatids in the synaptonemal complex is believed to be required in order for crossover events to occur. In diplotene, the pairs begin to separate. Chiasmata can be seen where crossovers have occurred. In diakinesis, the last stage of the first prophase, the chromosomes condense as they prepare to enter metaphase I. Meiosis I resumes after the long first prophase (Fig. 5). Metaphase I is followed by anaphase I and telophase I. The

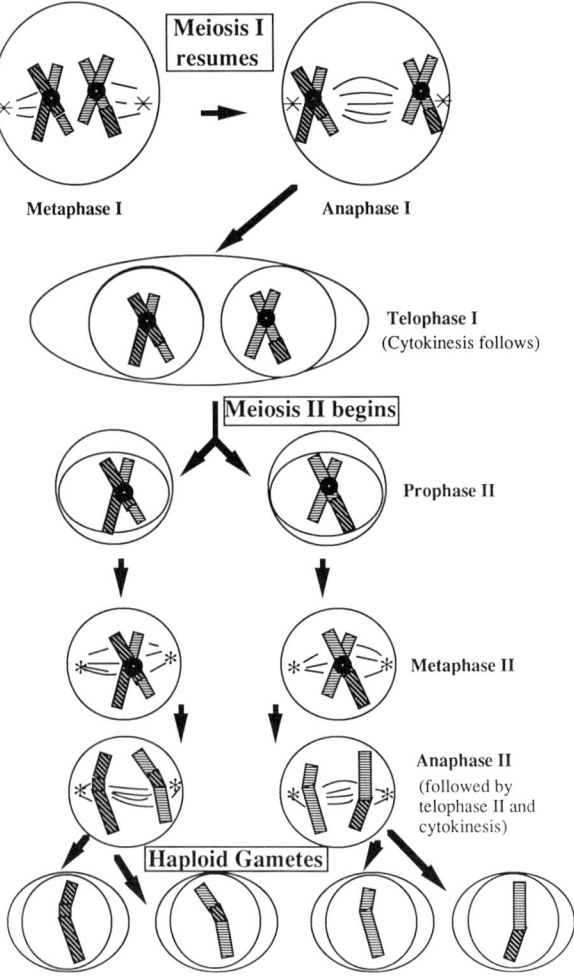

FIG. 5. After the five stages of meiotic prophase I are completed, the remainder of the meiotic process follows.

mitotic-like division of meiosis II quickly follows, but without an intervening replication of chromosomes. Thus, each diploid germ cell that originally enters meiosis yields four haploid cells. In the female, only one functional haploid ovum is formed as a result of meiosis. The rest of the daughter cells are smaller cells called polar bodies, which are nonfunctional and rapidly degenerate. In contrast, each spermatogonium gives rise to four haploid spermatozoa. To understand this, one must review the process of gamete formation in the two sexes.

DIFFERENCES IN MALE AND FEMALE GAMETE FORMATION

The process of meiosis in females and males differs considerably both in timing and in the number of actual gametes resulting from the meiotic divisions of each primordial germ cell. As mentioned, in females, only one functional gamete, the ovum, is produced. In males, four spermatozoa result from the meiosis of one spermatogonium.

Female gamete formation begins before birth. Primordial germ cells differentiate into oogonia, which early in fetal life undergo a number of mitotic divisions to develop into primary diploid oocytes. In the fifth prenatal month of life, primary oocytes complete the prophase of meiosis I. They remain arrested at this stage until just prior to ovulation, which begins at puberty. Women ordinarily ovulate only one oocyte every month until menopause, which in most cases occurs between the ages of 45 to 55 years, so the arrested stage of primary oocytes can represent a substantial period of time. At ovulation, the oocyte that is to be expelled from the ovary completes meiosis I and enters the metaphase stage of meiosis II. Meiosis II is not completed unless fertilization takes place.

The timing of the meiotic process in males is quite different from that of females. Whereas in females, the total number of oocytes is already fixed before birth, the male germ cells, spermatogonia, can increase their numbers from puberty to old age by undergoing mitoses. At the onset of puberty, a number of spermatogonia enter the meiotic process; however, others persist throughout reproductive life as unipotential stem cells that are capable of giving rise, via mitoses, to further spermatogonia. Spermatogonia that have entered the extended prophase of meiosis I are described as primary spermatocytes. The cells resulting from completion of meiosis I are secondary spermatocytes. These then enter meiosis II without interruption, and without any DNA replication, to yield their haploid progeny, the spermatids. Spermatids differentiate (without further division) into mature gametes, the spermatozoa (or sperm).

SEXUAL REPRODUCTION AS THE BASIS FOR GENETIC HETEROGENEITY

At fertilization, a sperm from a male and an ovum from a female fuse to form a diploid zygote. This cyclic alternation between the haploid and diploid state is the basis of sexual reproduction. As a result of the meiotic process that has already occurred, the chromosomes of spermatozoa and ova have already undergone genetic recombination, wherein parts of homologous maternal and paternal chromosomes have been exchanged. A further randomization of the genes of two individuals takes place when gametes fuse, because it is random as to which of the many different oocytes will be ovulated and which of the many different sperm will succeed in fertilizing the ovum. Thus, the entire process of sexual reproduction constitutes a unique and important mechanism whereby normal and rapid genetic changes can occur in a population from one generation to the next. The resultant genetic variation among individuals greatly increases the likelihood of survival of the species in a constantly changing environment.

GLOSSARY

Haploid cell   A cell carrying a single set of chromosomes.
Diploid cell   A cell carrying a double set of chromosomes.
Somatic cells   Cells of the body (not gametes).
Gametes or germ cells   Haploid cells specialized for sexual fusion.
Zygote   A fertilized egg, the result of fused gametes.
Homologue   One version (derived from either mother or father) of a pair of chromosomes.
Sister chromatids   Twin copies of a fully replicated chromosome.
Centromere   A region of the chromosome at which sister chromatids are joined.
Mitotic spindle   A structure composed of microtubules that aligns the replicated chromosomes in a plane during cell division.
Kinetochore   A structure near the centromere of the chromosome by means of which the chromosome binds to the mitotic spindle.
Meiosis   Division in which the chromosome complement is precisely halved.
Nondisjunction   An abnormal process during meiosis in which homologous chromosomes fail to separate.
Genetic recombination   The process by which crossing-over occurs between maternal and paternal chromatids during meiosis.
Chiasma   A point where a crossing-over between paternal and maternal chromatids has occurred during meiosis.
Leptotene, zygotene, pachytene, diplotene, diakinesis   Successive stages in the first meiotic division.
Synaptonemal complex   A structure that forms just before the pachytene stage of the first meiotic division; it keeps the homologous sister chromatids closely aligned.

Genes, Brain, and Behavior, edited by
P. R. McHugh and V. A. McKusick.
Raven Press, Ltd., New York © 1991.

Formal Genetics in Humans: Mendelian and Nonmendelian Inheritance

Reed E. Pyeritz

Department of Medicine and Pediatrics, Center for Medical Genetics, The Johns Hopkins University School of Medicine, Baltimore, Maryland 21205

Today and increasingly in the future, the basic principles of inheritance are indispensable equipment for anyone interested in understanding disorders of the nervous system. For the clinician, the educator, and the investigator alike, the general precepts of mendelism remain the foundation for understanding human inheritance. Unfortunately, what served as the "basic principles" of genetics in the early 1980s is both insufficient and, in some cases, incorrect.[1] This brief review discusses inheritance in the context of clinical medicine, a perspective that reveals numerous apparent violations of mendelian laws. The burden for the clinician and the investigator alike is to differentiate the situations actually due to novel genetic mechanisms that require a completely distinct interpretation and explanation.

MENDELIAN INHERITANCE

Mendel's Laws

In 1865, Gregor Mendel was fortunate in working with the garden pea, *Pisum sativum*, a simple diploid system that had easily and accurately assayable "characters" (*traits* or *phenotypes*, such as pod shape) that were determined each by a separate "factor" (first called a *gene* by Johannsen in 1909 [5]). Mendel was not burdened with the complexities of formal genetics in humans that would have likely prevented him from theorizing his *laws of inheritance* and, as some have suggested, "fudging" his data to confirm them (6).

Mendel promulgated three laws (7). The first stated, in essence, that it matters not from which parent a particular *allele* is inherited. In other words, from the fertilized zygote's perspective, both parents are equal. However, despite recent advances in fostering equality of the sexes, it is becoming increasingly certain that some genes behave differently depending on whether contributed by mother or by

---

[1] Recent reviews of many of the issues in this chapter provide considerably more detail and documentation (1–4).

father. The explanations for the exceptions to Mendel's First Law thus far involve *disomy* and *imprinting*, both discussed below.

The other two laws have held up much better and can be summarized in one phrase: *alleles segregate; nonalleles assort*. These principles are rooted in chromosome structure and meiosis, subjects discussed in the previous two chapters. Alleles segregate because they are on separate (but homologous) chromosomes and are drawn (segregate) to separate germ cells during the first meiotic division. Nonalleles (i.e., different genes) assort because which one of a pair of homologous chromosomes migrates to a given germ cell is purely a random event. This concept is simple enough for chromosomes, and even in terms of different genes on separate chromosomes. But genes on the same chromosome (*syntenic loci*) assort independently only if they are widely enough spaced for *genetic recombination* to be as likely to occur between them as not. When this pertains, the syntenic genes are said to be *unlinked*. However, when two genetic loci are close enough together for the chances for recombination at meiosis to be less than 50–50, then the genes do not assort independently and are said to be *linked*. Mendel was fortunate in having studied pea traits that were determined by unlinked genes. Linkage, while a true departure from mendelian law, has a ready explanation and is itself a principle that finds wide application in medical genetics.

Mendel also did not have to cope with three concepts that often befuddle interpretation of human inheritance patterns. *Pleiotropy*, *variability*, and *genetic heterogeneity* permeate all aspect of clinical genetics and will be discussed below.

Dominance and Recessiveness

These terms are used frequently in formal and informal discourse, often with disregard for accuracy. They are attributes of the phenotype, not the gene; an allele is not dominant or recessive. Second, these terms are utilitarian and empiric, not idealistic or immutable. Consider an *inborn error of metabolism*, due to deficiency of an enzyme activity. A functional ("normal" or "wild-type") allele is signified by + and a deleterious (mutant) allele by −. Whether the abnormal phenotype is dominant or recessive may depend largely on the level of enzyme activity when the individual is *homozygous* for both normal alleles ($+/+$). If this normal level of activity is far in excess of that needed to maintain metabolic homeostasis, even during periods of stress, then a partial reduction, as in a person *heterozygous* ($+/-$), may have little or no effect on homeostasis. The marked reduction in activity in homozygotes for the mutant allele ($-/-$) would be necessary to disrupt metabolism and produce the disease, which would be classified as a recessive phenotype. Most inborn errors of metabolism are of this type.

On the other hand, if the level of enzyme activity in the normal homozygote ($+/+$) is barely sufficient to maintain homeostasis, then a partial reduction in a heterozygote for a mutant allele ($+/-$) could produce a deleterious effect and a dominant phenotype. A few enzyme deficiency states are dominant (e.g., uroporphrinogen I synthetase deficiency in acute intermittent porphyria).

Dominance and recessiveness are determined by the sensitivity of the methods used to assay the phenotype. Years ago, the only phenotype associated with the HbS allele was sickle cell anemia, a condition of homozygotes (HbS/HbS) and one that satisfied all of the criteria listed below for an autosomal recessive trait. Subsequently, the obligate heterozygotes (genotype HbS/HbA; also called *carrier* and the phenotype is called *sickle cell trait*) were found to have an abnormal phenotype as well: some of their erythrocytes sickled when subjected to low oxygen tension; the amino acid substitution could be detected by electrophoresis; and clinically important pathology could occur during hypoxemic stress. Thus, by these criteria, sickle cell trait is a dominant phenotype.

Classification of Disease

Geneticists have been as guilty as specialists in any field of medicine in maintaining a typologic perspective, in which diseases are entities visited upon patients. In this view, the genes are the etiologic agents, and genetic diseases are those conditions due to disruptions of one locus (single gene disorders [8]), collections of loci on chromosomes (chromosomal disorders), or several loci that interact with external agents (multifactorial disorders). This ontologic scheme is deficient for numerous reasons that have been elegantly discussed by Childs (9).

As more has been learned about both etiology and pathogenesis of the diseases that have been classified neatly as single-gene, chromosomal, and multifactorial, sound empiric justification has emerged for revising not just terminology, but the mind-set of clinicians and investigators alike. Thus, some disorders caused by a mutation at a single locus are markedly affected by the genetic background or by manipulations of diet and might be thought of as multifactorial. Moreover, some disorders associated with identifiable deletions of specific chromosomal segments are clearly due to disruption of contiguous genes and are heritable according to mendelian principles.

In the following discussion, care has been taken to avoid reliance on a typologic classification of disorders, of causes, or of mechanisms of disease. For the student of human variation, the ontologic approach is a bit more arduous at the outset, but far more rewarding in the end.

Autosomal Dominant Inheritance

The characteristics of autosomal dominant inheritance in humans are:

- vertical pattern in a pedigree (multiple generations affected);
- heterozygotes for the mutant allele show an abnormal phenotype;
- males and females affected equally frequently and severely;

- only one parent needs to be affected for an offspring to be at risk for developing the phenotype;
- when an affected person mates with an unaffected one, each offspring has a 50% chance of inheriting the affected phenotype; this holds regardless of the sex of the affected parent; specifically, male-to-male transmission occurs;
- the frequency of sporadic cases is positively associated with the severity of the phenotype; more precisely, the greater the *reproductive fitness* of affected persons, the less likely any given case resulted from new mutation;
- on the average, the age of fathers of isolated (sporadic or new mutation) cases is advanced.

Figure 1 depicts a portion of an actual pedigree of a family with Huntington disease.

Autosomal dominant phenotypes are often:

- associated with malformations or other physical features;
- pleiotropic;
- variable;
- less severe than recessive ones;
- age dependent.

Sporadic Cases and Paternal Age Effect

A dominant phenotype that occurs in an offspring of two parents, neither of whom shows any trace of the phenotype, is termed a sporadic case. Although there

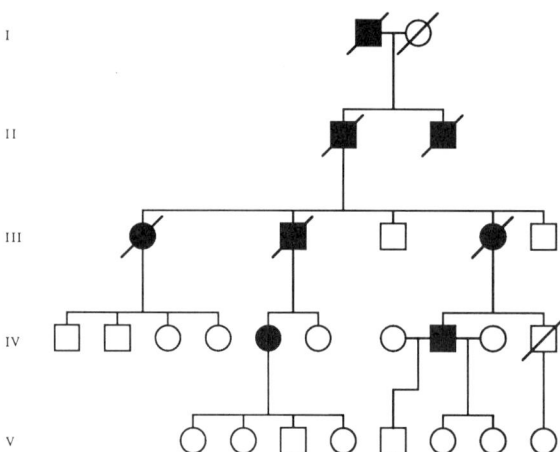

FIG. 1. Autosomal dominant inheritance. A pedigree showing segregation of Huntington disease in a portion of a large Maryland family (50). Assignment of phenotype was based on clinical signs, so that age dependency is evident.

are several reasons for misinterpretation, including genetic heterogeneity, nonpaternity, and nonpenetrance, true sporadic cases are caused by a new mutation at the locus causing the phenotype. The mutation may have occurred in a germ cell of either parent (and indeed mutations occur in gonads continuously), and by chance the mutated egg or sperm participated in the conception that led to the affected individual. For most dominant conditions, the average age of the fathers of sporadic cases, when corrected for maternal age, is greater than the age of fathers in general (10). This phenomenon has been explained by the continuous cycling of male spermatocytes; a mutation occurring at meiosis is perpetuated because one of the daughter cells returns to the pool of spermatocytes from which future sperm will emerge. In distinction, a female is born with a full complement of oocytes already part way through meiosis, and completion of the cycle for a given oocyte, even if a mutation occurs, does not return a defective genotype to the pool.

The frequency of any particular mutation is relatively constant in a population. If a mutation causes a severe, dominant phenotype incompatible with either survival (a true lethal) or reproduction (a genetic lethal), then that allele will not be perpetuated by passage from parent to offspring and will only arise through new mutation. On the other hand, a dominant phenotype with no impact on the ability of an affected person to reproduce (such as polydactyly) will be perpetuated by familial transmission; the proportion of cases due to a sporadic mutation would need to be low if the overall prevalence of the phenotype is to remain in equilibrium. An example of the latter is Huntington disease, in which people heterozygous for the mutation usually reproduce before signs of the disease appear. Few, if any, unequivocal examples of sporadic cases of Huntington disease have been identified.

An individual may develop an autosomal dominant phenotype because the defective allele arose by mutation, not in a parental germ cell, but in a somatic cell at an early embryonic stage. If the mutation occurred so early that all or most of the cells of the zygote that migrate to the embryo (as opposed to the placenta) contain the mutation, then the person at birth will be indistinguishable from someone who inherited the mutation from a parent. Obviously, the overall effect on the individual will depend on the developmental age at which the mutation occurs and whether cells of the particular organs involved in the phenotype develop from mutated cells. In addition, whether a condition that develops as a result of *somatic mutation* can be transmitted to the next generation will depend on whether the anlage cells of the gonads contain the mutation. A somatic mutation always produces *somatic mosaicism* in which some cells of the individual are different in genotype from the rest of the cells.

Germinal Mosaicism

In a person with somatic mosaicism, if the mutant allele does occur in some cells in a gonad, he or she might pass the condition to offspring. This situation is termed *germinal* (or *gonadal*) *mosaicism* and is of major importance in understanding etiology and in genetic counseling. Molecular genetic techniques, especially the ability to analyze DNA from single sperm (employing amplification of specific sequences by polymerase chain reaction [PCR]), have recently been used to demonstrate that germinal mosaicism is *not* necessarily rare (11). Conditions in which germinal mosaicism have now been documented include the X-linked disorders Duchenne muscular dystrophy (12) and hemophilia A (13), and autosomal dominant osteogenesis imperfecta type II (14).

The risk that a phenotypically normal mother or father, with germ-line mosaicism for a mutation that causes an autosomal dominant disorder, will have an affected offspring is proportional to the fraction of oocytes or spermatocytes carrying the mutation. This fraction is impossible to determine in women, but approaching routine determinability in men for those conditions with defined molecular defects.

Penetrance

The meaning of this concept is frequently mistaken and should be defined as the frequency (%) of appearance of a phenotype (dominant or recessive) when the mutant allele or alleles are present. For individuals, penetrance is an all-or-none phenomenon, that is, the phenotype is either present (penetrant) or not (nonpenetrant). Differences in expression of an allele are termed *variability* or *variable expressivity*, not incomplete penetrance. Nonpenetrance is illustrated in Fig. 2.

Nonpenetrance, in which the mutant allele is present in the individual without evident effect, has been thought to be rare. The potential causes of nonpenetrance are numerous and include some explanations not subjected to rigorous proof as yet.

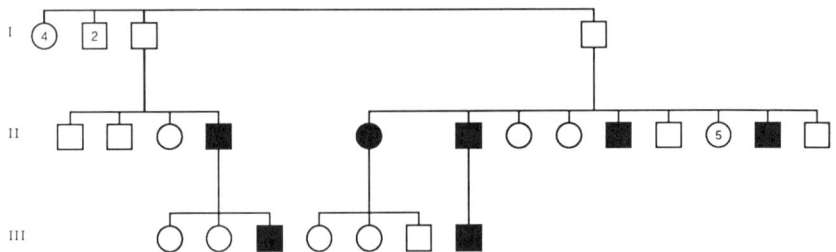

FIG. 2. Nonpenetrance of an autosomal dominant trait (51). This pedigree was reported by one of the founders of the field of dysmorphology, David W. Smith, and shows the segregation of ectrodactyly (congenital absence of some digits—often a so-called lobster-claw or split-hand deformity). If autosomal dominance is the correct interpretation for the etiology of this phenotype, the brothers in generation I who both have affected offspring must have been heterozygous, and hence nonpenetrant, for the mutation. One of their parents might have been as well, although no information on this point was presented and the pedigree has apparently never been revisited.

The ability to detect mutations in DNA holds promise for revealing a molecular basis for nonpenetrance.

The most frequent cause of apparent nonpenetrance is simply insensitive methods for detecting the phenotype. If this were the case in a parent of a child with a dominant condition, the parent would have a 50% chance at each subsequent conception of having another affected child. This fact emphasizes the need for careful, high-resolution scrutiny of both parents of a child with a condition that is known to be a mendelian dominant trait. One common cause in adult-onset neurologic diseases is the death of a person before he or she manifests the phenotype but after transmission of the mutant allele to offspring.

A reason for spurious nonpenetrance is *genetic heterogeneity*. For example, the family under consideration has an autosomal recessive or multifactorial condition that is difficult to distinguish from the phenotype of a recognized autosomal dominant condition.

Codominance

When both alleles are expressed in the heterozygote, as in blood group AB, in sickle trait (HbS/HbA), the major histocompatibility antigens, or in sickle-C disease (HbS/HbC), the phenotype is called codominant.

Incomplete Dominance

Human dominant traits are not true mendelian dominants (and are often called incomplete) in that the phenotype of the heterozygote is not the same as that in the homozygote. Mendel found for traits in peas that it made no difference whether the genotype was heterozygous or homozygous (e.g., $+/-$ or $-/-$) at a given locus; the trait determined by the $-$ allele was the same. This is not the case in humans, with one exception described in the next section.

Homozygosity for Alleles Causing Dominant Traits

In human dominant phenotypes, the homozygous state is almost always more severe, as in familial hypercholesterolemia (15), and often lethal, as in achondroplasia (16). Mating between parents both affected with an autosomal dominant form of Charcot-Marie-Tooth disease (17) or both affected with a distal myopathy (18) have been reported to produce presumed homozygotes for these disorders; the offspring were severely affected from early in life. Huntington disease is the first exception, in which individuals shown by DNA markers and linkage analysis to have inherited two copies of the mutant allele are not affected earlier or worse than their heterozygous parents and sibs (19,20).

Anticipation

This concept is defined as an apparent tendency of dominant phenotypes to appear more severely and at earlier ages in individuals of successive generations. In terms of genetic mechanisms, anticipation in an epiphenomenon. However, several mechanisms can explain the appearance of anticipation. *Variability* (which is defined in detail subsequently) may result in some offspring of a patient being more severely affected. Biased ascertainment is always a possibility because more severe cases are likely to be detected. Improved methods of detecting the condition provide a secular trend for increased ascertainment. Knowledge of genetics on the part of both investigators and families results in heightened alertness for the 50% probability of inheritance. Finally, there is good evidence for a *birth cohort effect* for some conditions, such as depression, in which the phenotype over time is displaying a decreased age of onset and increased population frequency (21,22). In a family, either of these trends can result in apparent anticipation.

Autosomal Recessive Inheritance

Characteristics of autosomal recessive inheritance in humans are:

- horizontal pattern in a pedigree (single generation affected);
- males and females affected equally frequently and severely;
- inheritance from both parents, each a heterozygote (*carrier*) and each usually clinically unaffected;
- each offspring of two carriers has a 25% chance of being affected, a 50% chance of being a carrier, and a 25% chance of inheriting neither mutant allele; thus, two-thirds of all clinically unaffected offspring are carriers;
- in matings between individuals, each with the same recessive phenotype, all their offspring will be affected;
- affected individuals who mate with unaffected individuals who are not carriers have only unaffected offspring;
- the rarer the recessive phenotype, the more likely the parents are to be *consanguineous*.

Figure 3 shows a characteristic pedigree in which an autosomal recessive condition, Friedreich ataxia, is present.

Autosomal recessive phenotypes are often:

- associated with deficient activity of enzymes and are thus termed inborn errors of metabolism;
- more severe than dominant conditions;
- less variable than dominant phenotypes;
- at this time, more easily recognized as genetically heterogeneous than dominant conditions;
- less age dependent than dominant conditions.

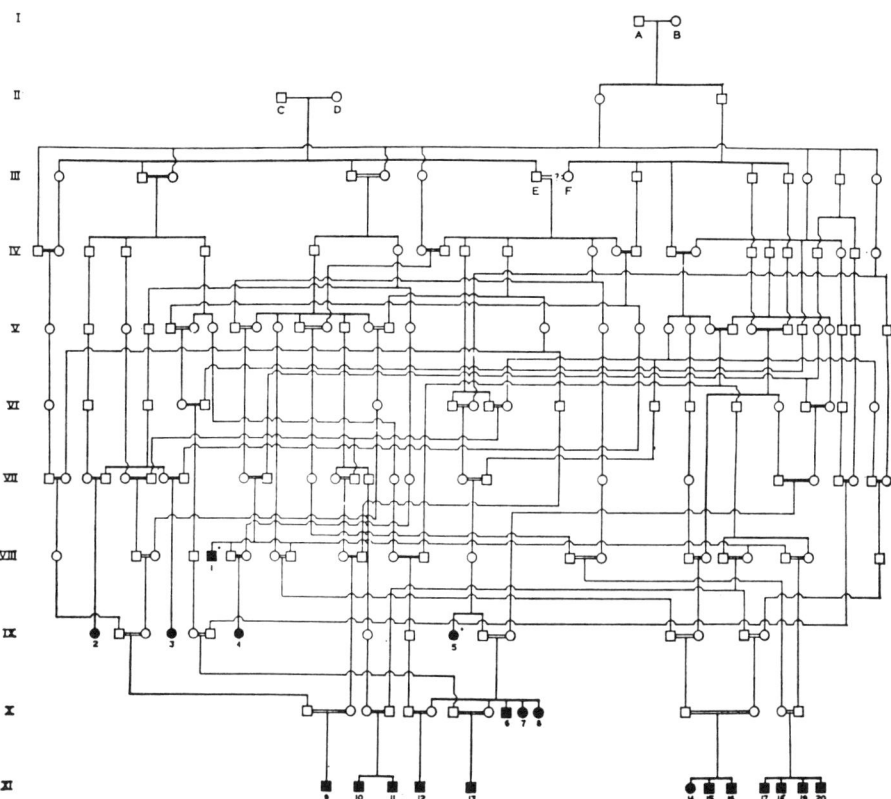

FIG. 3. Autosomal recessive inheritance. A pedigree showing segregation of spastic paraplegia with distal muscle wasting (the Troyer syndrome) in a large Amish kindred (52). Note that multiple sibships, but none of the parents of an affected child, are affected. Because of the social characteristics of this population, inbreeding is common, and most of the matings that produced affected children are clearly consanguineous, and all probably are.

Consanguinity

When an autosomal recessive condition is quite rare, the chance that the parents of cases are consanguineous is increased. As a result, the prevalence of rare recessive conditions is relatively high among inbred groups such as the Old-order Amish. When the autosomal recessive condition is common, then the chance of consanguinity between parents of cases is no higher than in the general population (about 0.5%).

Pseudodominance

When the frequency of a mutant allele is high, the chance that a homozygote will mate with a heterozygote is not insignificant. In such a family, successive generations might have the condition, and dominant inheritance might be suggested (Fig. 4).

Genetic Compound

An individual having two different mutant alleles at the same locus, as in HbS/HbC, is termed a genetic compound. The phenotype usually lies between those produced by the alleles in the homozygous state. Because of the large number of mutations possible in a given gene (the pervasiveness of genetic heterogeneity), many autosomal recessive phenotypes are likely due to genetic compounds, as in the thalassemias (23). Sickle cell disease is an exception. Consanguinity is strong presumptive evidence against a genetic compound.

Severity, Gene Frequency, and Selection

One teleologic reason why autosomal recessive disorders are, in general, more severe than dominant conditions is that persistence of recessive traits does not depend on reproduction of affected persons. Thus, an autosomal recessive condition can be a genetic lethal, yet the mutant allele will be perpetuated through clinically unaffected heterozygotes. In fact, the heterozygote frequency for some recessive conditions is so high that the mutant allele is *polymorphic* (present more commonly than could be due to recurrent mutation; arbitrarily taken as an allele frequency of 1%).

On the other hand, to the extent that some heterozygotes manifest the abnormal phenotype to a slight degree, carriers may be selected against in the evolutionary sense. This effect tends to reduce the frequency of the unfavorable allele in the population.

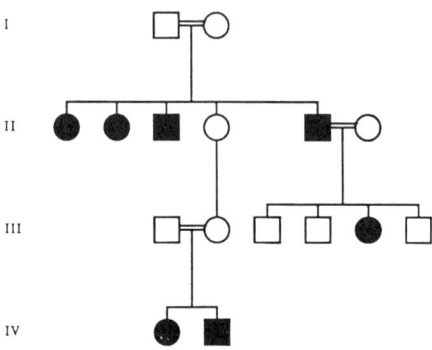

FIG. 4. Pseudodominance. At first glance, this pedigree suggests transmission of an autosomal dominance of Charcot-Marie-Tooth disease. Closer inspection shows multiple instances of "nonpenetrance," and even closer inspection reveals the high degree of consanguinity. In fact, in this Amish kindred, Charcot-Marie-Tooth disease is an autosomal recessive trait, and passage from parent to child occurs because an affected father (in generation VII) married a woman heterozygous for the mutant allele (53).

Human Genetic Variation—the Prevalence of Heterozygosity

The human genome is in a constant state of flux, with new mutations arising, many mutations disappearing after one or a few generations, and a few becoming fixed in the population due to selection or random drift (24). Upon first learning of the diagnosis of an autosomal recessive disorder in their child, parents express a range of emotions that usually include shock, anger, and guilt. To assist parents in coping with their feelings, one important message is often emphasized during genetic counseling. *All humans are heterozygous for alleles that, if present in homozygous form, would be lethal* (25). A rough estimate is 4–8 loci harboring lethal alleles. The first evidence with respect to specific loci is usually the birth of an affected offspring. Once the condition is diagnosed, then carrier status can often be determined in those who are not obligate heterozygotes.

X-Linked Inheritance

General characteristics of X-linked inheritance in humans include:

- no male-to-male transmission of the phenotype;
- unaffected males do not transmit the phenotype;
- all of the daughters of an affected male are heterozygous carriers;
- males are usually more severely affected than females;
- whether a heterozygous female is counted as affected—and whether the phenotype is called "recessive" or "dominant"—depends often on the sensitivity of the assay or the examination;
- some mothers of affected males will not be themselves heterozygotes (i.e., they will be homozygous normal); the proportion of heterozygous (carrier) mothers is negatively associated with the severity of the condition;
- heterozygous women transmit the mutant gene to one-half of sons, who are affected, and to one-half of daughters, who are heterozygotes;
- on average, the age of fathers of the first heterozygous woman in a pedigree is advanced;
- if an affected male mates with a heterozygous woman, half of their sons will be affected, giving the false impression of male-to-male transmission; one-half of the daughters of such matings will be affected as severely as the average hemizygous male; in small pedigrees, this pattern may simulate autosomal dominant inheritance.

The pedigree in Fig. 5 illustrates inheritance of a nonlethal X-linked disorder, one form of Charcot-Marie-Tooth disease.

Characteristics of X-linked inheritance depend on phenotypic severity. *When the disorder is a genetic lethal in males* (affected males do not reproduce, as in Duchenne muscular dystrophy), expect to observe about two-thirds of affected males

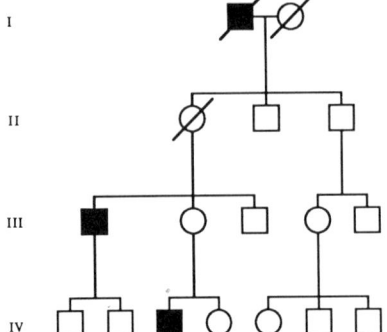

FIG. 5. X-linked inheritance. A pedigree showing segregation of Charcot-Marie-Tooth disease in males through carrier females.

have a carrier mother; the other third arise by new mutation in an X chromosome of the mother.

This has been the standard teaching, based on population genetic predictions. The hypothesis is now subject to confirmation by direct detection of the mutation in a mother and her parents. The pedigree shown in Fig. 6 illustrates a family with several men affected with Duchenne muscular dystrophy.

When the disorder is nearly always manifest in heterozygous females (also called X-linked dominant inheritance), expect to observe that females tend to be affected about twice as often as males and an affected female transmits the phenotype to half of her sons and half of her daughters, on the average.

Examples of conditions showing X-linked dominant inheritance are Coffin-Lowry syndrome and focal dermal hypoplasia (Goltz syndrome).

When the disorder is nearly always lethal in utero in hemizygous males (a form of X-linked dominant inheritance), expect to observe:

- only females are affected;
- an affected female transmits the disorder to one-half of her daughters;
- affected females have fewer sons than daughters;

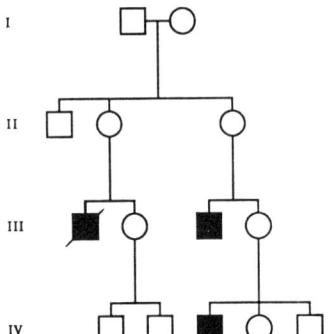

FIG. 6. X-linked inheritance of a lethal trait. A pedigree showing Duchenne muscular dystrophy, in which males do not live to reproduce. This is a lethal trait in the genetic trait because the affected individual does not pass the mutant allele to offspring.

- affected females show an increased frequency of spontaneous abortion, these losses being hemizygous males.

X-linked phenotypes are often:

- clinically variable, particularly in heterozygous females;
- suspected of being autosomal dominant with nonpenetrance.

Germinal mosaicism occurs in mothers of boys with X-linked conditions. The chance of such a mother having additional affected boy or heterozygous girl offspring depends on the fraction of her oocytes that carries the mutation. Presently, this fraction is impossible to determine. However, the presence of germinal mosaicism can be detected in a family, and this knowledge used for genetic counseling.

Y-Linked Inheritance

Characteristics of Y-linked (holandric) inheritance in humans include:

- only males affected;
- only male-to-male transmission.

Y-linked phenotypes are few, probably due to the relatively small number of genes present on this small chromosome. Genes specifying a testes-determining factor and influencing height are on the Y, as are genes controlling some aspects of spermatogenesis and tooth size. One gene in the sex-determining region encodes a protein that binds zinc and likely interacts with specific sequences of DNA (so-called finger protein) (26).

NONMENDELIAN INHERITANCE

As will be emphasized repeatedly in this book, nearly all human disease has some genetic factors important to etiology and pathogenesis. In most cases, especially in common diseases, the aberrant phenotype does not recur in families in patterns consistent with mendelian inheritance. Such diseases have been described as *multifactorial*, implying the importance of both multiple genes and environmental factors.

Recently, however, *somatic mosaicism, uniparental disomy*, and *mutations of the mitochondrial chromosome* have been recognized as additional important causes of disease with inheritance patterns that are not mendelian.

Somatic Mosaicism

Somatic mosaicism reflects heterogeneity of the genetic constitution of the cells of an organism. In all instances, this state arises from one or more mutations that occur after conception. Chromosomal aneuploidy or aberrations can occur as somatic mosaics. In some instances, the zygote begins life as an aneuploid cell, and during a later cell division, one of the daughter cell products contains a reversion to a normal chromosome constitution. In other instances, a chromosomally normal zygote undergoes a mitotic error and two chromosomally distinct cell lines emerge and persist. The resultant phenotype is an amalgam of the effects of the various cell lines present and determined in part by any inhomogeneity in tissue distribution of the chromosome abnormality. Thus, a patient with trisomy 21 in 50% of cells likely has, on average, a milder phenotype of the Down syndrome compared to a nonmosaic patient; the severity of mental retardation will be determined in part by the fraction of aneuploid cells in the central nervous system, a figure impossible to determine from karyotypic analysis of lymphocytes or dermal fibroblasts.

A particularly intriguing and relevant form of somatic mosaicism involves a mutation of one or a few contiguous genes. The mutation of an autosomal or sex-chromosomal gene occurs at any point after conception. The effect of the mutation and its mosaicism depends on:

- the type (i.e., regulatory, large deletion, etc.) of mutation;
- the type (i.e., regulatory, housekeeping, etc.) of gene(s);
- the specific locus or loci involved;
- whether the new mutation results in heterozygosity at the locus or has occurred serendipitously at a locus that already had the other allele mutated and transmitted through mendelian inheritance;
- the stage of development at which the mutation occurs;
- the specific cell types that differentiate from the mutated cell;
- the fate of the specific cell types (i.e., mixing with unmutated cells, *in vivo* selection for or against their propagation).

Potential results on phenotype are wideranging (27). If the mutation occurred very early and the derivative cells populated the part of the zygote that became the embryo, then the phenotype might be indistinguishable from an embryo that inherited the same mutation from a parent. Alternatively, if only the placenta receives the mutation, there may be no phenotypic effect on the embryo. Some human disease that affects only discrete parts of the body (e.g., hemihypertrophy, segmental neurofibromatosis) may be due to somatic mutations. Most human neoplasia involves somatic mutation of chromosomes, individual loci, or both.

As noted above, whether or not a person with a disorder due to a somatic mutation can pass the mutation to offspring depends on the presence of *germinal mosaicism*.

Uniparental Disomy

Except for mature germ cells, all cells of the human body are *disomic*, in that both members of each chromosome pair are present in each cell, for a total of 46. In the usual case, one of the chromosomes of each pair originated from the mother and one from the father. When *both* of the chromosomes of a given pair originated from one parent (and none from the other parent), the total chromosome number is still 46, but the cells are uniparental disomic for two of the complement. A special case, called *isodisomy*, occurs when the two chromosomes from the same parent are *identical* (28). These possibilities are illustrated in Fig. 7.

Depending on the mechanism for generating the disomic state (depicted in Fig. 8), one or two spontaneous pathologic events are necessary. These events can occur at either stage of meiosis or during mitosis in the embryo. Only in the past few years has evidence begun to accumulate that these various events do occur. The most convincing proof of mitotic (somatic) errors comes from the molecular analysis of neoplastic tissue, especially retinoblastoma (29). Germinal errors account for two unrelated examples of children with cystic fibrosis and growth retardation. In both cases, the children inherited both chromosomes 7 from their mother; these chromosomes were shown by analysis of RFLPs to be identical and therefore an example of isodisomy (30,31). Their fathers were not carriers for the cystic fibrosis mutation and their mothers were; they happened to be isodisomic for the chromosome 7 of their mothers that carried the cystic fibrosis allele. The cause of their short stature is unclear, but may be due to homozygosity for another mutant allele of this chromosome, or because inheriting some portion of chromosome 7 from the father may be essential for normal development. This latter phenomenon is an example of *imprinting* (discussed in the next section).

Uniparental disomy should be suspected when a patient has:

- more than one autosomal recessive disorder;
- an autosomal recessive disorder and additional phenotypic abnormalities not usually present in the mendelian condition;
- an autosomal recessive disorder for which only one parent is heterozygous;
- a female with an X-linked recessive disorder.

Imprinting

This term has several meanings in biology. In the genetic sense, imprinting refers to germ line-specific modifications of parental genetic contributions to the zygote. The net result is differential expression of (potentially identical) genetic information inherited from the mother compared with that from the father (32). This phenomenon probably accounts for some of the phenotypic effects of uniparental disomy and is a clear violation of Mendel's First Law; for some loci, it indeed *is* important from which parent a particular allele is inherited.

Considerable evidence for imprinting is accumulating through studies of experimental animals (33). The mechanisms by which imprinting occurs are being explored and may well involve DNA methylation and other processes that regulate gene expression (32,34). At this stage of understanding, the following points seem clear. Imprinting affects both the embryo and the placenta. Defects in imprinting can have diffuse but major impact on growth and development. Both maternal and

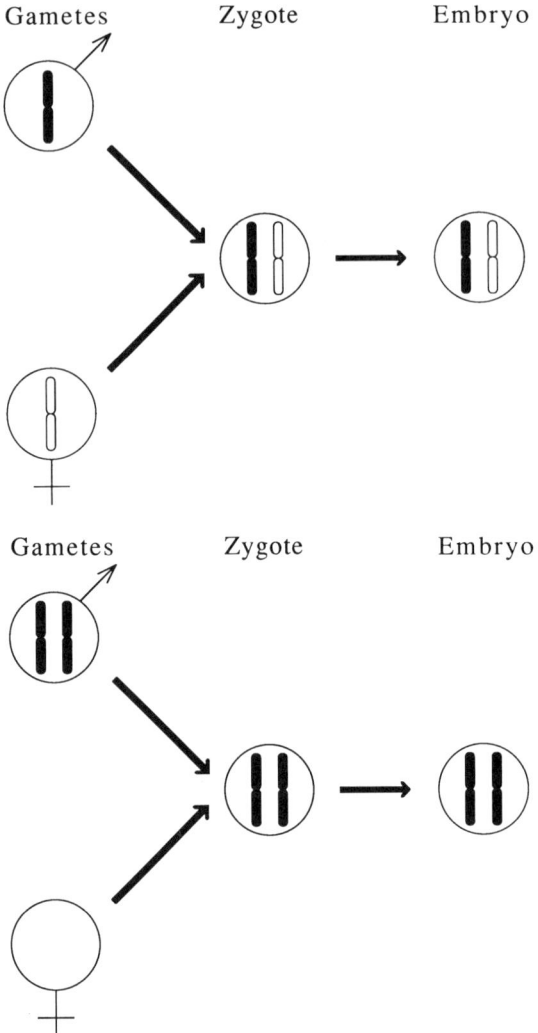

FIG. 7. Biparental disomy and uniparental disomy. **Top:** Normal gametogenesis and assortment of chromosomes at meiosis coupled with normal fertilization and mitosis produce the desired embryo, which is characterized by biparental disomy. **Bottom:** One mechanism for achieving uniparental isodisomy requires two errors. An error in separation of chromosomes at the second stage of meiosis produces a male (in this illustration) gamete with two identical copies of the same chromosome. If this gamete then fertilizes an egg that lacks the same chromosome present in two copies in the sperm (i.e., a nullisomic egg), the zygote will contain the correct number of chromosomes, but will suffer from at least two deleterious effects: some mutant alleles on the chromosome will be homozygous, and the zygote will lack a maternal contribution for that chromosome (30).

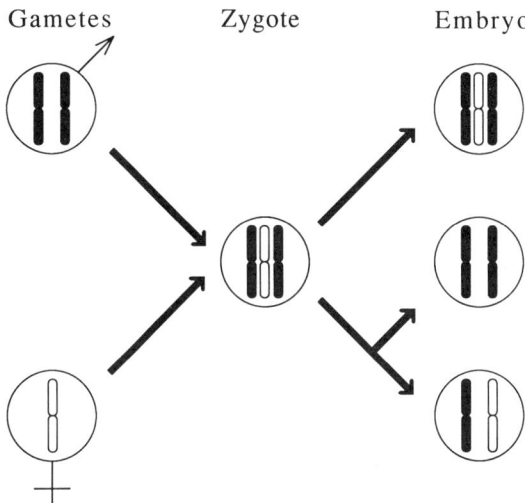

FIG. 8. Uniparental disomy. Various mechanisms, in addition to that in Fig. 7, bottom, are depicted by which uniparental disomy might arise, with some leading to isodisomy (30). Some mechanisms involve postfertilization errors.

paternal contributions of certain regions of the genome are essential and in some ways complementary. Imprinting is not a permanent change, as it is specified by the gonad. Thus, an alteration dictated by the ovary as a gene passes from mother to son will have that particular imprint removed when the same gene passes through the son's testes.

Several well-studied examples of parental effect on phenotype might be explained by imprinting. Offspring of mothers affected by myotonic dystrophy stand a 50-50 chance of inheriting the condition, but about one-half of those children who do develop a severe, early-onset form of the disease; this does not occur to the offspring of affected fathers (35). Contrarily, offspring of fathers with Huntington disease who inherit the mutant allele develop the disease, on average, at an earlier age than the offspring of affected mothers (36). The affected offspring of mothers with neurofibromatosis (NF I) tend to have a more severe phenotype than if the father contributes the mutant gene (37).

Mitochondrial Inheritance

The mitochondrial chromosome (mtDNA) is a circle of double-stranded DNA consisting of 16,569 nucleotide pairs, the exact sequence for which is known. Although each chromosome is relatively small, because each mitochondrion has several chromosomes and each cell has thousands of mitochondria, mtDNA may account for 0.3% of total cellular DNA. The mtDNA encodes its own set of transfer RNAs, has several nuances in its genetic code compared with nuclear chromosomes, and encodes 13 proteins that are translated within the mitochondrion. All of these proteins function, along with many other proteins encoded by the nuclear chromosomes and imported from the cytoplasm, in oxidative phosphorylation reactions (38).

The following are the expected characteristics of a mutation in one of the structural genes of mtDNA:

- the phenotype should include a defect in oxidative phosphorylation;
- different tissues should express an abnormal phenotype in proportion to their dependency on oxidative phosphorylation;
- a somatic mutation in an individual mtDNA would never be recognized because its effect would be diluted by the immense number of normal mtDNAs.

The inheritance pattern of a disorder due to a mutation of the mitochondrial chromosome, Leber hereditary optic neuropathy (39), is shown in Fig. 9.

Mitochondria, and hence mtDNA, are inherited from the oocyte. Because the father contributes virtually none of this pool of mtDNA genes, the inheritance is termed *maternal* or *cytoplasmic*, and males do not pass any mtDNA mutations they might have to their offspring.

The following are the expected characteristics of maternal inheritance:

- males and females generally affected equally frequently and severely;
- males do not transmit the phenotype to offspring;
- all of the offspring of a woman may be affected;
- a high degree of variability in phenotype is not unusual because each oocyte contains a mixture of both mutant and wild-type mtDNAs; the phenotype in the offspring depends on the partitioning of the mutant mtDNA within the zygote.

In addition to Leber hereditary optic neuropathy, a form of ocular myopathy and a form of myoclonic epilepsy with ragged red fiber myopathy result from mutations of mtDNA.

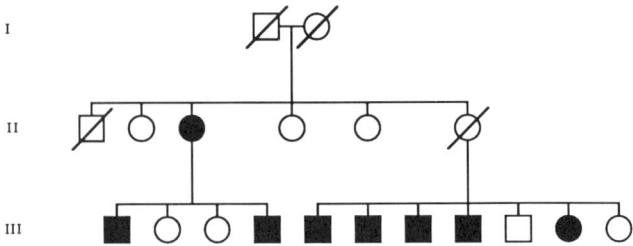

FIG. 9. Mitochondrial inheritance. A pedigree showing "maternal" or "cytoplasmic" inheritance of Leber optic atrophy (39). Note that not all offspring of an affected woman express the disease in this family; this apparent lack of penetrance can be due to age dependency, variability in expression of the mutation, passage of variable numbers of mutant mitochondrial genomes to an egg, and random variation in segregation of mutant and nonmutant mitochondrial genomes within the cytoplasm of the fertilized egg.

PRINCIPLES OF CLINICAL GENETICS

Three principles have a major role in understanding inheritance in humans, especially as viewed in a clinical setting. Each of these concepts is an old one, dating from the early part of this century.

Pleiotropy

A given allele (whether mutant or wild-type) may have multiple phenotypic effects (40). The lists of signs and symptoms that can be constructed for any human hereditary disorder is a testament to pleiotropy.

Von Recklinghausen NF I exemplifies pleiotropy (Table 1). The gene has been localized to a narrow region of chromosome 17 (17q11.2), but neither the defect nor the function of the unmutated locus has been defined (41). This basic information is important in this context because *the closer the basic defect is approached, the better pleiotropy is understood*. At this stage, knowing little of either cause or pathogenesis of NF I interferes with deciding if a clinical manifestation is due directly to gene action (or inaction) or the result of a long chain of events stemming from a remote event. For example, most observers conclude that benign tumors (neurofibroma, Lisch nodules, and optic glioma) are a direct result of the NF-I mutation. Scoliosis develops in about 10% of patients who have otherwise unremarkable vertebral columns; this may represent a primary manifestation of the NF-I gene

TABLE 1. *Pleiotropic manifestations of von Recklinghausen NF-I*

Abnormal pigmentation
  Axillary and other freckling
  Café au lait macules
Neurofibromas
  Cutaneous
  Deep
  Ocular
Skeletal
  Reduced stature
  Macrocephaly
  Scoliosis
  Pseudoarthrosis
Intellectual
  Retardation
  Learning disabilities
Tumors
  Benign
    Optic gliomas
    Meningiomas
  Malignant
    Pheochromocytoma
    Neuroblastoma

by a mechanism as yet uncertain. Alternatively, paraspinal neurofibromas may distort vertebrae and produce scoliosis by a mechanism so remote from the gene as to represent an epiphenomenon. Particularly important yet enigmatic examples of pleiotropy are mental retardation and learning disabilities; it will be enlightening to understand how the NF-I mutation produces these manifestations.

Variability

This principle, also called variable expression, is quantitative and qualitative differences in phenotype between individuals having the same allele. The simplicity of this definition belies the extent of ignorance about the mechanisms that account for variability.

Evidence of variability abounds in nearly all hereditary conditions. Variability can be classified as:

- nonpenetrance of individual manifestations or of the entire phenotype;
- severity of individual manifestations or of the entire phenotype;
- frequency of occurrence of cyclic or episodic events;
- age of onset of the first evidence of the phenotype or of specific manifestations.

NF-I illustrates each of these points. Whereas most patients have café au lait macules and Lisch nodules, some escape cutaneous neurofibromas and many escape optic gliomas. It takes little experience with NF-I before the wide range of severity present, even among relatives, becomes evident. Certain manifestations, such as seizures, glaucoma, and neurocutaneous pain, are cyclic and largely unpredictable. The age of appearance of individual manifestations is highly variable; café au lait macules usually emerge early, scoliosis in childhood, and cutaneous neurofibromas later in life, but there is wide deviation even among relatives.

The causes of variability have been explored to only limited degrees in humans. Table 2 lists some of the numerous potential explanations. Variability may lead to overlap with the "normal" distribution of a particular manifestation or of the entire phenotype. This is more likely the further removed the manifestation is from the basic defect.

In general, the shorter the pathogenetic tree between the basic defect and the phenotypic manifestation, the less the variability.

Genetic Heterogeneity

Two unrelated people may have abnormal phenotypes that are indistinguishable clinically, but that are due to fundamentally different mutations. The individuals are said to be *genocopies* of one another, and the principle illustrates genetic heterogeneity. The mutations may be subtly distinct, involving different nucleotide changes within the same gene; if the functional effect on the gene product (such as a structural protein or enzyme) is the same, it is not at all surprising that the phe-

TABLE 2. Potential causes of variability

Genetic background
Age dependency
Sex influence and sex limitation
Maternal factors
   Mitochondrial inheritance
   Intrauterine environment
Genetic heterogeneity (pseudovariability)
Variation in X-inactivation—heterozygotes for X-linked loci
Endogenous complementation—heterozygotes for X-linked loci
Modifying loci
   Hypostasis and epistasis—regulation of expression
   Loci not having physical interaction
Gene alteration
   Somatic mutation
   Amplification
   Transpositions—position effects
Exogenous or ecologic factors
   Ecology—temperature, diet
   Phenocopy
     Teratogens
   Medical intervention
   Chance

notypes are identical. However, the more intriguing examples of heterogeneity involve fundamentally distinct mutations, especially at different loci (42).

Genetic heterogeneity can be detected by a wide variety of techniques, including many widely available to clinicians (Table 3). An example of how astute bedside observation can reveal heterogeneity of cause is the differentiation of homocystinuria from the Marfan syndrome. Until the early 1960s, all patients who had the typical bodily habitus, dislocated lenses, and cardiovascular problems were labeled as having the Marfan syndrome. McKusick and colleagues (43), on learning that patients with a newly discovered inborn error of amino acid metabolism, homo-

TABLE 3. Methods for detecting genetic heterogeneity

Differences in clinical manifestations
   Severity
   Age of onset
Genetic analysis
   Chance matings between affected individuals
   Mode of inheritance
   Linkage analysis
   Differences in manifestations in heterozygotes
   Complementation in cell culture
   Restriction site polymorphism linkage analysis
   Nucleotide sequence of the gene
Biochemical analysis
   Constituents of tissue, plasma, etc.
   Enzyme assay
   Protein characterization, e.g., differences in cross-reacting material status

cystinuria, were often retarded, developed strokes at early ages, and developed ectopia lentis, immediately collected urine from their large clinic population of Marfan patients and screened for homocysteine. They found that indeed a small fraction of these patients did not have the Marfan syndrome, but a syndrome later shown to be due to deficiency of cystathionine beta-synthase deficiency. In retrospect, differentiating these syndromes seems trivial, because vascular occlusive events, retardation, and autosomal recessive inheritance are inconsistent with the Marfan syndrome, and aortic root aneurysm, limber joints, and autosomal dominant inheritance are not manifestations of homocystinuria. However, one or two patients a year are still referred to the Johns Hopkins Center for Medical Genetics for management of the Marfan syndrome, only to be found affected by homocystinuria (44). This approach for detecting heterogeneity is limited by the extensive and intrinsic variability of phenotypes. Thus, as *intra*familial variation becomes extensive; the reliability of detecting heterogeneity of cause based on *inter*familial variability becomes unacceptably low. Nonetheless, it is well worth scrutinizing familiar diseases for unambiguous phenotypic evidence of differences in cause among patients and families. Different inheritance patterns are a reliable marker, and a substantial list of neurologic disorders is obviously heterogeneous by this benchmark (Table 4).

At a biochemical level, homocystinuria itself is readily demonstrated to be heterogeneous. Some patients respond to large doses of pyridoxine, a cofactor for cystathionine beta-synthase, by markedly improving metabolism of sulfurated amino acids. If therapy is begun early in life, clinical sequelae such as displacement of the ocular lenses and retardation can be prevented (45). However, only about one-half of patients respond biochemically, and hence clinically, to pharmacologic therapy

TABLE 4. *Genetic heterogeneity, detectable by inheritance pattern, of selected neurologic disorders*

Disorder	Inheritance patterns
Hereditary optic neuropathy	AD, AR, M
Primary microcephaly	AD, AR, XL
Myoclonic epilepsy	AD, AR, XL, M
Cerebellar ataxia and retinitis pigmentosa	AD, AR
Cerebellar ataxia and optic atrophy	AD, AR
Hereditary sensory neuropathy	AD, AR
Hereditary motor and sensory neuropathy (Charcot-Marie-Tooth disease)	AD, AR, XL
Scapuloperoneal muscular atrophy	AD, AR, XL
Juvenile spinal muscular atrophy (Kugelberg-Welander disease)	AD, AR, XL
Amyotrophic lateral sclerosis	AD, AR
Hereditary spastic paraplegia	AD, AR, XL
Dystonia musculorum deformans	AD, AR, XL
Myotonia congenita	AD, AR
Adrenoleukodystrophy	AD, AR

AD, autosomal dominant; AR, autosomal recessive; M, maternal; XL, X-linked.

(46). The *in vivo* assays of the effectiveness of pyridoxine are recapitulated *in vitro* by direct analysis of enzyme activities, kinetics, and binding constants, thus demonstrating considerable heterogeneity at the protein level (47).

At a nucleic acid level, any disease-causing gene that has been cloned has been shown to be heterogeneous in terms of defects, except for the sickle cell mutation at the beta-globin locus. Some disorders have remarkably few mutations that account for most cases, with cystic fibrosis being an instructive, recent example (48). Others, such as Duchenne and Becker muscular dystrophies, are caused by a host of different mutations at the same locus (49).

In all aspects of medical genetics, from clinical service and clinical investigation to molecular analysis of etiology, it is important to remember: *Genetic heterogeneity is the rule, rather than the exception.*

GLOSSARY OF GENETIC TERMS

Allele One of two or more alternate forms of a gene at a given locus.

Ascertainment The manner in which individuals with a trait or condition come to medical attention.

Clone In a cellular sense, a population of cells derived from a single precursor cell by repeated mitoses and all having the same genotype. In molecular terms, a homogeneous population of DNA molecules derived from a single messenger RNA molecule (hence a clone of DNA complementary to the mRNA and designated cDNA), or from a single genomic DNA fragment. The cloned sequence is usually contained within a vector molecule (phage or plasmid), which provides a means of replication.

Codominance Expression of both alleles in the heterozygote.

Complementary base sequence A linear array of nucleotide base pairs (either RNA or DNA), the sequence of which is determined by a second array (strand) of nucleotides, the sequence being determined by hydrogen bonding between adenosine and thymine (A-T) and guanine and cytosine (G-C).

Compound An individual heterozygous for two mutant alleles at the same locus, as in hemoglobinS/hemoglobinC. Distinct from an individual doubly heterozygous at two loci, as A/a, B/b.

Congenital Present at birth; does not imply heritable.

Contiguous gene syndrome A syndrome resulting from a small chromosomal deletion involving several genes related only in that they lie next to one another. Variability between two unrelated individuals with the same general spectrum of clinical manifestations, or the same apparent deletion visible at the light microscopic level, is due in part to submicroscopic differences in the extent of the deletion.

Diploid Having two complete sets of homologous chromosomes. One set is termed haploid and the number of chromosomes in the set is designated N; a diploid individual has 2N chromosomes.

Dominant Strictly, referring to a phenotype, due to the action of a particular allele, that is invariant whether the allele is homozygous or heterozygous; in human genetics, most dominant phenotypes are "incomplete," that is, the heterozygote is affected, but the homozygote is even more affected.

Gene The unit of heredity, in most instances, a region of the chromosomal DNA in which a particular polypeptide chain or function is encoded.

Genome The total genetic endowment of a cell or an individual.

Genotype The genetic constitution, either at one specific locus or for an entire cell or organism. In the general sense, synonymous with genome.

Haploid Having one set of chromosomes, the number of chromosomes being designated N. The usual state of the gametes of diploid organisms.

Heterozygous Having two different alleles at a given locus.

Homozygous Having identical alleles at a given locus.

Imprinting The differential modification of the paternal and maternal genetic contributions to the zygote, resulting in the differential expression of parental alleles. The mechanism(s) is unknown, but may involve DNA methylation.

Independent assortment The random distribution of chromosomes (first stage of meiosis) and chromatids (second stage of meiosis) to gametes. Chromatid assortment, coupled with recombination, results in the random distribution of nonalleles, except when linkage reduces the chance of recombination between two loci.

Lethal In the genetic sense, failure to reproduce; due to infertility or mortality before reproduction.

Linkage Failure of two loci on a chromosome to assort independently in apparent violation of mendelian law; a statistical concept, based on close physical proximity of loci in all situations studied. Loci that are widely spaced (unlinked) assort independently because of recombination.

Locus The site on a chromosome occupied by a gene.

Mendelian Referring to inheritance patterns that conform to the laws proposed by Gregor Mendel in 1865. In simplest terms, "Alleles segregate; nonalleles assort."

Methylation Addition of a methyl ($-CH_3$) moiety to the nucleoside cytosine of a DNA molecule; methylated cytosine mimics thymine and becomes a potential site for mutation. Methylation likely has a role in gene regulation and may produce some instances of imprinting.

Meiosis The process occurring during gametogenesis by which the diploid chromosome number (2N) is reduced to N, as found in the sperm and ova. The word is the same as miosis, meaning a reduction in size. By convention, miosis is used for small pupils and meiosis for the genetic process.

Mitochondrial inheritance Transmission of a phenotype-producing (disease-causing) mutation of a mitochondrial chromosome. Both sexes are equally frequently and severely affected, but mothers transmit the mutant mitochrondrial chromosomes to all of their offspring, whereas affected fathers transmit the mutation to none of their offspring. Also called "maternal" or "cytoplasmic inheritance."

Mitosis The process of cell division in somatic tissue, during which chromosome replication and division insures a 2N diploid complement in each of two daughter cells.

Multifactorial Determination of a phenotype by genetic and nongenetic inheritance factors. Polygenic refers just to multiple genetic factors.

Mutation Any permanent change in a gene.

Penetrance An attribute of a phenotype that is expressed. If the phenotype is always expressed whenever the responsible allele is present, the trait is fully penetrant; if the phenotype is expressed only in some individuals having the requisite genotype, the trait is incompletely penetrant; if the trait is not expressed at all, it is nonpenetrant.

Phenotype The observable characteristics of a cell or organism.

Pleiotropy Multiple (perhaps seemingly unrelated) phenotypic effects caused by one gene.

Polymorphism Regarding genes, any allele of a set of two or more alleles, the rarest of which occurs at a frequency greater than can be maintained by new mutation and genetic drift alone; arbitrarily taken to be a frequency of 0.01 (1%).

Recessive A characteristic of a phenotypic trait that is expressed only when the responsible gene is homozygous.

Recombination The process by which genes on the same chromosome end up on separate (but homologous) chromosomes in the subsequent generation is crossing over. Recombination is the consequence of crossing over and reflected in assortment of nonallelic genes.

Segregation In an organism that is heterozygous at a given locus, the separation of the two alleles at meiosis and distribution to two different gametes.

Somatic recombination Any process by which genes are reorganized within the genome of any somatic cell. A change is heritable only in the daughter cells of the cell in which the recombination occurs; in other words, a clone with a genotype different from the rest of the organism is established.

Syntenic Referring to loci located on the same chromosome; they need not be linked.

Wild type Referring to a genetic locus or an allele that specifies a phenotype that predominates in natural populations or that is designated as normal.

REFERENCES

1. Vogel, F., and Motulsky, A. G. (1986): Formal genetics of man. In: *Human Genetics*, 2nd ed., pp. 111–227. Springer-Verlag, New York.
2. McKusick, V. A. (1986, 1987, 1988): The morbid anatomy of the human genome: a review of gene mapping in clinical medicine. (4 parts). *Medicine*, 65:1–33; 66:1–63; 66:237–296; 67:1–19.
3. Beaudet, A. L., Scriver, C. R., Sly, W. S., and Valle, D. (1989): Genetics and biochemistry of variant human phenotypes. In: *The Metabolic Basis of Inherited Disease*, 6th ed., edited by C. R. Scriver, A. L. Beaudet, W. S. Sly, and D. Valle, pp. 3–53. McGraw-Hill, New York.
4. Skinner, R. (1983): Unifactorial inheritance. In: *Principles and Practice of Medical Genetics*, edited by A. E. H. Emery, and D. L. Rimoin, pp. 65–74. Churchill Livingstone, New York.
5. Johannsen, W. (1909): *Elemente der exakten Erblichkeitslehre*. Fischer, Jena.

6. Orel, V. (1984): *Mendel*. Oxford University Press, London.
7. Mendel, G. (1865): Experiments on plant-hybridization. *Verh naturf Ver in Brunn*. Abhandlungen, iv. A more accessible presentation is: Mendel, G. (1865): *Experiments on Plant Hybridisation*, edited by J. H. Bennett, with notes by R. A. Fisher. Edinburgh, Oliver and Boyd.
8. McKusick, V. A. (1989): *Mendelian Inheritance in Man*, 8th ed. Johns Hopkins University Press, Baltimore.
9. Childs, B. (1981): Genetic factors in human disease. In: *Genetic Issues in Pediatrics*, edited by M. M. Kaback, pp. 3–16. Year Book Medical, Chicago.
10. Penrose, L. S. (1955): Parental age and mutation. *Lancet*, 2:312–313.
11. Boehnke, M., Arnheim, N., Li, H., and Collins, F. S. (1989): Fine structure genetic mapping of human chromosomes using the polymerase chain reaction on single sperm: experimental design considerations. *Am. J. Hum. Genet.*, 45:21–32.
12. Darras, B. T., Blattner, P., Harper, J. F., Spiro, A. J., Alter, S., and Francke, U. (1988): Intragenic deletions in 21 Duchenne muscular dystrophy (DMD)/Becker muscular dystrophy (BMD) families studied with the dystrophin cDNA: location of breakpoints on *Hin*dIII and *Bgl*II exon-containing fragment maps, meiotic and mitotic origin of the mutations. *Am. J. Hum. Genet.*, 43:620–629.
13. Higuchi, M., Kochhan, L., and Olek, K. (1988): A somatic mosaic for hemophilia A detected at the DNA level. *Mol. Biol. Med.*, 5:23–27.
14. Byers, P. H., Tsipouras, P., Bonadio, J. F., Starman, B. J., and Schwartz, R. C. (1988): Perinatal lethal osteogenesis imperfecta (OI type II): a biochemically heterogeneous disorder usually due to new mutations in the genes for type I collagen. *Am. J. Hum. Genet.*, 42:237–248.
15. Goldstein, J. L., and Brown, M. S. (1989): Familial hypercholesterolemia. In: *The Metabolic Basis of Inherited Disease*, 6th ed., edited by C. R. Scriver, A. L. Beaudet, W. S. Sly, and D. Valle, pp. 1215–1250. McGraw-Hill, New York.
16. Hall, J. G., Dorst, J. P., Taybi, H., Scott, C. I., Jr., Langer, L. O., Jr., and McKusick, V. A. (1969): Two probable cases of homozygosity for the achondroplasia gene. *Birth Defects*, 5(4):24–34.
17. Killian, J. M., and Kloepfer, J. W. (1979): Homozygous expression of a dominant gene for Charcot-Marie-Tooth neuropathy. *Ann. Neurol.*, 5:515–22.
18. Welander, L. (1957): Homozygous appearance of distal myopathy. *Acta Genet. Stat. Med.*, 7:321–325.
19. Wexler, N. S., Young, A. B., Tanzi, R. E., et al. (1987): Homozygotes for Huntington's disease. *Nature*, 326:194–197.
20. Myers, R. H., Leavitt, J., Farrer, L. A., et al. (1989): Homozygote for Huntington disease. *Am. J. Hum. Genet.*, 45:615–618.
21. Gershon, E. S., Hamovit, J. H., Guroff, J. J., and Nurnberger, J. I. (1987): Birth-cohort changes in manic and depressive disorders in relatives of bipolar and schizoaffective patients. *Arch. Gen. Psychiatr.*, 44:314–319.
22. Lavori, P. W., Klerman, G. L., Keller, M. B., Reich, T., Rice, J., and Endicott, J. (1987): Age-period-cohort analysis of secular trends in onset of major depression: findings in siblings of patients with major affective disorder. *J. Psychiatr. Res.*, 21:23–35.
23. Antonarakis, S. E., Kazazian, H. H., Jr., and Orkin, S. H. (1985): DNA polymorphism and molecular pathology of the human globin gene clusters. *Hum. Genet.*, 69:1–14.
24. Muller, H. J. (1950): Our load of mutations. *Am. J. Hum. Genet.*, 2:111–176.
25. Harris, H. (1969): Enzyme and protein polymorphism in human populations. *Br. Med. Bull.*, 25:5–13.
26. Page, D. C., Mosher, R., Simpson, E. M., et al. (1987): The sex determining region of the human Y chromosome encodes a finger protein. *Cell*, 51:1091–1104.
27. Hall, J. G. (1988): Somatic mosaicism: observations related to clinical genetics. *Am. J. Hum. Genet.*, 43:355–363.
28. Engel, E. (1980): A new genetic concept: uniparental disomy and its potential effect, isodisomy. *Am. J. Med. Genet.*, 6:137–43.
29. Cavenee, W. K., Dryja, T. P., Phillips, R. A., et al. (1983): Expression of recessive alleles by chromosomal mechanisms in retinoblastoma. *Nature*, 305:779–784.
30. Spence, J. E., Perciaccante, R. G., Greig, G. M., et al. (1988): Uniparental disomy as a mechanism for human genetic disease. *Am. J. Hum. Genet.*, 42:217–226.
31. Voss, R., Ben-Simon, E., Avital, A., et al. (1989): Isodisomy of chromosome 7 in a patient with cystic fibrosis: could uniparental disomy be common in humans. *Am. J. Hum. Genet.*, 45:373–380.

32. Holliday, R. (1989): A different kind of inheritance. *Sci. Am.*, June: 60–73.
33. Cattanach, B. M., and Kirk, M. (1985): Differential activity of maternally and paternally derived chromosome regions in mice. *Nature*, 315:496–498.
34. Cedar, H. (1988): DNA methylation and gene activity. *Cell*, 53:3–4.
35. Harper, P. S. (1979): *Myotonic Dystrophy*, pp. 200–204. W. B. Saunders, Philadelphia.
36. Reik, W. (1988): Genomic imprinting: a possible mechanism for the parental origin effect in Huntington's chorea. *J. Med. Genet.*, 25:805–808.
37. Miller, M., and Hall, J. G. (1978): Possible maternal effect on severity of neurofibromatosis. *Lancet*, 2:1071–1073.
38. Wallace, D. C. (1986): Mitochondrial genes and disease. *Hosp. Prac.*, 15:77–92.
39. Wallace, D. C., Singh, G., Lott, M. T., et al. (1988): Mitochondrial DNA mutation associated with Leber's hereditary optic neuropathy. *Science*, 242:1427–1430.
40. Pyeritz, R. E. (1989): Pleiotropy revisited: molecular explanations of a classic concept. *Am. J. Med. Genet.*, 34:124–134.
41. Collins, F. S., Ponder, B. A. J., Seizinger, B. R., and Epstein, C. J. (1989): The von Recklinghausen neurofibromatosis region on chromosome 17—genetic and physical maps come into focus. *Am. J. Hum. Genet.*, 44:1–5.
42. Childs, B., and Der Kaloustian, V. M. (1968): Genetic heterogeneity. *N. Engl. J. Med.*, 279:1205–1212.
43. Schimke, R. N., McKusick, V. A., Huang, T., and Pollack, A. D. (1965): Homocystinuria. *JAMA*, 193:711–715.
44. Pyeritz, R. E. (1987): Marfan syndrome and homocystinuria. In: *Clinical Studies in Medical Biochemistry*, edited by R. Glew and S. Peters, pp. 155–166. Oxford University Press, New York.
45. Valle, D., Pai, G. S., Thomas, G. H., and Pyeritz, R. E. (1980): Homocystinuria due to cystathionine beta-synthase deficiency: clinical manifestations and therapy. *Johns Hopkins Med. J.*, 146:110–117.
46. Mudd, S. H., Skovby, F., Levy, H. L., et al. (1985): The natural history of homocystinuria due to cystathionine beta-synthase deficiency. *Am. J. Hum. Genet.*, 36:1–31.
47. Skovby, F., Kraus, J. P., and Rosenberg, L. E. (1984): Homocystinuria: biogenesis of cystathionine beta-synthase subunits in cultured fibroblasts and in an in vitro translation system programmed with fibroblast messenger RNA. *Am. J. Hum. Genet.*, 36:452–459.
48. Kerem, B., Rommens, J. M., Buchanan, J. A., et al. (1989): Identification of the cystic fibrosis gene: genetic analysis. *Science*, 245:1073–1080.
49. Koenig, M., Beggs, A. H., Moyer, M., et al. (1989): The molecular basis for Duchenne versus Becker muscular dystrophy: correlation of severity with type of deletion. *Am. J. Hum. Genet.*, 45:498–506.
50. Folstein, S. E., Phillips, J. A. III, Meyers, D. A., et al. (1985): Huntington's disease: two families with differing clinical features show linkage to the G8 probe. *Science*, 229:776–779.
51. Smith, D. W. (1966): Dysmorphology (teratology). *J. Pediatr.*, 69:1150–1169.
52. Cross, H. E., and McKusick, V. A. (1967): The Troyer syndrome. *Arch. Neurol.*, 16:473–485.
53. Beighton, P. H. (1971): Recessively inherited Charcot-Marie-Tooth syndrome in identical twins. *Birth Defects*, 7(2):105.

Genes, Brain, and Behavior, edited by
P. R. McHugh and V. A. McKusick.
Raven Press, Ltd., New York © 1991.

The Search for the Genetic Defects in Huntington's Disease and Familial Alzheimer's Disease

James F. Gusella

Molecular Neurogenetics Laboratory, Massachusetts General Hospital, and Department of Genetics, Harvard University, Boston, Massachusetts 02114

A traditional method for studying inherited diseases has been the attempted identification of a protein defect, usually via enzyme activity measurements or structural analyses. It has been most successful for "loss of function" mutations, which are typically transmitted as recessive disorders. When the defective protein is known, cloning of the disease gene has become a relatively straightforward matter in most cases. Unfortunately, for the majority of neurogenetic disorders of dominant inheritance, it has not been possible to find the protein defect directly due to the complexity of the brain and often the abundance of secondary changes in the disorder. In recent years, an alternative indirect strategy based on DNA variations has evolved for approaching such disorders via the chromosomal location of their genetic defect rather than through a knowledge of the defective protein involved.

Genetic linkage studies, in which the alleles of individual polymorphic DNA markers are traced through several generations of families with a given heritable disorder, can establish the chromosomal location of the gene defect (1). Two genes located close to each other on a chromosome will display a correlated pattern of inheritance because they are physically linked as part of the chromosomal material and are not far enough apart to be randomized with respect to each other by recombination events during meiosis. Consequently tracing a polymorphic DNA marker through a family acts as a way of tracking the entire chromosomal region around that DNA segment. Detection of a DNA polymorphism showing a correlated pattern of inheritance with the disease in a given family then implies that the genetic defect causing the disorder is located somewhere in the chromosomal vicinity of the DNA marker. Knowledge of the location of the genetic defect provides a potential handle for isolating the disease gene and characterizing its product in the absence of any knowledge of its biochemical function. The degree to which attempts to identify the disease gene by this approach can be successful depends in part on the particular chromosomal region involved and to a greater extent on the nature of the disorder under investigation. We have concentrated on two neurodegenerative disorders that present very different problems: Huntington's disease (HD) and Alzheimer's disease (AD). This report will review the current status of our efforts in these disorders.

HD

HD is a progressive neurodegenerative disorder in which a dominant gene defect causes motor abnormalities, personality changes, and cognitive decline (2). The principal manifestation of the disorder is chorea, uncontrolled dance-like movements that ultimately consume all parts of the body. The onset of HD typically occurs between 35 and 50 years of age, but virtually all carriers of the defective gene eventually develop the disorder. Neuropathologic studies have demonstrated the loss of specific striatal neurons in HD, but the biochemical cause of the cell death is not known. There is no effective treatment for preventing the onset of HD or for delaying its progression.

The disease gene causing HD was the first autosomal genetic defect mapped using only the DNA marker approach. In 1983, we demonstrated that alleles of the DNA marker *D4S10*, located on chromosome 4, displayed the same pattern of inheritance as the HD defect in a single American family and a very large Venezuelan pedigree (3,4). Later, the DNA marker was localized to the terminal cytogenetic band on the short arm (4p16) by *in situ* hybridization and by analysis of children with 4p depletions causing Wolf-Hirschhorn syndrome (5-9). The identification of extensive DNA variation in the *D4S10* segment has subsequently improved the marker to the point where it can be traced effectively in most HD families. In no case did HD within a family fail to display genetic linkage with this marker, suggesting that all families with the disorder have a mutation in the same gene (10). About 4% of the time, the expected marker allele for *D4S10* fails to travel with the HD gene through meiosis, indicating the rare occurrence of a recombination event between the two. This suggests that the HD gene is probably a few million base pairs away from the *D4S10* segment.

Since 1984, we have participated in a multigroup collaborative effort (D. Housman, Massachusetts Institute of Technology; A.-M. Frischauf and H. Lehrach, Imperial Cancer Research Fund; F. Collins, University of Michigan; J. Gusella, Massachusetts General Hospital; J. Wasmuth, University of California, Irvine) catalyzed by the Hereditary Disease Foundation to identify the HD gene based on its chromosomal location. A combination of somatic cell genetic mapping, genetic linkage mapping, and pulsed field gel mapping has been applied to the problem and produced detailed maps of the terminal band of the chromosome, but the HD gene has not yet been identified.

Crucial to the fine mapping of the HD region were the isolation of large numbers of additional DNA probes from the chromosome and the ability to map them rapidly. Consequently, the development of regional somatic cell hybrid mapping panels that specifically divided the 4p16 band into smaller regions (11,12) was essential for the next step in more precisely localizing HD. These panels indicate that *D4S10* is actually located in the proximal portion of the terminal 4p16.3 subband (Fig. 1). Genetic linkage studies of HD families with DNA markers from the

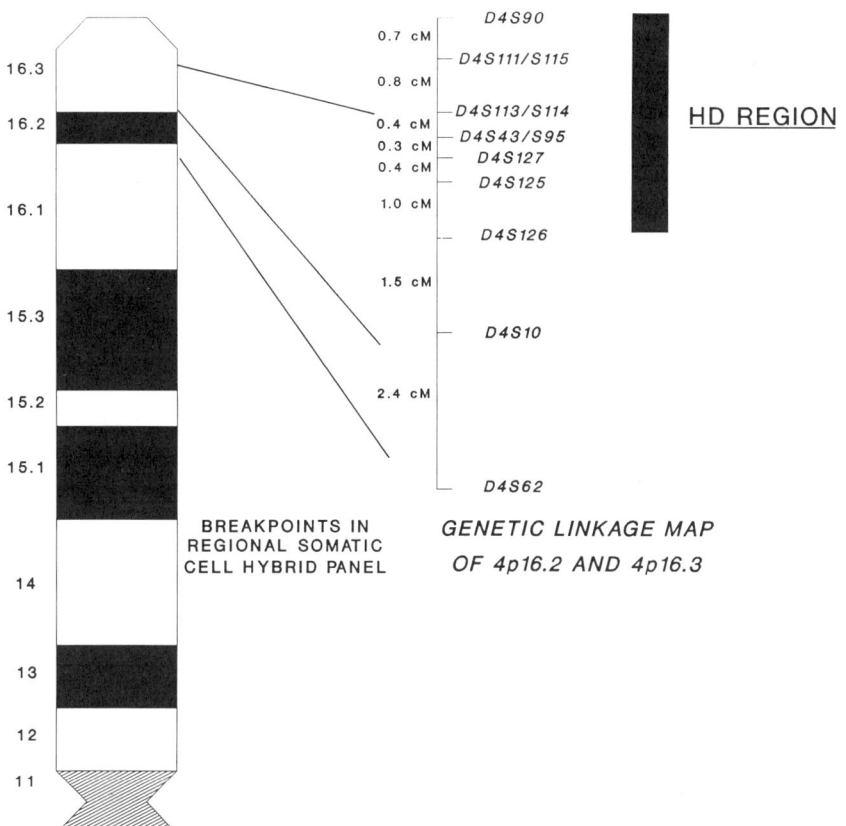

FIG. 1. The short arm of chromosome 4 is shown with a detailed genetic linkage map of the 4p16.2 and 4p16.3 bands. Loci were also oriented by the somatic cell hybrid mapping panel with breakpoints in chromosome 4 shown. The HD gene has been placed distal to *D4S126*, with favored locations either distal to *D4S90* or between *D4S126* and *D4S115*.

more proximal 4p16.1 and 4p16.2 subbands demonstrated that these segments displayed more recombination with HD than did *D4S10*, leading to the conclusion that HD lies within 4p16.3, between *D4S10* and the telomere of the chromosome 4 short arm (13). 4p16.3 is approximately 3% of chromosome 4 and therefore is expected to contain about 6 million base pairs of DNA.

A large number of new DNA markers have been mapped to 4p16.3 despite its small size because of the importance of developing a complete map of the region to find HD (12,14–18). Although these were initially assigned to the 4p16.3 band using the somatic cell hybrid panels, resolution of the order of the markers required a combination of genetic and fine structure physical mapping. The genetic mapping was carried out by finding DNA polymorphisms for each of the segments and then tracing these variations through reference families in which rare recombinations between loci provide a basis for establishing their order. Detailed linkage maps of

4p16.3 have been constructed and indicate that about 6% recombination occurs within the region and that we have markers spaced every 0.5% recombination in the critical HD region (18,19) (see Fig. 1).

Fine structure physical mapping of DNA probes from 4p16.3 has been achieved by using pulsed field gel electrophoresis to produce a long-range restriction map using restriction enzymes that cut human DNA on average every 100,000 to 1,000,000 bp. The current map spans 5.5×10^6 bp of DNA, the vast majority of what 4p16.3 is expected to contain, but has two gaps of indeterminate size, one in proximal 4p16.3 and one in distal 4p16.3, as defined by an interstitial deletion breakpoint occurring within 4p16.3 in a 4p⁻ patient (20).

Unfortunately, the precise position of the HD gene on either the physical or genetic maps has not been established with certainty. Since there is no chromosomal rearrangement associated with HD, the only method of defining the position of the disease gene is to examine those rare cases in which a recombination event has occurred within 4p16.3 in an HD family and to determine which markers have displayed recombination with the disease in these cases. This analysis has, however, produced conflicting results, with some events suggesting that the HD defect is located telomeric to all markers tested, in the final few hundred thousand base pairs of the chromosomal DNA, while others suggest a more proximal location, between *D4S10* and the marker *D4S115* (19,21,22) (see Fig. 1).

While it is conceivable that in different families the location of the actual mutated site differs by as much as 1.5×10^6 bp, it is also possible that one or the other of the classes of recombination events represents something other than a simple meiotic exchange. If double recombination or gene conversion were to occur frequently in this region, then such apparently conflicting results could arise. The best method for resolving which events were not single recombinations would be to have a highly informative DNA marker located at the telomere itself so that it *must* flank the HD gene with respect to the more proximal markers. Bates et al. (22) recently isolated a yeast artificial chromosome containing the terminal 125,000 bp of an HD chromosome 4, suggesting that the development of a telomeric polymorphism and resolution of this issue may be possible.

Whichever of the two candidate regions contains the HD gene, it will be necessary to identify genes within these regions as HD candidates without any guidance as to the biochemical nature of the defect. However, regardless of the pathway involved, it is likely that HD represents a "gain of function" mutation, since we have been able to demonstrate that there is no apparent difference in onset or expression of the disorder in HD homozygotes, who possess two copies of the HD gene and no copy of the normal allele, relative to HD heterozygotes who possess one of each (23). Thus, two doses of the HD gene are no more deleterious than one, and in typical HD heterozygotes, the normal counterpart of the HD gene does nothing to slow the course of the disorder. By analogy with mutations of this type in *Drosophila*, it is conceivable that HD causes inappropriate expression in the striatum of an otherwise normal protein that should be produced in smaller amounts or should be restricted to another tissue. Beyond obvious structural changes in the genomic

DNA or corresponding cDNA for a candidate gene, this putative altered pattern of expression of the HD gene represents the only ready means of implicating a particular candidate as the likely site of the HD defect before proceeding to DNA sequence analysis to identify the mutation itself. Ultimately, since there is no biochemical or neuronal culture assay for the effects of the HD gene, it may be necessary to use transgenic technologies to reproduce part of the HD phenotype in an experimental animal by using a cloned candidate gene in order to guarantee that the disease gene has indeed been identified. Fortunately, since HD has a completely dominant phenotype in humans, there is reason to hope that simple introduction of the disease gene into the germ line of an experimental animal may be sufficient to create an animal model of the disorder.

AD

AD is a far greater public health problem than HD, but is a much more difficult disorder in which to apply the genetic linkage strategy (24). Like HD, AD is a late-onset disorder with symptoms typically appearing after the age of 70. The predominant clinical feature of AD is a progressive dementia, but the disorder is most reliably identified by its neuropathologic effects, the formation of neuritic plaques containing insoluble amyloid deposits and of intracellular neurofibrillary tangles. Most cases of AD do not show clear heritability, but a small subset of cases are clustered in large pedigrees where they appear to display autosomal dominant inheritance. This form of the disorder has been termed familial AD (FAD) and has provided the basis for attempting the genetic linkage strategy (25). In the most extensive pedigrees, FAD usually shows early onset of symptoms in the fourth to sixth decades, but is clinically and neuropathologically indistinguishable from the later onset AD.

The neuropathologic hallmarks of AD and FAD, amyloid plaques and neurofibrillary tangles, have also been reported in a separate genetic disorder, Down syndrome, in which the cause is known. Down syndrome is a common birth defect, involving a constellation of symptoms including mental retardation, in which the abnormalities can all be attributed to an extra third copy of chromosome 21. Consequently, when we began our linkage analysis of FAD, we first targeted markers from this chromosome. In early 1987, we presented evidence that in four large FAD pedigrees, the FAD gene was linked to two DNA markers (*D21S1/S11* and *D21S16*) on the proximal long arm of chromosome 21 (21q) (25) (see Fig. 2). Simultaneously, several groups including our own isolated the gene encoding the protein precursor (APP) of the peptide found in AD amyloid plaques and showed that it mapped on chromosome 21q (26–28). However, we and others soon discovered that the straightforward scenario that a mutation in the APP gene was the cause of FAD was incorrect, since this locus displayed frequent recombination with the FAD gene and was therefore not located close to the genetic defect (29,30). Instead, the FAD gene appeared to be closer to the centromere of the chromosome, far from the more distal region associated with the typical features of Down syndrome (Fig. 2).

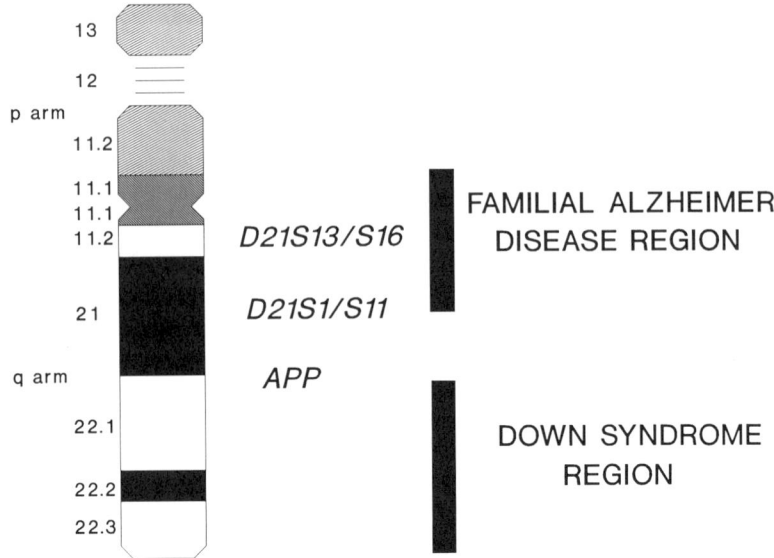

FIG. 2. The APP gene is located in the middle of the chromosome 21 long arm, at the upper end of the obligate Down syndrome region. Markers linked to FAD place the genetic defect in this disorder proximal to *D21S1/S11*, and possibly above *D21S13/S16* as well, far from the APP locus.

Further progress toward precisely localizing the genetic defect in FAD and ultimately isolating it has been hampered by the very nature of the disorder (31). Unlike HD, AD is not a genetically homogeneous disorder with all affected individuals apparently having a genetic defect at one location in the genome that displays clear-cut dominant inheritance and high penetrance. Instead, AD consists of a mixture of types of cases, with some displaying dominant inheritance, others being most consistent with either reduced penetrance or some other mode of inheritance, and still others appearing to be sporadic, with no obvious genetic component. Unfortunately, there are no means for unequivocally distinguishing the category into which any individual case should be placed, even within a pedigree where the inherited form of the disorder is present. Consequently, recombination events in AD pedigrees cannot be used to place the defect with certainty since any individual crossover event can usually be alternatively explained as a misclassification of a single AD case into the genetic category.

Beyond the problems of categorization of AD cases into genetic and nongenetic categories, there is a greater difficulty in the linkage strategy for localizing FAD. Although the linkage of FAD to 21q has been confirmed by Goate et al. (32), two others have failed to confirm the result. Schellenberg et al. (33), using mainly families of Volga-German origin exclude proximal 21q as the site of the defect, and Pericak-Vance et al. (34), using late onset pedigrees, report similar conclusions. Thus, in addition to the heterogeneity entailed by genetic and nongenetic cases, the genetic category itself appears to be heterogeneous, with some families having a defect on chromosome 21 and others presumably carrying a gene defect at one or more other locations in the genome, although none of these have yet been found. Unfortunately, individual FAD families are almost invariably too small to categorize cleanly into 21-linked or non-21-linked groups, casting further doubt on any recombination event detected in such a pedigree with respect to its use for precise localization of the FAD defect.

Clearly, the major obstacle to overcome if the linkage strategy is to be effective in permitting isolation of a FAD gene is the paucity of large multigenerational FAD pedigrees that can be unequivocally classified with respect to chromosome-21 linkage. This lack of family material results partly from the relatively advanced onset of the disorder and the short subsequent life span of its victims, which assures that at any given time a family will have few living affected individuals, rarely in different generations. Either ascertainment of additional large families or the accumulation over time of newly affected individuals within families already identified could eventually overcome this difficulty. However, a more immediate solution could be achieved if a diagnostic test were developed to predict the occurrence of AD in individuals before the onset of clinical signs. Such a test would immediately increase the informativeness of existing FAD pedigrees that typically contain many "at risk" family members who have not yet reached the age of onset.

The current inability to narrow the location of the FAD defect on chromosome 21 to a region smaller than about 10^7 bp dictates that the search for the disease is unlikely to be successful in the near future unless an obvious structural abnormality or alteration in expression of a specific 21q gene is seen in FAD. Several groups are currently generating long-range restriction maps of the FAD region and isolating candidate cDNAs, but to date no flagrant abnormality has revealed itself. In the absence of better definition of the FAD region by genetic analysis, it seems particularly important to pursue those biochemical and neuropathologic studies that might implicate a particular protein or pathway as the probable sight of the primary defect. Such a clue from the neurobiology of the disorder could provide an assay for more rapid screening of the many candidate genes that are likely to populate the candidate FAD region.

ACKNOWLEDGMENTS

The author wishes to acknowledge the assistance and helpful discussions provided by the many collaborators who have been essential to our work in both HD and AD. This work is supported by grants NS22031, NS16367 (Huntington's Disease Center Without Walls) and AG06865 from the National Institutes of Health, and by grants from the Hereditary Disease Foundation, the Huntington's Disease Society of America, and the American Health Assistance Foundation.

REFERENCES

1. Gusella, J. F. (1986): DNA polymorphism and human disease. *Annu. Rev. Biochem.*, 55:831–854.
2. Martin, J. B., and Gusella, J. F. (1986): Huntington's disease: pathogenesis and management. *N. Engl. J. Med.*, 315:1267–1276.

3. Gusella, J. F., Wexler, N. S., Conneally, P. M., et al. (1983): A polymorphic DNA marker genetically linked to Huntington's disease. *Nature*, 306:234–238.
4. Gusella, J. F., Tanzi, R. E., Anderson, M. A., et al. (1984): DNA markers for nervous system diseases. *Science*, 225:1320–1326.
5. Zabel, B. U., Naylor, S. L., Sakaguchi, A. Y., and Gusella, J. F. (1986): Mapping of the DNA locus D4S10 and the linked Huntington's disease gene to 4p16-p15. *Cytogenet. Cell Genet.*, 42:187–191.
6. Magenis, R. E., Gusella, J., Weliky, K., et al. (1986): Huntington disease-linked restriction fragment length polymorphism localized within band p16.1 of chromosome 4 by in situ hybridization. *Am. J. Hum. Genet.*, 39:383–392.
7. Wang, H. S., Greenberg, C. R., Hewitt, J., Kalousek, D., and Hayden, M. R. (1986): Subregional assignment of the linked marker G8 (D4S10) for Huntington's disease to chromosome 4p16.1-16.3. *Am. J. Hum. Genet.*, 39:392–396.
8. Landegent, J. E., Jansen in de Wal., N., Fisser-Groen, Y. M., Bakker, E., Van der Ploeg, M., and Pearson, P. L. (1986): Fine mapping of the Huntington disease linked D4S10 locus by non-radioactive in situ hybridization. *Hum. Genet.*, 73:354–357.
9. Gusella, J. F., Tanzi, R. E., Bader, P. I., et al. (1985): Deletion of Huntington's disease-linked G8(D4S10) locus in Wolf-Hirschhorn syndrome. *Nature*, 318:75–78.
10. Conneally, P. M., Haines, J., Tanzi, R., et al. (1989): No evidence of linkage heterogeneity between Huntington disease (HD) and G8 (D4S10). *Genomics*, 5:304–308.
11. MacDonald, M. E., Anderson, M. A., Gilliam, T. C., et al. (1987): A somatic cell hybrid panel for localizing DNA segments near the Huntington's disease gene. *Genomics*, 1:29–34.
12. Smith, B., Skarecky, D., Bengtsson, U., Magenis, R. E., Carpenter, N., and Wasmuth, J. J. (1988): Isolation of DNA markers in the direction of the Huntington disease gene from the G8 locus. *Am. J. Hum. Genet.*, 42:335–344.
13. Gilliam, T. C., Tanzi, R. E., Haines, J. L., et al. (1987): Localization of the Huntington's disease gene to a small segment of chromosome 4 flanked by D4S10 and the telomere. *Cell*, 50:565–571.
14. Gilliam, T. C., Bucan, M., MacDonald, M. E., et al. (1987): A DNA segment encoding two genes very tightly linked to Huntington's disease. *Science*, 238:950–952.
15. Wasmuth, J. J., Hewitt, J., Smith, B. (1988): A highly polymorphic locus very tightly linked to the Huntington's disease. *Nature*, 332:734–736.
16. Pohl, T. M., Zimmer, M., MacDonald, M. E., et al. (1988): Construction of a NotI linking library and isolation of new markers close to the Huntington's disease gene. *Nucleic Acids Res.*, 16:9185–9198.
17. Whaley, W. L., Michiels, F., MacDonald, M. E., et al. (1988): Mapping of D4S98/S114/S113 confines the Huntington's defect to a reduced physical region at the telomere of chromosome 4. *Nucleic Acids Res.*, 16:11769–11780.
18. Youngman, S., Sarfarazi, M., Bucan, M., et al. (1989): A new DNA marker [D4S90] is located terminally on the short arm of chromosome 4, close to the Huntington's disease gene. *Genomics*, 5:802–809.
19. MacDonald, M. E., Haines, J. L., Zimmer, M., et al. (1989): Recombination events suggest possible locations for the Huntington's disease gene. *Neuron*, 3:183–190.
20. Bucan, M., Zimmer, M., Whaley, W. L., et al. (1990): Physical maps of 4p16.3, the area expected to contain the Huntington's disease mutation. *Genomics*, 6:1–15.
21. Robbins, C., Theilman, J., Youngman, S., et al. (1989): Evidence from family studies that the gene causing Huntington disease is telomeric to *D4S95* and *D4S90*. *Am J. Hum. Genet.*, 44:422–425.
22. Bates, G. P., MacDonald, M. E., Baxendale, S., et al. (1990): A YAC telomere clone spanning a favoured location of the Huntington's disease gene. *Am. J. Hum. Genet.*, 46:762–775.
23. Wexler, N. S., Young, A. B., Tanzi, R. E., et al. (1987): Homozygotes for Huntington's disease. *Nature*, 326:194–197.
24. Katzman, R. (1986): Alzheimer's disease. *N. Engl. J. Med.*, 314:964–973.
25. St George-Hyslop, P. H., Tanzi, R. E., Polinsky, R. J., et al. (1987): The genetic defect causing familial Alzheimer's disease maps on chromosome 21. *Science*, 235:885–890.
26. Kang, J., Lemaire, H. G., Unterbeck, A., et al. (1987): The precursor of Alzheimer's disease amyloid A4 protein resembles a cell-surface receptor. *Nature*, 325:733–736.
27. Tanzi, R. E., Gusella, J. F., Watkins, P. C., et al. (1987): The amyloid beta protein gene: cDNA cloning, mRNA distribution, and genetic linkage near the Alzheimer locus. *Science*, 235:880–884.
28. Goldgaber, D., Lerman, M. I., McBride, O. W., Saffiotti, U., and Gajdusek, D. C. (1987): Characterization and chromosomal localization of a cDNA encoding brain amyloid of Alzheimer's disease. *Science*, 235:877–880.

29. Tanzi, R. E., St. George-Hyslop, P. H., Haines, J. L., et al. (1987): The genetic defect in familial Alzheimer disease is not tightly linked to the amyloid beta protein gene. *Nature*, 329:156–157.
30. Van Broeckhoven, C., Genthe, A. M., Vandenberghe, A., et al. (1987): Failure of familial Alzheimer's disease to segregate with the A4-amyloid gene in several European families. *Nature*, 329: 153–155.
31. St. George-Hyslop, P. H., Myers, R. H., Haines, J. L., et al. (1989): Familial Alzheimer's disease: progress and problems. *Neurobiol. Aging*, 10:417–425.
32. Goate, A., Haynes, A. R., Owen, M. J., et al. (1989): Predisposing locus for Alzheimer's disease on chromosome 21. *Lancet*, 1:352–354.
33. Schellenberg, G. D., Bird, T. D., Wijsman, E. M., et al. (1988): Absence of linkage of chromosome 21q21 markers to familial Alzheimer's disease. *Science*, 241:1507–1510.
34. Pericak-Vance, M. A., Yamaoka, L. H., Haynes, C. S., et al. (1988): Genetic linkage studies in Alzheimer's disease families. *Exp. Neurol.*, 102:271–279.

Genes, Brain, and Behavior, edited by
P. R. McHugh and V. A. McKusick.
Raven Press, Ltd., New York © 1991.

Down Syndrome and the Trisomy 16 Mouse: Impact of Gene Imbalance on Brain Development and Aging

*†‡§Joseph T. Coyle, †**Mary Lou Oster-Granite, **Roger Reeves,
*Christine Hohmann, *Patrizia Corsi, and **John Gearhart

*Departments of *Psychiatry, †Neuroscience, ‡Pharmacology, and §Pediatrics, and
**The Developmental Genetics Laboratory of the Department of Physiology,
The Johns Hopkins University School of Medicine,
Baltimore, Maryland 21205*

For those individuals who survive the neonatal period, mental retardation is an invariable consequence of aneuploidy of the autosomes (25). Heller (30) estimated that individuals with chromosomal abnormalities accounted for up to 30% of the chronically institutionalized patients in the United States, primarily because of mental retardation. The most common human chromosomal abnormality observed in this group is trisomy of chromosome 21 (HSA 21), which results in Down syndrome (DS). Ninety to ninety-five percent of the cases of DS result from miotic nondisjunction, 4% to 6% from chromosomal translocations, and 1% from mitotic nondisjunction of cells within the early embryo, which results in mosaicism (34).

Mental retardation is the most consistent feature of DS. Surveys reveal that the intelligence quotient is typically in the range of moderately retarded, with some individuals exhibiting severe mental retardation, and a few functioning in the range of normal (2). Whether the severity of mental retardation is a consequence of institutional care and may be moderated by more intense early stimulation and specialized training remains an important question. In mosaics, the intelligence is dependent on the proportion of euploid cells present within the individual, since mosaic DS individuals have significantly higher intelligence quotients than completely trisomic individuals (20). The DS individual suffers from a variety of other CNS abnormalities, including an increased incidence of seizure disorders and abnormalities of neuromuscular tone, audiovestibular function, and visual acuity (42). These additional congenital abnormalities may exacerbate the intrinsic cognitive limitations of the DS individual.

Although a number of structural and cellular abnormalities have been described in the brains of DS individuals, as reviewed below, the precise genetic mechanisms responsible for the developmental abnormalities of the brain and the consequent mental retardation remain poorly understood. In fact, DS can be viewed as a paradigmatic disorder for a much wider range of neuropsychiatric disorders in which the fundamental genetic problem involves gene imbalance and not mutant genes. Thus, the fundamental neurobiologic question with regard to DS is how having an extra copy of genes located on HSA 21, or a portion of it, affects neuronal generation, differentiation, function, and aging in the brain.

NEUROPATHOLOGY OF THE DOWN'S BRAIN

Abnormalities of Neurogenesis

Several studies have reported substantial structural abnormalities in the brains of DS individuals. For example, Whalley (69) found that the average weight of the DS brain was 24% less than that of brains from control adults. The frontal lobes, operculum, and superior temporal gyrus appear to be reduced in size and exhibit altered convolutional patterns. Furthermore, there appears to be a hypoplasia of important structures, including the cerebrum (11,23) and cerebellum (27). Davidoff (17) described abnormality in the convolutional structure of the cerebral hemispheres in DS individuals, with narrowed superior temporal gyrus, shallow primary sulci, and a decreased number of secondary sulci. Such alterations would result in a reduction of the cortical surface area.

A number of microscopic abnormalities have also been described in DS brains, although none of these are considered pathognomonic. Reduction in the total number and density of neurons in the cerebellum, the cerebral cortex, and in the collicular nuclei, have been described. Galaburda and Kemper (23) observed a selective depletion of granule cells from the cortical layers II and III. Similarly, Colon (11) found decreased nuclear size and a reduction of 49% in the neuron populations in five cortical areas sampled in two adolescent DS brains. In support of this, Ross et al. (57) described a reduction in density of cortical granule cells primarily involving aspinous stellate cells. An interesting microscopic abnormality noted by Norman (46) was the uneven neuronal density resulting in heterotopias in both the cerebral cortex and the cerebellum. Furthermore, Golgi staining techniques have revealed abnormal patterns of dendrites, reduction in the number of spines, and dystrophic spines, the primary neuronal structure for synaptic contacts (43,44,51).

Alzheimer's Disease and DS

DS individuals invariably develop the pathologic stigmata of Alzheimer's disease (AD) by mid-adulthood. This relationship was first described over 60 years ago (67). Wisniewski et al. (71), in a systematic investigation of the brains of 100 institutionalized DS individuals, found that the neuropathology of AD, including plaques and tangles, occurred in the brains of all DS patients who survived into the fourth decade. Studies by Ball and Nuttal (1) demonstrated that the hippocampal distribution of neurofibrillary tangles and granulovacular degeneration was indistinguishable from that which occurred in AD. Furthermore, Glenner and Wong (26) purified amyloid protein, the major component of neuritic plaques, from the brains of both aged DS individuals and patients with pathologically confirmed AD, and demonstrated that the amino acid sequence of amyloid peptide was virtually identical from the two sources.

During the past decade, unequivocal evidence has accrued from postmortem analyses of the brains of individuals dying with AD that specific neuronal systems are selectively vulnerable (15). Among these, the basal forebrain cholinergic projections to the cerebral cortex and the limbic system appear to be particularly affected, as evidenced by striking decline in the presynaptic cholinergic markers, including choline acetyltransferase (ChAT), acetylcholinesterase (AChE), choline high-affinity uptake, and the ability to synthesize and release acetylcholine (18,64). Furthermore, histologic studies of the basal forebrain indicate that the large cholinergic neurons either degenerate or undergo striking atrophy (50).

Less consistent reductions have been found for the presynaptic markers for noradrenergic neurons innervating the cortex in AD (16); loss of noradrenergic perikarya in the locus coeruleus is particularly striking in those patients with an early age of onset of AD, compared to those affected later in life (5). Nevertheless, most studies have not revealed a significant decrease in CSF levels of 3-methoxy-4-hydroxy phenylglycol, a metabolite of norepinephrine related to its release (22). The raphe serotonergic neurons are inconsistently affected in AD, although the nigral striatal dopaminergic pathway appears to be relatively spared in AD.

Markers for several neuronal systems intrinsic to the cerebral cortex and hippocampus are not consistently or invariably reduced in AD. Neuronal systems examined include GABAergic neurons (18) and those containing a variety of peptides, including cholecystokinin, vasoactive intestinal peptide, neuropeptide Y(NPY), and arginine vasopressin (58–60). Furthermore, muscarinic receptors, which are presumably localized on cortical and hippocampal neurons innervated by cholinergic afferents, are also not reduced (18).

In light of the fact that DS individuals invariably develop the neuropathology of AD, it was of interest to determine whether DS individuals with AD pathology have the same neuronal systems affected. Limited postmortem synaptic neurochemical studies indicate reductions in the presynaptic marker for cholinergic neurons in the temporal cortex and a reduction in norepinephrine levels in the hypothalamus of aged DS individuals. These alterations appear to be specific since the levels of thyrotropin-releasing hormone, luteinizing hormone-releasing hormone, and substance P were not reduced in the DS cases nor the AD cases (72,73).

Since DS is the only situation in which the risk for AD can be predicted with certainty, it is possible to determine the sequence of events associated with pathogenesis of AD. In studies by Wisniewski et al. (71), the neuropathologic stigmata diagnostic for AD appeared as early as the third decade of life and affected virtually all DS individuals by the fourth decade of life. More recently, utilizing immunochemical procedures, Rumble et al. (61) have documented the early appearance of amyloid peptide in the brains of DS individuals with a time course that has phase shifted by nearly 40 years, as compared to euploid individuals. The relationship between these changes and the neurotransmitter deficits of AD remains less precisely defined. Thus, Casanova et al. (9) reported a reduced complement of basal forebrain, presumably cholinergic, perikarya in the brains of DS individuals examined in childhood and early adulthood. In contrast, Kish et al. (35) did not observe significant reductions in presynaptic markers for cholinergic neurons in the cortex, limbic system, and several other brain regions, in the brains of DS individuals who died before the period of risk for AD pathology. However, since experimental studies indicate collateral innervation of the neocortex from surviving basal forebrain cholinergic neurons after partial neonatal lesion of the complex, these results may not be contradictory (33).

GENETICS OF DS

The Genetic Determinants of DS

While fully 95% of DS results from miotic nondisjunction of HSA 21 during the formation of the ovum, which results in triplication of HSA 21 in the affected offspring, there remains considerable debate about whether all genes on HSA 21 or one or more critical genes are responsible for the DS phenotype. This controversy centers on which features are critical for the DS phenotype. Do these include mental retardation, facial features, dermatoglyphic abnormalities, and endocardial cushion defects and risk for AD? Studies of isolated cases of partial translocation of distal end of HSA 21, resulting in triplication of only a portion of the chromosome, suggest that many of the features of DS occur in individuals who have suffered from triplication of only the distal one-quarter of HSA 21 at Q 22.3 (37,52). However, it remains to be determined whether these cases will ultimately develop the pathology of AD since genes implicated in the cause of AD are located more proximally (see below).

Genetic Homology Between HSA 21 and Mouse Chromosome 16

Mapping of cloned genes and anonymous segments localized on HSA 21 to the mouse genome has revealed a growing degree of homology between a major portion of the long arm of HSA 21 and the distal end of mouse chromosome 16 (MMU 16). Thus, six genes and two anonymous DNA segments located on HSA 21 map to the distal end of MMU 16 (13,53,56). More impressively, where they have been established, the precise sequential relationships among these genes and their localization on the two chromosomes are identical (Fig. 1). Thus, it would appear that this segment of DNA has remained relatively well preserved in the evolutionary diversion between mouse and human, suggesting that intervening genes yet to be identified and mapped will also be shared in this portion of HSA 21 and MMU 16. Of further note is the fact the gene encoding the amyloid precursor protein (APP),

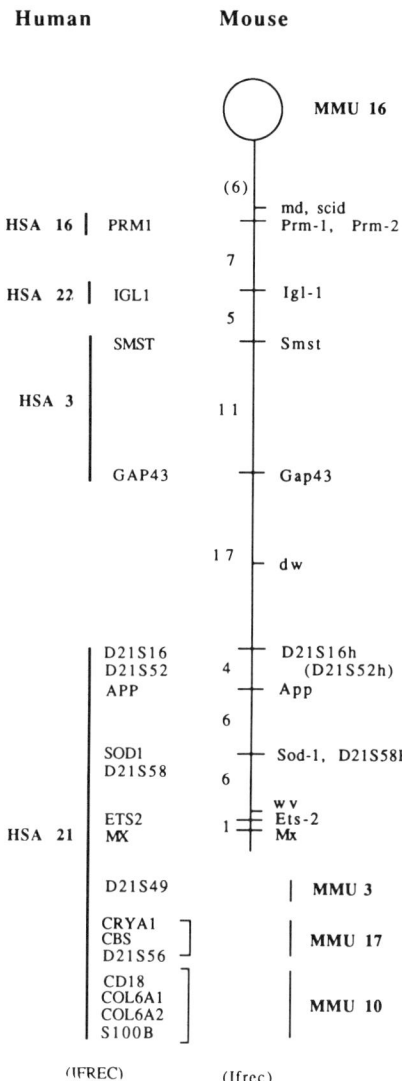

FIG. 1. Schematic representation of gene localization on the human genome of genes mapped to mouse chromosome 16. Derivation of these maps has been reviewed recently (8,40,54). Homology between HSA21 and MMU3 is from Burmeister et al. (7). SMST, pre-pro-somatostatin; GAP43, growth association protein; D21S16h and D21S52h, anonymous sequences; APP, amyloid precursor protein; PRGS, phosphoribosyl glycinamide synthetase; SOD-1, superoxide dismutase; Mx, influenza virus resistance; ETS2, chicken leukemia protooncogene; CRYA1, alpha-crystallin lens protein; CBS, cystathionine β-synthetase; COL6A1 and COL6A2, collagen types 1 and 2; S100, beta subunit of S100 protein; IFREC, interferon receptor; md, mahoganoid; Prm-1 and Prm-2, protamine-1 and -2; Akv-2, endogenous ecotropic pro-virus; Igl-1, immunoglobulin light chain; Bst, belly spot and tail; Mtv-6, endogenous mouse mammary tumor virus sequence; Mtv-6r, MTV regulatory locus; dw, dwarf; wv, weaver.

which is thought to play the critical role in the vulnerability of DS to AD pathology (49), is located in this region on HSA 21 and MMU 16 (56). In addition, two anonymous segments of DNA linked to one dominantly inherited form of AD (66) also map to both HSA 21 and MMU 16.

Nevertheless, MMU 16 is substantially larger than HSA 21 and genes located on the proximal segment of MMU 16 have been mapped to HSA 3, 22, and 16 (55). Furthermore, genes mapped to the distal part of HSA 21 Q 22.2→TER have been mapped to MMU 3, 17, and 10. The reason why genes located between HSA q 11 to mid-q 22.2 remain grouped together across the evolutionary gap from mouse to human remains unclear but suggests the existence of important regulatory relationships that might be disrupted by physical separation.

The Trisomy 16 Mouse

Based on the marked degree of homology between a major portion of the long arm of HSA 21 and the distal end of MMU 16, mice with trisomy for MMU 16 (Ts 16) should provide an informative genetic model for studying the neurobiologic consequences of triplication of a number of genes involved in DS. A special breeding scheme has been devised that results in mice with Ts 16 (24). When male mice with balanced bilateral Robertsonian translocations of MMU 16 (e.g., the fusion of MMU 16 with another chromosome) are mated with normal females, approximately one-third of the progeny surviving to 15 days gestation have Ts 16, whereas the two-thirds are euploid (e.g., a normal complement of chromosomes). The limitation of this model for DS has become apparent with the demonstration that several genes located on the distal end of the long arm of HSA 21, which are thought by some to be essential for the DS phenotype, are not located on MMU 16 (Fig. 1) and the fact that genes located on other human chromosomes map to the proximal end of MMU 16 (24). Analysis of the effects of triplication of genes unrelated to HSA 21, and therefore to DS, might nevertheless be informative with regard to understanding the genetic mechanisms and the functional consequences of triplication of specific genes.

NEUROBIOLOGY OF THE Ts 16 MOUSE

Neurotransmitter Abnormalities in the Ts 16 Mouse

While the Ts 16 mouse offers important opportunities for defining the neurobiologic consequences of specific genes triplicated on MMU 16, it also provides a paradigm for defining and exploring mechanisms involved in the more indirect or secondary consequences of specific gene triplication. Since postmortem studies have demonstrated selective vulnerabilities of certain neurotransmitter systems in AD and in DS with AD pathology, it was of interest to determine the effects of Ts 16 on the developmental expression of several neurotransmitter systems in the embryonic brain. Initial studies employed quantitative synaptic neurochemical analyses on whole brain or brain bisected into forebrain and hindbrain, with euploid littermates serving as controls.

These studies (65), which have been independently corroborated (48), reveal reductions in the presynaptic markers for noradrenergic and serotonergic neurons and brainstem cholinergic neurons at 15 days gestation in the Ts 16 mouse (Table 1). At this point in development, basal forebrain cholinergic neurons have not yet developed axons to innervate forebrain regions (32); thus, brainstem cholinergic

TABLE 1. *Comparisons of DS, Ts 16 mouse, and Ts 19 mouse synaptic neurochemistry*

	DS	Ts 16	Ts 19
Brain weight	D	D	D
Brain protein	D	D	D
ChAT			
Striatum	N	N	D
Midbrain	D	D	N
Glutamate decarboxylase	N	N	D
Serotonin	–	D/N	N
Dopamine	N	N	D
Norepinephrine	D	D	D

Findings for DS reflect postmortem analyses performed on aged DS individuals with Alzheimer's pathology (12). The findings for Ts 16 and Ts 19 mouse fetuses were obtained at 15 to 18 days gestation (36,62,65). D, decreased; N, within normal limits.

markers were presumably localized to the nuclear components of the basal forebrain complex. In contrast, presynaptic markers for the GABAergic and dopaminergic neurons were not significantly reduced in the fetal Ts 16 brain (65). Thus, the developmental deficits appear to exhibit some degree of neuronal selectivity.

Aneuploidy invariably results in brain hypoplasia, which raises the question whether the synaptic neurochemical deficits were a specific consequence of triplication of genes located on MMU 16 and possibly shared with HSA 21. To address this concern, similar studies were carried out on mice with trisomy of chromosome 19 (Ts 19) and their euploid littermates since MMU 19 encodes for completely different genes than those located on MMU 16. Ts 19 was associated with brain hypoplasia as was the case for Ts16. However, the synaptic neurochemical analysis revealed a considerably different profile of neuronal developmental deficits (62). Thus, the specific activity of choline acetyltransferase, the presynaptic marker for cholinergic neurons, was reduced in the forebrain but not in the brainstem. The specific activity of glutamate decarboxylase was significantly reduced in brain as was also the case for presynaptic markers for dopaminergic neurons, whereas the presynaptic marker for noradrenergic neurons was reduced. Thus, the synaptic neurochemical analysis of Ts 19 revealed developmental impairments in the expression of several neurotransmitter systems, but the ones affected were in all cases different from those affected in Ts 16, except for the noradrenergic system.

Because of the central role of basal forebrain cholinergic vulnerability in AD and DS with AD pathology, the basis for reduced ChAT activity in the brainstem was examined to determine whether this resulted from an impairment in the neurogenesis of the basal forebrain (68). [^{3}H]Thymidine autoradiography was combined with AChE histochemistry to determine both the time course of neurogenesis as well as the total complement of neurons in the basal forebrain expressing cholinergic markers. These studies revealed that fewer AChE-positive neuronal perikarya were labeled with [^{3}H]thymidine at later gestational dates in the anterior aspects of the basal forebrain in Ts 16 as compared to the euploid littermates. Quantitative analysis demonstrated that the total number of AChE-positive neurons in the basal forebrain of the Ts 16 fetus was reduced by approximately 40% as compared to its euploid littermates (68). These results are consistent with an impairment in the neurogenesis of basal forebrain cholinergic neurons in Ts 16, analogous to the reduced complement of these neurons observed in the brains of young DS individuals (9). Alternatively, the Ts 16 neurons may suffer from a failure to express cholinergic markers in neurons that normally express these characteristics in the euploid condition.

Restorative Effects of Nerve Growth Factor

Considerable evidence has accumulated that the basal forebrain cholinergic neurons are dependent on nerve growth factor (NGF), a trophic factor originally identified as critical for the survival of peripheral primary sensory afferents and sympathetic neurons (41), for their differentiation, expression of cholinergic characteristics, and even survival (70). Basal forebrain cholinergic neurons richly express NGF receptors (6) and retrogradely transport NGF from target sites of innervation in the cerebral cortex and hippocampal formation (63). Interference with the retrograde transport of NGF to the cholinergic perikarya results in atrophy and degeneration of the basal forebrain cholinergic neurons (28,38,70). For these reasons, investigators have speculated that pathologic alterations of basal forebrain cholinergic neurons in AD may reflect in part a disruption on NGF trophic processes or that NGF treatment might reverse or attenuate the degeneration of these cholinergic neurons in AD (19).

Since the Ts 16 mouse exhibits an impairment in the development of the basal forebrain cholinergic system, perhaps analogous to DS and its vulnerability to AD, the effects of NGF on primary cultures of the basal forebrain from Ts 16 and littermate controls were examined in primary cultures with immunocytochemical visualization of ChAT used to identify cholinergic neurons (12). Culture for 7 days in completely defined medium, which does not contain serum or embryonic extracts, resulted in very clearcut differences between Ts 16 and euploid littermate control basal forebrain cholinergic neurons. Although plated under the same conditions as the euploid littermates, the Ts 16 cultures exhibited significantly fewer ChAT-positive neurons than the euploid littermates (Table 2). Furthermore, Ts 16 cholinergic neurons had smaller cell bodies, emitted fewer neuritic processes that were significantly shorter and exhibited fewer bifurcations than the euploid cholinergic neurons. Notably, the cholinergic axons in Ts 16 were thin and smooth in contrast to the thicker varicosity-punctuated axons of the euploid cholinergic neurons.

As previously reported from studies in the rat (29), addition of maximally stimulatory concentrations of NGF to the culture medium resulted in a significant increase in the length and number of bifurcations of the euploid cholinergic neurons although it did not affect either their number or their perikaryal size. In contrast, not only did NGF treatment markedly augment the length and complexity of the neuritic arbor of Ts 16 cholinergic neurons but it also increased the number and the peri-

TABLE 2. Effects of β-NGF on Ts 16 basal forebrain cholinergic neurons in culture

	Percentage of euploid control	
	Ts 16	Ts 16 + β-NGF
Number of bipolar neurons	61[a]	78[b]
Surface area	94	120[b]
Neurite length	54[a]	119[b]
ChAT activity	65[a]	154[b]

The basal forebrains were obtained from Ts 16 fetuses and euploid littermates at 15 days gestation, disaggregated with papain and grown for 7 days in completely defined medium in the absence or presence of 100 mg/ml of β-NGF. Cholinergic neurons were identified by ChAT immunocytochemistry (Corsi and Coyle, *submitted*).
[a] $p<0.05$ versus euploid.
[b] $p<0.05$ versus Ts 16.

karyal size of the basal forebrain cholinergic neurons. In fact, most of these parameters were restored to the range of values obtained for the euploid cholinergic neurons cultured in the absence of added NGF.

These findings suggest that there is a deficit either in the synthesis of endogenous NGF or in the ability of the cholinergic neurons to respond to NGF in Ts 16. Notably, the quantitative deficits in the basal forebrain cholinergic system observed in primary culture mirror the findings *in vivo* with regard to fewer cholinergic neurons and reduced activity of ChAT in Ts 16. The fact that NGF can restore many of these parameters to normal in this genetic model for DS/AD lends further support to the hypothesized therapeutic effects of NGF receptor agonists in DS and, possibly, in AD (19).

Amyloid Precursor Protein Gene Expression in Ts 16 Mouse

The gene encoding for amyloid precursor protein (APP) is located both on HSA 21 and MMU 16 (56). Amyloid, the major extracellular component of the senile plaque in the brains of individuals with AD and of DS individuals with AD pathology, is a proteolytic degradation product of this cell surface protein. *In situ* hybridization studies have revealed in the mouse that while APP is expressed in many cell types, relatively high levels of expression are observed in the brain (4). Regions such as the cerebral cortex and limbic structures, which are particularly vulnerable to senile plaque formation in AD, exhibit disproportionately large amounts of mRNA encoding APP. Developmental studies in the mouse indicate significant levels of the APP mRNA as early as embryonic day 11 in the mouse brain, with nearly two-thirds of the adult values obtained by embryonic day 15, when normalized against ribosomal RNA (47).

Comparison of the mRNA amounts for APP in the Ts 16 fetal brain to that of its euploid littermate at embryonic day 15 has revealed nearly a twofold elevation in the Ts 16 brain when normalized against beta actin mRNA, a protein whose gene is not localized to MMU 16. *In situ* hybridization studies to sections prepared from embryonic day 15 forebrains confirm a marked overexpression of the APP mRNA in Ts 16 as compared to euploid littermates. Regional analysis indicates that the overexpression of APP mRNA occurs in a regional- and possibly a cellular-specific fashion so that cells that normally express APP synthesize more of the transcript under the condition in which the gene is triplicated. However, the degree of overexpression does not appear to be directly linked to gene dosage (1.5-fold increase) but rather twofold or more.

At least three forms of post-transcriptionally modified APP have been characterized, which contain 695, 751, or 770 amino acids. All three are encoded by the APP gene on HSA 21 or MMU 16 (45). While the smaller 695 amino acid form lacking the Kunitz protease inhibitor insert appears to be particularly expressed in forebrain neurons, it is unclear at present how triplication of the APP gene affects the differential expression of these APP forms. Nevertheless, the results observed with the Ts 16 mouse brain are consistent with those reported for postmortem analysis of DS brains. Furthermore, the overexpression of APP likely accounts for the early accumulation of amyloid peptide in the DS brain (61).

Neuropeptide Expression in Ts 16 Mouse Brain

The gene encoding for pre-pro-somatostatin (ppSS) is located on HSA 3 in humans, but maps to the proximal end of MMU 16 (39). Although triplication of ppSS gene is not directly involved in DS pathology, it is likely that the gene encoding for one or more neuropeptides may be ultimately mapped to HSA 21 because of the large number of neuropeptides identified in brain (>40). Thus, the Ts 16 mouse provides a heuristically valuable paradigm for examining the consequences of triplication of a gene encoding for a neuropeptide.

Northern blot analysis revealed that ppSS transcripts are detectable in mouse fetal brain as early as embryonic day 11, whereas nearly 60% of the adult level is achieved by embryonic day 15 (47). Studies exploiting immunocytochemical visualization of somatostatin in cortex, as well as *in situ* hybridization for ppSS transcripts in cortex, indicate that somatostatin expression occurs predominantly after birth with a peak density of positive neurons between 2 and 3 weeks postnatally, followed by a modest decline (4,21). Quantitative Northern blot analysis of Ts 16 whole brain at embryonic day 15 as compared to the euploid littermate has revealed a 50% elevation of the ppSS mRNA in the Ts 16 brain. At this point in time, *in situ* hybridization for ppSS transcripts in forebrain sections of Ts 16 and euploid littermates confirmed an increased hybridization signal overlying the primordial amygdala-pyriform cortex in Ts 16. However, at this early stage of development, it is difficult to determine whether neurons that normally express somatostatin have increased levels of ppSS transcripts or whether transcripts are present in cells that do not ordinarily express somatostatin.

Since the Ts 16 mouse does not survive to birth, studies have been carried out utilizing primary cultures of the embryonic cerebral cortex to "rescue" Ts 16 neurons in order to follow their further differentiation. Following 7 days of culture in completely defined medium, disaggregated cortex obtained from Ts 16 and euploid littermates at 15 days gestation were immunocytochemically stained for presynaptic neurotransmitter markers and counterstained for Nissl substance to identify all neurons (10). The percentage of cortical neurons that were GABAergic did not differ between Ts 16 and euploid littermates, consistent with previous synaptic neurochemical results in Ts 16 fetuses (65). Similarly, there were no differences in the percentage of cortical neurons immunostained for NPY in the cultures. In contrast, immunohistochemical staining for somatostatin revealed a highly significant increase in the percentage of neurons expressing somatostatin, which over four experiments ranged from 140% to 190% of that of the euploid cortical cultures (Table 3). Since somatostatin is generally colocalized to GABAergic and NPY expressing neurons in cortex, this increase in the number of somatostatin immunoreactive cells appears to be specific.

As neuronal differentiation is affected by tissue culture conditions, we have also exploited brain transplantation to rescue Ts 16 fetal cortex through implantation into neonatal euploid mouse cortex. Preliminary results indicate an increased density of somatostatin-expressing cells 2 weeks after transplantation of 15-day gestational Ts 16 cortex in comparison to euploid littermate cortex when assessed by *in situ* hybridization (31). Thus, the presence of an extra copy of the ppSS gene in Ts 16 results not simply in the overexpression of its transcripts, as well as the product somatostatin, but the ppSS gene appears to be expressed in cells, presumably neurons, that do not ordinarily express it in the cerebral cortex. While these findings are subject to alternative interpretations, they do suggest that dose imbalance for a neuropeptide gene may have important consequences with regard to altered patterns of neuronal innervation.

CONCLUSION

DS is the most common, genetically identified cause of mental retardation. Furthermore, DS is associated with the inevitable appearance in midlife of the pathologic stigmata of AD, the most common cause of cognitive deterioration in the

TABLE 3. *Neurotransmitter marker expression in Ts 16 cortical cultures*

	Percentage of neurons	
	Ts 16	Euploid
Somatostatin	1.5 ± 0.2^a	0.8 ± 0.1
Glutamate decarboxylase	4.6 ± 0.5	4.7 ± 0.5
NPY	0.6 ± 0.2	0.5 ± 0.2

Cerebral cortices from 15-day gestational and euploid littermate fetuses were disaggregated, plated at a density of 700,000 cells/well, and cultured for 7 days. The cells were fixed, immunocytochemically stained for the marker, and then counterstained for Nissl substance (10).
$^a p<0.01$.

elderly. The abnormalities in brain development in DS and its vulnerability to AD pathology reflect the consequences of disregulation of normal gene expression due to the presence of extra copies of genes located on HSA 21. A murine model of DS, involving triplication of MMU 16, a chromosome that shares important genetic homology to HSA 21, demonstrates a number of developmental neurobiologic similarities to DS, including overexpression of APP, the source of amyloid in neuritic plaques. Exploitation of animal models that involve triplication of specific genes or groups of genes located on HSA 21 should elucidate how imbalance in gene number affects expression in brain and contributes to the DS phenotype. Such an understanding could lead to therapeutic strategies to correct abnormal gene expression in DS or its consequences, such as impaired basal forebrain cholinergic development. However, DS is paradigmatic of a range of neuropsychiatric disorders that are due to gene imbalance and not due to mutant genes, including one form of schizophrenia. Thus, the mechanisms and principles elucidated in these studies have broader implications for the pathogenesis of neuropsychiatric disorders.

REFERENCES

1. Ball, M. U., and Nuttal, K. (1981): Topography of neurofibrillary tangles and granulovacuoles in hippocampi of patients with Down syndrome: quantitative comparison with normal aging and Alzheimer's disease. *J. Neuropathol. Appl. Neurobiol.*, 7:13–20.
2. Benda, C. E. (1969): *Down's Anomaly*, 2nd ed., Grune and Stratton, New York.
3. Bendotti, C., Forloni, G. L., Morgan, R. A., et al. (1988): Neuroanatomical localization and quantification of cerebrovascular amyloid peptide RNA following *in situ* hybridization in the brains of normal, aneuploid, and experimentally lesioned mice. *PNAS*, 85:3628–3632.
4. Bendotti, C., Hohmann, C., Forloni, G., Reeves, R., Coyle, J. T., and Oster-Granite, M. L. (1990): Developmental expression of somatostatin in mouse brain: II. *In situ* hybridization. *Dev. Brain Res.*, 53:26–39.
5. Bondareff, W., Mountjoy, C. Q., and Roth, M. (1982): Selective loss of neurons of origin of adrenergic projection to cerebral cortex (nucleus locus coeruleus) in senile dementia. *Neurology*, 32:164–168.
6. Buck, C. R., Martinez, H. J., Black, I. B., and Chao, M. V. (1987): Developmentally regulated expression of nerve growth factor receptor gene in the periphery and brain. *Proc. Natl. Acad. Sci. USA*, 84:3060–3063.
7. Burmeister, M., Kim, S. W., deLange, T., et al. (1989): The fine structure map of the distal long arm of chromosome 21: hot spots of recombination and homology to several mouse chromosomes. *Am. J. Hum. Genet.*, 45:A133.
8. Carritt, B., and Litt, M. (1989): Report of the committee on the genetic constitution of chromosomes 20 and 21. Human Gene Mapping 10: Tenth International Workshop on Human Gene Mapping. *Cytogenet. Cell Genet.*, 51:358–371.
9. Casanova, M. F., Walker, L. C., Whitehouse, P. J., and Price, D. L. (1985): Abnormalities of the nucleus basalis in Down syndrome. *Ann. Neurol.*, 18:310–314.
10. Caserta, M. T., Corsi, P., Oster-Granite, M. L., and Coyle, J. T. (1990): Increased number of somatostatin-immunoreactive neurons in primary cultures of trisomy 16 mouse neocortex. *Mol. Brain Res.*, 7:269–272.
11. Colon, E. J. (1972): The structure of the cerebral cortex in Down syndrome. *Neuropediatrics*, 3: 362–376.
12. Corsi, P., Sweeney, J. E., and Coyle, J. T. (1989): Nerve growth factor stimulates basal forebrain cholinergic neuronal differentiation in trisomy 16 mice. *Soc. Neurosci. Abst.*, 15:707.
13. Cox, D. R., and Epstein, C. J. (1985): Comparative gene mapping of human chromosome 21 and mouse chromosome 16. *Ann. NY Acad. Sci.*, 450:169–177.

14. Coyle, J. T., Oster-Granite, M. L., and Gearhart, J. D. (1986): The neurobiologic consequences of Down syndrome. *Brain Res. Bull.*, 16:773–787.
15. Coyle, J. T., Price, D. L., and DeLong, M. R. (1983): Alzheimer's disease: a disorder of cortical cholinergic innervation. *Science*, 219:1184–1190.
16. Cross, A. J., Crow, T. J., Perry, E. K., Perry, R. H., Blessed, G., and Tomlinson, B. E. (1981): Reduced dopamine beta-hydroxylase activity in Alzheimer's disease. *Br. Med. J.*, 282:93–94.
17. Davidoff, L. M. (1928): The brain in mongolian idiocy. *Arch. Neurol. Psychiatr.*, 20:1229–1257.
18. Davies, P. (1979): Neurotransmitter-related enzymes in senile dementia of the Alzheimer's type. *Brain Res.*, 171:319–327.
19. Fisher, W., Wictorim, K., Bjorklund, A., Williams, L. P., Varon, S., and Gage, F. (1987): Amelioration of cholinergic neuron atrophy and spatial memory impairment in aged rats by nerve growth factor. *Nature*, 329:65–68.
20. Fishler, K., Koch, R., and Donnell, G. N. (1976): Comparison of mental development in individuals with mosaic and trisomy 21 Down's syndrome. *Pediatrics*, 58:744–748.
21. Forloni, G., Hohmann, C., and Coyle, J. T. (1990): Developmental expression of somatostatin in mouse brain. I. Immunocytochemical studies. *Dev. Brain Res.*, 53:6–25.
22. Francis, P. T., Palmer, A. M., Sims, N. R., et al. (1985): Neurochemical studies on early onset Alzheimer's disease: possible influence on treatment. *N. Engl. J. Med.*, 313:7–10.
23. Galaburda, A. M., and Kemper, T. L. (1979): Down syndrome: is there a missing population of neurons? *Neurology*, 29:569–570.
24. Gearhart, J. D., Davisson, M. T., and Oster-Granite, M. L. (1986): Autosomal aneuploidy in mice: generation and developmental consequences. *Brain Res. Bull.*, 16:789–801.
25. Gilbert, E. F., and Opitz, J. M. (1982): Developmental and other pathological changes in syndromes caused by chromosome abnormalities. *Perspect. Pediatr. Pathol.*, 7:1–63.
26. Glenner, G. G., and Wong, C. W. (1984): Alzheimer's disease and Down syndrome: sharing of a unique cerebrovascular amyloid fibril protein. *Biochem. Biophys. Res. Commun.*, 122:1131–1135.
27. Gullotta, F., and Rehder, H. (1974): Chromosomal anomalies and central nervous system. *Beitr. Pathol. Bild.*, 152:74–80.
28. Hefti, F. (1986): Nerve growth factor (NGF) promotes survival of septal cholinergic neurons after fimbrial transection. *J. Neurosci.*, 6:2155–2162.
29. Hefti, F., Hartikka, J., Eckenstein, F., Grahn, H., Heuman, R., and Schwab, M. E. (1985): Nerve growth factor increases choline acetyltransferase but not survival or fiber outgrowth of cultured fetal septal cholinergic neurons. *Neuroscience*, 14:56–68.
30. Heller, J. H. (1969): Human chromosome abnormalities as related to physical and mental dysfunction. *J. Hered.*, 60:239–252.
31. Hohmann, C., Capone, G., Oster-Granite, M. L., and Coyle, J. T. (1990): Transplantation of brain tissue from murine trisomy 16 into euploid hosts: effects of gene imbalance on brain development. In: *Progress in Brain Research, Vol. 82*, edited by S. B. Dunnett and S.-J. Richards, pp. 203–214. Elsevier, Amsterdam.
32. Hohmann, C., and Ebner, F. F. (1985): Development of cholinergic markers in mouse forebrain I. Choline acetyltransferase enzyme activity and acetylcholinesterase histochemistry. *Dev. Brain Res.*, 23:225–241.
33. Hohmann, C. F., Wenk, G. L., Lowenstein, P., Brown, M. E., and Coyle, J. T. (1987): Age-related recurrence of basal forebrain lesion-induced cholinergic deficits. *Neurosci. Lett.*, 82:253–259.
34. Hook, E. B. (1981): Down syndrome: its frequency in human populations and some factors pertinent to variations in rates. In: *Trisomy 21 (Down Syndrome): Research Perspectives*, edited by F. F. de la Cruz and P. S. Gerald, pp. 3–68. University Park Press, Baltimore.
35. Kish, S., Karlinsky, H., Becker, L., et al. (1989): Down's syndrome individuals begin life with normal levels of brain cholinergic markers. *J. Neurochem.*, 52:1183–1187.
36. Kiss, J., Schlumpf, M., and Balazs, R. (1989): Selective retardation of the development of the basal forebrain cholinergic and pontine catecholaminergic nuclei in the brain of trisomy 16 mouse, an animal model of Down's syndrome. *Dev. Brain Res.*, 50:251–264.
37. Kornberg, J. R., Pulst, S. M., Neve, R. L., and West, R. (1989): The Alzheimer amyloid precursor protein maps to human chromosome 21 bands q 21.105–q 21.05. *Genomics*, 5:124–127.
38. Kromer, L. F. (1987): Nerve growth factor treatment after brain injury prevents neuronal death. *Science*, 235:214–216.
39. Lalley, P. A., Davisson, M. T., Graves, J. A. M., et al. (1988): Report on the committee on comparative mapping. *Cytogenet. Cell Genet.*, 49:227–235.

40. Lalley, P. A., Davisson, M. T., Graves, J. A. M., et al. (1989): Report of the committee on comparative mapping. Human Gene Mapping 10: Tenth International Workshop on Human Gene Mapping. *Cytogenet. Cell Genet.*, 51:503–532.
41. Levi-Montalcini, R. (1987): The nerve growth factor: thirty-five years later. *EMBO*, 6:1145–1154.
42. Loesch-Mdzewska, D. (1968): Some aspects of the neurology of Down syndrome. *J. Ment. Defic. Res.*, 12:237–244.
43. Marin-Padilla, M. (1972): Structural abnormalities of the cerebral cortex in human chromosomal aberrations: A Golgi study. *Brain Res.*, 44:625–629.
44. Marin-Padilla, M. (1976): Pyramidal cell abnormalities in the motor cortex of a child with Down syndrome. *J. Comp. Neurol.*, 167:63–82.
45. Muller-Hill, B., and Beyreuther, K. (1989): Molecular biology of Alzheimer's disease. *Annu. Rev. Biochem*, 58:287–307.
46. Norman, R. M. (1971): Malformations of the nervous system, birth injury, and diseases in early life. In: *Greenfield's Neuropathology*, edited by W. Blackwood and J. A. N. Corsellis, pp. 324–337. Edward Arnold Publishers, London.
47. O'Hara, B. F., Fisher, S., Oster-Granite, M. L., Gearhart, J. D., and Reeves, R. H. (1989): Developmental expression of the amyloid precursor protein, growth-associated protein 43, and somatostatin in normal and trisomy 16 mice. *Dev. Brain Res.*, 49:300–304.
48. Ozand, P. T., Hawkins, R. L., Collins, R. M., Jr., Reed, W. D., Baab, P. J., and Oster-Granite, M. L. (1984): Neurochemical changes in murine trisomy 16: delay in cholinergic and catecholaminergic systems. *J. Neurochem.*, 43:401–408.
49. Patterson, D., Gardiner, K., Kao, F.-T., Tanzi, R., Watkins, P., and Gusella, J. F. (1988): The mapping of the gene encoding the beta amyloid precursor protein and its relationship to the Down syndrome region of chromosome 21. *Proc. Natl. Acad. Sci. USA*, 85:8266–8270.
50. Price, D. L., Whitehouse, P. J., Struble, R. G., et al. (1982): Basal forebrain cholinergic systems in Alzheimer's disease and related dementias. *Neurosci. Comment.*, 1:84–92.
51. Purpura, D. P. (1975): Normal and aberrant neuronal development in the cerebral cortex of human fetus and young infant. In: *Brain Mechanisms in Mental Retardation*, edited by N. A. Buchwald and M. A. B. Brazier, pp. 141–169. Academic Press, New York.
52. Rahmani, Z., Blouin, J.-L., Creau-Goldberg, N., et al. (1989): Critical role of the D21S55 region on chromosome 21 in the pathogenesis of Down syndrome. *Proc. Natl. Acad. Sci. USA*, 86:5958–5962.
53. Reeves, R. H., Gallahan, D., O'Hara, B. F., Callahan, R., and Gearhart, J. D. (1987): Genetic mapping of *Prm-1, Igl-1, Smst, Mtv-6, Sod-1* and *Ets-2*, and localization of the Down syndrome region on mouse chromosome 16. *Cytogenet. Cell Genet.*, 44:76–81.
54. Reeves, R. H., Gearhart, J. D., Hecht, N. B., Yelick, P., Johnson, P., and O'Brien, S. J. (1989): The gene encoding protamine 1 is located on human chromosome 16, and near the proximal end of mouse chromosome 16 where it is tightly linked to the gene encoding protamine 2. *J. Hered.*, 80:442–446.
55. Reeves, R. H., Gearhart, J. G., and Littlefield, J. W. (1986): Genetic basis for a mouse model of Down syndrome. *Brain Res. Bull.*, 16:803–814.
56. Reeves, R. H., Robakis, N. K., Oster-Granite, M. L., Wisniewski, H. M., Coyle, J. T., and Gearhart, J. D. (1987): Genetic linkage in the mouse of genes involved in Down syndrome and Alzheimer's disease in man. *Mol. Brain Res.*, 2:215–221.
57. Ross, M. H., Galaburda, A. M., and Kemper, T. L. (1984): Down's syndrome: is there a decreased population of neurons? *Neurology*, 34:909–916.
58. Rosser, M., Emson, P. C., Mountjoy, C. Q., Roth, M., and Iversen, L. L. (1980): Reduced amounts of immunoreactive somatostatin in the temporal cortex in senile dementia of the Alzheimer's type. *Neurosci. Lett.*, 20:373–377.
59. Rossor, M., Fahrenkrug, J., Emson, P., Mountjoy, C., Iversen, L., and Roth, M. (1980): Reduced cortical choline acetyltransferase activity in senile dementia of Alzheimer type is not accompanied by changes in vasoactive intestinal polypeptide. *Brain Res.*, 201:249–253.
60. Rossor, M., Iversen, L. L., Mountjoy, C. Q., Roth, M., Hawthorn, J., Ang, V. Y., and Jenkins, J. S. (1980): Arginine vasopressin and choline acetyltransferase in the brains of patients with Alzheimer type senile dementia. *Lancet*, 2:1367–1368.
61. Rumble, B., Retallack, R., Hilbrich, C., et al. (1989): Amyloid A4 protein and its precursor in Down's syndrome and Alzheimer's disease. *N Engl. J. Med.*, 320:1446–1452.
62. Saltarelli, M. D., Forloni, G. L., Oster-Granite, M. L., Gearhart, J. D., and Coyle, J. T. (1987) Neurochemical characterization of embryonic brain development in trisomy 19 (Ts19) mice: impli-

cations of selective deficits observed for abnormal neural development in aneuploidy. *Dev. Genet.*, 8:267–279.
63. Seiler, M., and Schwab, M. E. (1984): Specific retrograde transport of nerve growth factor from neocortex to nucleus basalis in rat. *Brain Res.*, 300:33–39.
64. Sims, N. R., Bowen, D. M., Allen, S. J., et al. (1983): Presynaptic cholinergic dysfunction in patients with dementia. *J. Neurochem.*, 40:53–509.
65. Singer, H. S., Tiemeyer, M., Hedreen, J. C., Gearhart, J., and Coyle, J. T. (1984): Morphologic and neurochemical studies of embryonic brain development in murine trisomy 16. *Dev. Brain Res.*, 15:155–166.
66. St. George-Hyslop, P. H., Tanzi, R. E., Polinsky, R. J., et al. (1987): The gene causing familial Alzheimer's disease maps on chromosome 21. *Science*, 235:885–890.
67. Struwe, F. (1929): Histopathologische Untersuchungen uber Entstehung und Wesen der senile Plaques. *Zeitbild Gesch. Neurol. Psychiatry*, 122:291–306.
68. Sweeney, J. E., Hohmann, C. F., Oster-Granite, M. L., and Coyle, J. T. (1989): Neurogenesis of the basal forebrain in euploid and trisomy 16 mice: an animal model for developmental disorders in Down syndrome. *Neuroscience*, 31:413–425.
69. Whalley, L. J. (1982): The dementia of Down's syndrome and its relevance to aetiological studies of Alzheimer's disease. *Ann. NY Acad. Sci.*, 396:39–54.
70. Williams, L. R., Varon, S., Peterson, G. M., et al. (1986): Continuous infusion of nerve growth factor prevents basal forebrain neuronal death after fimbria fornix transection. *Proc. Natl. Acad. Sci. USA*, 83:9231–9235.
71. Wisniewski, K. E., Wisniewski, H. M., and Wen, G. Y. (1985): Occurrence of neuropathological changes and dementia of Alzheimer's disease in Down's syndrome. *Ann. Neurol.*, 17:278–282.
72. Yates, C. M., Harmar, A. J., Rosie, R., et al. (1983): Thyrotropin-releasing hormone, luteinizing hormone-releasing hormone, and substance P immunoreactivity in post-mortem brain from cases of Alzheimer-type dementia and Down's syndrome. *Brain Res.*, 258:45–52.
73. Yates, C. M., Simpson, J., Gordon, A., et al. (1983): Catecholaminergic and cholinergic enzymes in presenile and senile Alzheimer's like disease and Down syndrome. *Brain Res.*, 280:119–126.

Genes, Brain, and Behavior, edited by
P. R. McHugh and V. A. McKusick.
Raven Press, Ltd., New York © 1991.

Mitochondrial Genes and Neuromuscular Disease

Douglas C. Wallace

Departments of Biochemistry, Pediatrics, and Neurology, Emory University School of Medicine, Atlanta, Georgia 30322

ATP PRODUCTION AND THE MITOCHONDRIAL DNA

The mitochondria produce most of our cellular energy. This energy is synthesized in the form of ATP by the process of oxidative phosphorylation (OXPHOS). Each human cell has hundreds of mitochondria and each mitochondrion contains multiple small circular DNAs, the mitochondrial DNA (mtDNA).

Each mtDNA codes for 13 genes essential for OXPHOS energy production. In addition, the mtDNA encodes the rRNAs and tRNAs used in mitochondrial protein synthesis (1). We now know that mutations in the mtDNA cause hereditary diseases of the central nervous system and muscle through starving the cells for energy (48).

Mitochondrial OXPHOS consists of five enzyme complexes (I through V) located within the mitochondrial inner membrane. Complexes I, II, III, and IV form the electron transport chain by which NADH generated from the oxidation of organic acids and fats is oxidized by Complex I (NADH: ubiquinone oxidoreductase) and succinate is oxidized by Complex II (succinate: ubiquinone oxidoreductase). The electrons from both complexes are transferred to ubiquinone (Coenzyme Q [CoQ]). From there they are transferred to Complex III (ubiquinol: cytochrome c oxidoreductase), then to cytochrome c, then to Complex IV (cytochrome c oxidase), and finally to $1/2$ O_2 to form H_2O. In the process, protons are pumped out of the mitochondrion to form an electrochemical gradient. The potential energy stored in this gradient is used by Complex V (ATP synthase) to condense ADP + Pi to form ATP. The resulting matrix ATP is exchanged for cytosolic ADP by the adenine nucleotide translocator (ANT) (38,45,47).

Each OXPHOS complex is composed of multiple polypeptides, some derived from the mtDNA and others derived from the nuclear DNA. Complex I encompasses seven mtDNA subunits (ND 1, 2, 3, 4L, 4, 5, 6) and over 19 nuclear subunits; Complex II, four nuclear subunits; Complex III, one mtDNA subunit (cytb) and about nine nuclear subunits; Complex IV, three mtDNA subunits (COI, II, III) and about 10 nuclear subunits; and Complex V, two mtDNA subunits (ATPase 6 and 8) and 10 nuclear subunits. The mtDNA replicates in a unique manner using two separate origins, one for the G-rich heavy (H)-strand and one for the C-rich light (L)-strand. The two origins are separated by two-thirds of the genome so that replication is bidirectional but asynchronous (38).

The extrachromosomal location of the mtDNA and its high copy number results in the mtDNA having five unique genetic characteristics (48). First, the mtDNA is maternally inherited. MtDNA is transmitted from mother to all of her children, but only daughters can pass the mtDNA to the next generation. Males make no contribution to the mtDNA of their offspring (5,8). Second, the mtDNA can undergo replicative segregation. Each cell contains thousands of mtDNAs (40). If the cytoplasm contains a mixture of mutant and wild-type (normal) mtDNAs (heteroplasmy), then the proportion of mutant mtDNAs can drift along mitotic and meiotic lineages. This occurs because mtDNAs are distributed randomly to the daughter cells during cytokinesis (46). Third, mtDNA mutants show threshold expression. In cells harboring mutant mtDNAs, the reduction in cellular energy production will be a product of the severity of the mutation and the proportion of mutant mtDNAs. Since different tissues and organs rely on mitochondrial energy production to varying extents, a particular mtDNA genotype will have deleterious effects on tissues requiring a higher mitochondrial energy output (threshold), but will not affect tissues with a lower mitochondrial energy threshold. The brain is most sensitive to energy deficiency followed by skeletal muscle, heart, kidney, liver, etc. Hence, the majority of the diseases will affect brain and muscle and the greater the severity of the mtDNA defect, the more tissues that will be affected (38,45,47). Fifth, the mtDNA has a high mutation rate, about 10- to 20-fold greater than nuclear genes that function in the same enzyme complex. Hence, gene for gene, deleterious OXPHOS mutations will be much more common in mtDNA genes than in nDNA genes (21,22,25).

OXPHOS DISEASES OF THE mtDNA

Disease producing mutations of the mtDNA can be of three types: missense mutations (point mutations that alter an amino acid), protein synthesis mutations (point mutations in rRNA or tRNA genes), and insertion-deletion mutations. Severe mutations are generally heteroplasmic, since they are lethal when homoplasmic.

Leber's hereditary optic neuropathy (LHON) is an example of a mild missense mutation (51). LHON is maternally inherited (Fig. 1) and presents as a rapid onset, bilateral, loss of central vision after puberty. Patients frequently have cardiac dysrhythmias and show presymptomatic retinal changes such as tortuous blood vessels and microangiopathy (38,47).

About two-thirds of LHON cases are caused by a G to A base substitution at nucleotide pair (np) 11778 in the mtDNA sequence. This changes the 340th amino acid in the ND4 gene from an arginine to a histidine (51). This mutation was shown to cause LHON because it was found in the majority of LHON patients, was not found in normal controls, changed an amino acid that is conserved throughout

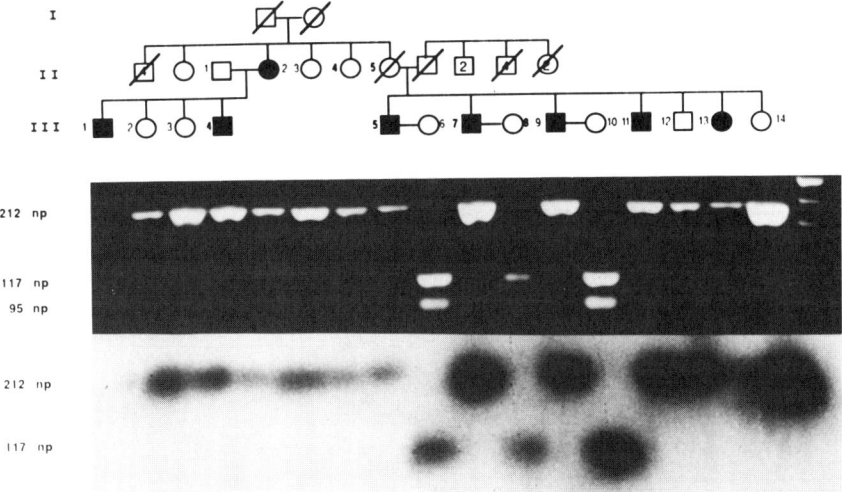

FIG. 1. The maternal transmission of LHON and the maternal inheritance of the ND4 mutation (51). **Top:** Three-generation Georgia LHON pedigree. *Solid symbols* indicate central vision loss; *open symbols* no vision loss. Numbers in symbols indicate number of individuals. Individuals III-6, III-8, and III-10 are spouses not related to blind family members through the maternal lineage. All affected individuals are related through females II-2 and II-5. **Middle:** SfaNI digestion of the 212 np PCR fragment surrounding the mutant nucleotide at np 11778. All maternal lineage relatives have the LHON mutation eliminating the SfaNI site. Their 212 bp fragment remains undigested. Spouse controls III-6, III-8, and III-10 have the normal sequence and retained the site. Their 212 np fragment is cut into 117 and 95 np fragments. **Bottom:** Southern blot of middle panel hybridized to an internal mtDNA oligonucleotide probe. Hybridization confirmed that the fragments have the appropriate origin. (From ref. 51.)

mtDNA evolution from protists and fungi to humans (51), and has occurred multiple times in the human population and in every case given rise to the same disease (41). The LHON mutation eliminates an SfaNI restriction site in the patient's mtDNA. This provides an accurate and rapid molecular genetic test for individuals harboring the mutation. The region surrounding the mutation is amplified using the polymerase chain reaction (PCR) in a 212 bp fragment. This fragment is then digested with SfaNI and the products separated on an agarose gel. If the fragment is cut in two, then the individual has the normal sequence. If it remains uncut, the patient carries the mutation (51) (Fig. 1).

In large LHON pedigrees with many affected individuals, the mutant mtDNA predominates in maternal relatives (Fig. 1). These individuals are viable since the mutation only partially reduces mitochondrial Complex-I activity. Hence, in homoplasmic individuals only cells highly reliant on OXPHOS energy, the optic nerve and heart conduction system, are affected (51). In singleton cases, unaffected maternal lineage relatives can be heteroplasmic (12,17) (Fig. 2). Possibly, these are new mutations that have recently become enriched by replicative segregation and thus were detected in the first individual to manifest symptoms. In most individuals, the presence of normal mtDNA in heteroplasmic cells should elevate mitochondrial

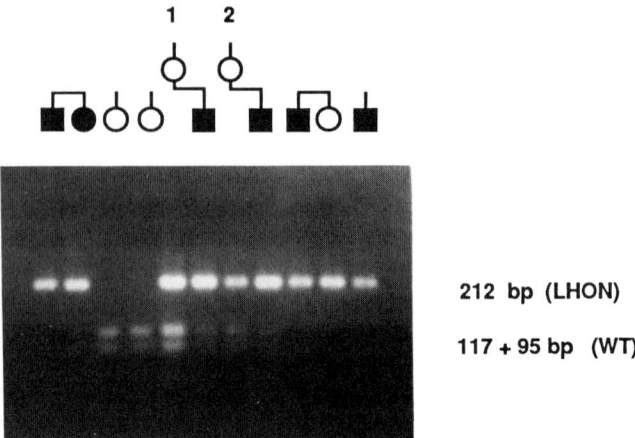

SFA N1 digest of PCR-mtDNA

FIG. 2. Heteroplasmic segregation at nt11778 in Leber's optic atrophy. Heteroplasmy of the LHON mutation (17). *Solid symbols*, central vision loss; *open symbols*, no vision loss. Counting from left: lanes 1+2, LHON siblings homoplasmic for mutant mtDNA; lanes 3+4, independent controls homoplasmic for normal (WT) mtDNA; lanes 5+6 and 7+8, mother and blind son, both heteroplasmic for normal and mutant mtDNAs, two independent tests; lanes 9+10, LHON patient and unaffected sister homoplasmic for mutant mtDNA; and lane 11, LHON patient homoplasmic for mutant mtDNA.

energy production sufficiently to mask all clinical manifestations. Since the proportion of mutant mtDNAs can shift rapidly between generations and even within individuals, it is important that each maternal relative be tested for heteroplasmy before predicting his or her potential for vision loss (17).

Maternally inherited retinitis pigmentosa with bone-spicule formation has also been associated with a missense mutation (11). Maternal relatives also manifest ataxia, seizures, dementia, proximal neurogenic muscle weakness, sensory neuropathy, developmental delay, but no overt mitochondrial myopathy. This disease is the result of a T to G transversion at np 8993, which changes a conserved leucine at position 156 of the ATPase 6 subunit to an arginine. The mutation creates an AvaI site providing a simple molecular test, and it is heteroplasmic with the proportion of mutant mtDNAs correlating with the severity of the disease (11).

Myoclonic epilepsy and ragged-red fiber disease (MERRF) is caused by a mtDNA protein synthesis mutation (37,54). The most prominent feature of MERRF patients is an uncontrolled and debilitating myoclonic jerking. On muscle biopsy, these patients also have mitochondrial myopathy. They exhibit a ragged deterioration of the type-I (oxidative) skeletal muscle fibers, while the type-II (glycolytic) fibers are unaffected. The type-I fibers also have large aggregates of highly abnormal mitochondria, frequently bearing paracrystalline arrays, that stain red with Gomori modified trichrome stain and are thus designated ragged-red muscle fibers.

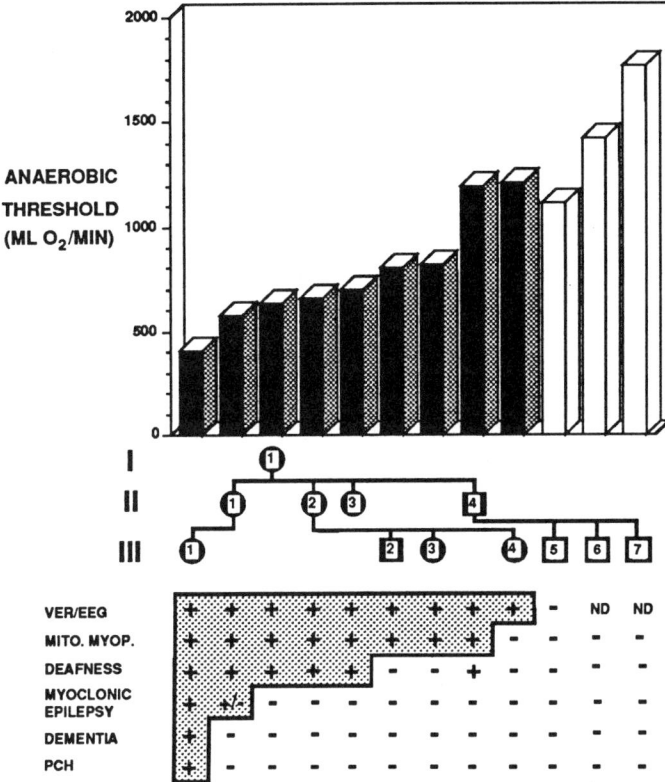

FIG. 3. Maternal MERRF pedigree showing variable phenotypic expression and impaired oxidative work capacity (38,54). **Middle panel:** Pedigree showing maternal inheritance. *Filled symbols*, patients with two or more disease manifestations. *Open symbols*, normal. *Upper panel:* Anaerobic threshold (Θan), the transition point from aerobic energy production to anaerobic energy production with increasing muscle work. Patients are arranged from low to high anaerobic threshold rather than by age. **Lower panel:** Variable clinical manifestations. +, aberrations present; −, aberrations absent; +/−, rare aberration. VER, visual evoked response; EEG, electroencephalogram; Mito. Myop., mitochondrial myopathy; PCH, primary central hypoventilation.

Other symptoms include aberrations of the visual evoked response (VER) and electroencephalographic (EEG) readings, bilateral sensory neural hearing loss, dementia, hypoventilation, and cardiomyopathy (31).

Extensive analysis of a large MERRF pedigree has shown that this disease conforms to all of the characteristics of a heteroplasmic point mutation (Fig. 3). The disease is maternally inherited with everyone on the maternal lineage being affected to some degree (54). The severity of the disease varies among maternal lineage relatives with the VER and EEG aberrations being found in all family members, ragged-red fibers found in most, deafness in half, and debilitating epilepsy and dementia found in only the most severely affected. Affected individuals have a deficiency in their ability to perform oxidative muscle work as indicated by reduced anaerobic threshold (Fig. 3) and to generate high energy phosphate compounds. These defects are associated with deficiencies in muscle mitochondrial respiratory Complexes I and IV (Fig. 4) that correlate with a relative reduction in synthesis of the higher molecular weight mitochondrial translation products (52), most of which are subunits of Complexes I and IV.

The severity of the Complex-I and -IV defects are directly proportional to the severity of the patient's clinical symptoms, as expected for a heteroplasmic mtDNA mutation segregating along the maternal lineage. As the patients' ATP-generating capacity declines, progressively more organ thresholds will be traversed (54).

Extensive restriction analysis has ruled out insertion-deletion mutations as the cause of MERRF (49,50,54), but direct sequencing of PCR-amplified MERRF patient mtDNA revealed an A to G transition at np 8344, which causes the disease (37). The mutation alters a conserved nucleotide in the TψC loop of the tRNA^{Lys} gene (Fig. 5), was present in three independent MERRF families but not in 75 controls, was heteroplasmic, and the proportion of mutant and wild-type mtDNAs correlated with the severity of the disease when family members of comparable ages were compared. The mutation creates a restriction site for the enzyme CViJI providing a simple molecular diagnostic test and greater than 70% to 80% of the patient's mtDNAs must be mutant before they exhibit any clinical manifestations. This implies that the mutation has a relatively mild effect on tRNA^{Lys} function (37).

The ocular myopathies are frequently caused by mtDNA insertion-deletion mutations (38). They are characterized by ophthalmoplegia, ptosis, and mitochondrial

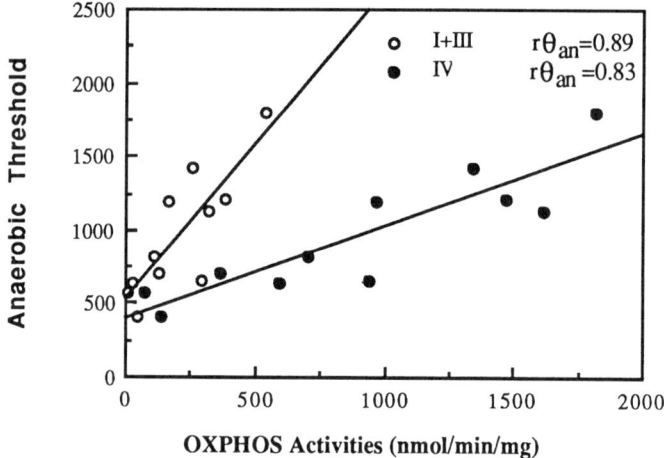

FIG. 4. Correlation between MERRF patient anaerobic threshold and OXPHOS enzyme defect (54). Specific activities of muscle mitochondria respiratory Complexes I + III (rotenone-sensitive NADH-cytochrome c oxidoreductase) and IV (cytochrome c oxidase) are shown, both assayed using sonicated mitochondria. Additional enzyme data in 54. rθan, correlation coefficient relative to anaerobic threshold.

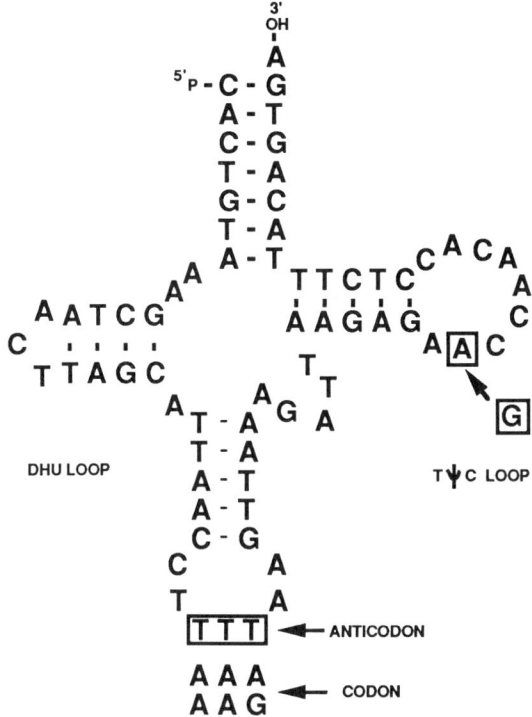

FIG. 5. A mutation at np 8344 that causes MERRF. The normal tRNA sequence is shown. The affected nucleotides, A for normal and G for patient, are surrounded by boxes. The mutation creates a CViJI restriction site (PuGCPy) permitting its ready detection (37).

myopathy (chronic external opthalmoplegia plus [CEOP]), but can also manifest more severe symptoms including lactic acidosis, retinitis pigmentosa, cerebellar ataxia, elevated cerebral spinal fluid protein, and heart conduction defects (Kearns-Sayre syndrome).

In one informative CEOP case, the 61-year-old female proband was admitted to the intensive care unit with respiratory failure requiring mechanical ventilation and manifesting ptosis and ophthalmoplegia. Muscle biopsy revealed mitochondrial myopathy and biochemical analysis of muscle mitochondria revealed a 50% reduction in respiratory Complexes II through V and an absence of Complex I. The proband's siblings had no evidence of comparable disease and muscle biopsy of two sisters revealed no pathology or OXPHOS deficiency (39).

Analysis of the muscle mtDNAs of the proband revealed heteroplasmy with 50% of the molecules having a 4977 np deletion spanning nps 13466 to 8469 of the mtDNA sequence (Fig. 6). No deleted molecules could be detected in the muscle mtDNAs of her two sisters. The proband's mtDNA breakpoint occurred two base pairs outside of an exact 13 bp direct repeat with the sequence 5′ACCTC-CCTCACCA3′. These repeats are located at np 8470 to 8482 and 13447 to 13459

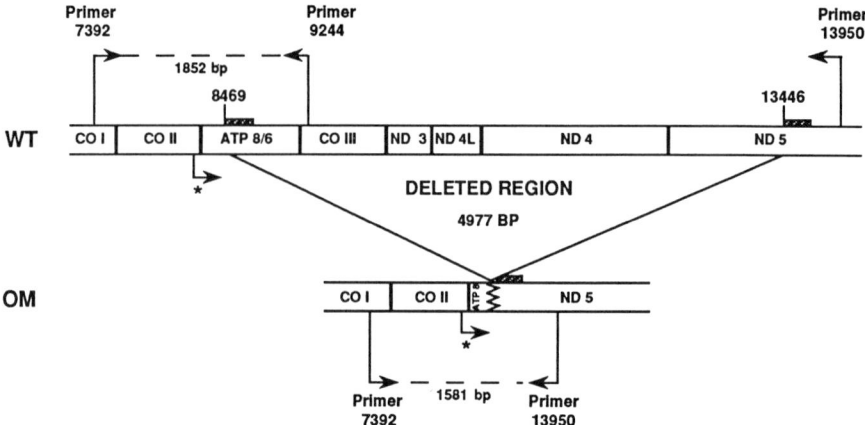

FIG. 6. Map of the most common ocular myopathy deletion and the PCR primers used for direct molecular identification and sequencing of the deletion (39). WT, normal mtDNA molecule from wild-type individual. *Shaded boxes* above map at np 8469 and 13446 show direct 13 bp repeats. OM, deleted mtDNA molecule from ocular myopathy patient, jagged line indicates breakpoint. Polypeptide genes are defined in text, intervening tRNAs are COI-(Ser)-COII-(Lys)-ATP8-ATP6-COIII-(Gly)-ND3-(Arg)-ND4L-ND4-(His)-(Ser)-(Leu)-ND5. Primers for PCR diagnosis and sequencing are positioned on maps. Primer with asterisks (np 8282) was used for direct sequencing.

(Fig. 7). Because this breakpoint occurred outside of the direct repeat, it was apparent that relative to the direction of the H-strand replication, the deleted molecule retained the upstream 13447 to 13459 repeat and lost the downstream 8470 to 8482 repeat. This suggests that this deletion and possibly other mtDNA deletions may be the product of slip-replication errors that occur during the protracted period of mtDNA replication when the parental H-strand remains single stranded (39). This hypothesis is supported by the accumulating evidence that about 30% of all deletions occur at this 13 np repeat and that a variety of other deletions also include direct repeats (9,10,14,15,18,20,23,24,32,34).

To detect this mtDNA deletion in other tissues of the proband, a PCR strategy

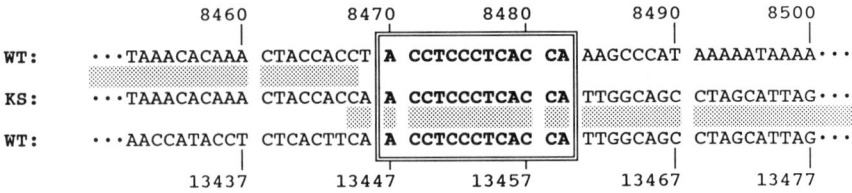

FIG. 7. Sequence homology of the common deletion breakpont in ocular pathway. Alignment of ocular myopathy deletion and normal mtDNA sequences (39). Sequence homology is indicated by shading. Nucleotide positions are numbered according to the master sequence (1). The 13 bp direct repeat is highlighted by boldface letters and outlining. The nucleotide break that permitted identification of the retained repeat sequence occurs at np 13445 and is shown by shading.

was developed for simultaneously assaying for normal and deleted molecules in small tissue samples. PCR permits selective amplification of specific regions of the mtDNA. Opposing pairs of primers are prepared homologous to sequences flanking the region of interest and the intervening sequence is synthesized using a heat-stable DNA polymerase and deoxyribonucleotides through repeated cycles of DNA denaturation, primer annealing, and primer extension. To amplify the normal mtDNA, one primer was used outside the deleted region starting at np 7392 and a second primer inside the deleted region starting at np 9244 (Fig. 6). Only normal molecules have both primer binding sites and amplification on normal mtDNAs generates a 1852 bp fragment. To identify the deleted molecules, a third primer was employed starting at np 13950 and opposing the primer at 7392. In normal mtDNAs, the 7392 and 13950 primers are too far apart to generate a product. However, in the deleted molecule, these primers are brought together and will generate a 1581 bp fragment. When these three primers were added to proband's muscle DNA, both the normal fragment and the deletion fragments were observed. This confirmed that the muscle was heteroplasmic for normal and deleted molecules. By contrast, when the three primers were added to blood cell DNA, only the normal fragment was found (39). This implies that the patient was a mosaic with some cells having deleted molecules and others not. The absence of affected maternal relatives and the mosaic cellular distribution of the patient's mtDNAs raises the possibility that the deletion occurred during the proband's development after the separation of her myogenic and hemopoietic cell lineages. MtDNA analysis of autopsy tissues of a Kearns-Sayre patient indicated a broad tissue distribution of deleted molecules (36). The contrast in distribution of deleted molecules in CEOP and Kearns-Sayre syndrome suggests that the severity of the disease may be a product of when in development the deletion occurred.

The absence of respiratory Complex I, but retention of partial activities for Complexes II through V in the proband, suggested that electron flow and hence energy production were blocked at NADH oxidation, the first step in the pathway. In an effort to bypass this block, the patient was fed succinate and CoQ. Succinate donates electrons to Complex II and CoQ collects the electrons and passes them on down the pathway. Within a week, the respiratory failure of the patient resolved and she was discharged from the hospital. She remained stable on this therapy regime for 2 months until she decided to stop taking the medication. Within a week, she was readmitted to the intensive care unit with respiratory failure. Readministration of the medication again led to resolution of the symptoms (39). These results are consistent with the conclusion that her primary defect was in respiratory Complex I and indicates that at least some of these diseases will be amenable to rational metabolic therapy.

MOLECULAR GENETICS OF nDNA OXPHOS GENES

While it is now established that mtDNA mutations can cause neuromuscular disease, it is still unclear why some organs are more affected than others. These organ-specific thresholds are not a product of differences in the mtDNA, since the mtDNA is the same in all tissues. Thus, the differences must be generated through differential expression of nuclear OXPHOS genes.

To obtain insight into tissue OXPHOS differences, two of the most important nuclear-encoded OXPHOS genes were cloned and analyzed: the ATP synthase β subunit (ATPsynβ), which is the catalytic subunit of the ATP synthase (Complex V) (53), and the heart-skeletal muscle isoform of the adenine nucleotide translocator (ANT) (ANT1) (21).

ATPsynβ is a single-copy nuclear gene located on human chromosome 12 (Table 1). It has 10 exons and CpG-rich regions surrounding the first exon. Promoter-like elements (22,25) include a cluster of four CCAAT boxes adjacent to the transcription start site, plus an additional CCAAT site, two Sp1 sites and a Z-DNA region further upstream. The gene also contains an Sp1 site at the beginning of the first intron, a "CCArGG"-like element often associated with muscle gene expression in the fourth intron, and multiple other putative transcription elements. Comparison of the ATPsynβ gene sequence with that of ANT1 revealed an identical 13 np element about 500 np 5' to the initiation codon in both genes. This element was designated the OXBOX (22).

Analysis of the ATPsynβ expression in different tissues revealed very high mRNA levels in heart, lower levels in skeletal muscle, and the lowest levels in liver, kidney, and brain. Hence, this gene is induced in heart and muscle, consistent with the higher OXPHOS enzyme levels in these tissues (22).

ANT1 (21) is one of three ANT isoforms. ANT2 was isolated from a fibroblast library (2) and ANT3 from liver (13) and heart-liver libraries (29). All three ANT coding regions are equally divergent and appear to have evolved from the triplication of an ancestral gene about 275 million years ago during the radiation of the reptiles (21).

ANT1 has four exons and a CpG island that encompasses the 5' nontranslated region, first exon and intron. Promoter elements 5' to the transcription initiation site include a single CCAAT, TATA, and OXBOX element as well as three Sp1 sites at the beginning of the first intron (6,16) (Table 1). ANT1 is located on chromosome 4 and its mRNA is abundant in heart, less abundant in muscle, but barely detectable in liver, kidney, or brain. ANT2 is expressed in all tissues (16). ANT3 has been reported to be expressed in smooth muscle (29) and has the same gene structure as ANT1 but lacks obvious OXBOX, CCAAT, and TATA promoter elements (6).

The high mRNA levels of both ATPsynβ and ANT1 in heart and muscle imply that these genes are coordinately regulated at the transcription level. Since these genes share the unique OXBOX, it is possible that this element contributes to their high expression in heart and muscle. Three Complex IV nDNA subunits, VIa, VIIa, and VIII also have heart-specific isoforms (4,7,30,33,35,42,44). Possibly, these genes also share some common transcription factors.

These studies indicate that mitochondrial energy production can be regulated by nuclear OXPHOS genes in at least two major ways: variation in the transcription rate of pivotal single-copy OXPHOS genes like the ATPsynβ and tissue-specific and developmental stage-specific expression of functionally related isoforms like the ANT and cytochrome c oxidase subunits.

TABLE 1. *OXPHOS gene structure and expression*

Gene	Chromosome no.	CpG island	No. of exons	Promoter				Intron 1	mRNA level
				OXBOX	Sp1	CCAAT	TATA	Sp1	
ATPsynβ	12	+	10	1	2	5	0	1	H>M>L,K
ANT1	4	+	4	1	0	1	1	2	H>M>>L,K,B

Genomic elements and chromosomal assignment of the ATPsynβ and ANT1 genes (16,22). The OXBOX cis-element is 5'GGCTCTAAAGAGG. For mRNA levels: H, heart; M, muscle; L, liver; K, kidney; and B, brain.

However, other parameters are also clearly involved in the differential sensitivity of tissues to OXPHOS defects. These might include buffering of the effect of partial OXPHOS deficiency in tissues like the heart by excess ATP-generating capacity or the ability of some tissues to switch to a glycolytic metabolism as mitochondrial ATP production declines (55).

OXPHOS DISEASES OF THE nDNA

Since most of the OXPHOS genes are encoded by the nucleus, it is likely that many OXPHOS deficiency diseases are due to nuclear mutations. Analysis of ATP-synβ and ANT gene structure and expression is beginning to provide insights into this class of diseases as well.

The most common presentation of putative nuclear OXPHOS diseases is lethal or transient respiratory deficiency in the neonatal and early childhood periods (38). One case of lethal infantile mitochondrial disease associated with heart and skeletal muscle Complex-I and -IV deficiency has the characteristics to be expected for a nuclear isoform gene mutation (58).

The proband had good vital signs at birth, but his sucking response was weak and he experienced a sudden loss of consciousness at 1 month. Biochemical analysis revealed an elevated serum lactic acid. The child continued to decline over the next 3 months with hypotonia, progressive enlargement of heart, and a metabolic acidosis that could not be controlled even using peritoneal dialysis. At 4 months the child died of respiratory and cardiac failure. Pathological analysis at autopsy of skeletal muscle revealed ragged-red muscle fibers, severe degeneration of skeletal muscle sarcomeres, and a generalized proliferation of mitochondria that lacked mitochondrial inner membranes. The heart cells were swollen with their contractile elements pushed to the side of the cell and the interior of the cardiac myocytes were filled with mitochondria. The liver had large accumulations of fat droplets, but the remaining tissues did not show significant pathological abnormalities.

Analysis of mitochondrial OXPHOS levels for heart, skeletal muscle, liver, kidney, and brain revealed a complete absence of Complexes I and IV in heart and muscle but normal activities in brain and kidney. Liver levels were partially reduced, but this was probably the result of enzyme inhibition due to the excessive lipid deposition in this tissue. Respiratory Complex-III levels were normal for all tissues (Fig. 8). Analysis of cytochrome levels in heart, muscle, brain, and kidney revealed that the cytochrome b levels associated with Complex III were normal in all tissues, but that the cytochromes $a + a_3$ associated with Complex IV were completely absent in heart and muscle although normal in brain and kidney. Hence, this child died of a tissue-specific OXPHOS deficiency involving the heart and skeletal muscle (58).

Comparison of the proband with his parents permitted exclusion of a mtDNA mutation. The parents were phenotypically normal. Analysis of parental muscle biopsies revealed no pathology and their mitochondria contained normal levels of

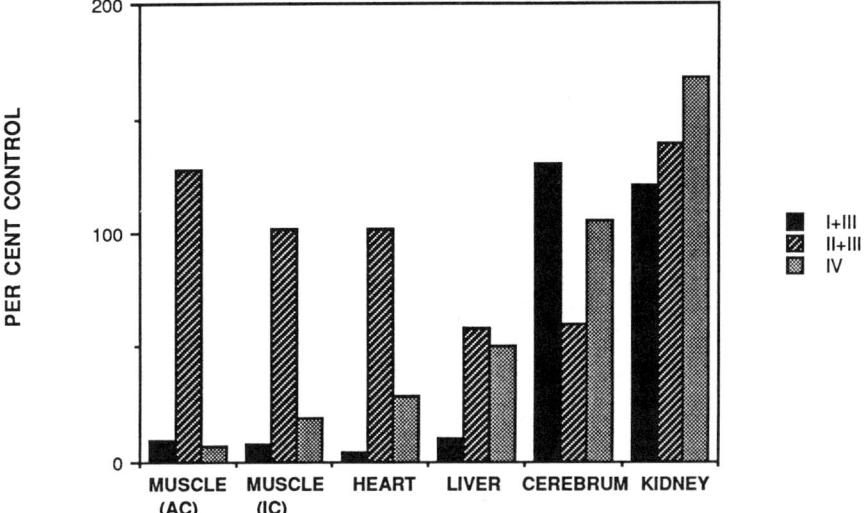

FIG. 8. Specific activities of mitochondrial respiratory complexes in various organs of a lethal infantile mitochondrial disease patient (58). Complex I+III (rotenone-sensitive NADH-cytochrome c oxidoreductase), Complex II+III (antimycin A-sensitive succinate-cytochrome c oxidoreductase) and Complex IV (cytochrome c oxidase). Since the Complex-II+III activities are normal, the reduced Complex I+III must be due to a Complex-I deficiency. Values are presented as percentage of adult controls (AC) and infant controls (IC) (58).

the respiratory complexes and their cytochromes. Analysis of the mtDNAs and mitochondrial translation products of the proband and his parents ruled out mtDNA insertion-deletion mutations and gave no indication of altered mtDNA gene products. Consequently, a mtDNA mutation was unlikely since a point mutation that was sufficiently severe to give total respiratory deficiency in the proband should have affected the mother. The only mechanism by which the mother could have been spared would be if the mutation were heteroplasmic. However, a heteroplasmic mtDNA mutation would have given intermediate enzyme levels in the proband's tissues, not the complete absence of activity in heart and muscle, but normal activity in brain and kidney. Hence, this disease was probably the product of a recessive mutation in the heart-skeletal muscle isoform of a nuclear OXPHOS polypeptide (58).

OVERVIEW OF OXPHOS DISEASES

These cases have revealed three major classes of OXPHOS diseases (Table 2). The first are the mtDNA point mutations. These are transmitted through the germ line and thus are maternally inherited. The mutations can either be mild as in LHON or severe as in MERRF. The mild mutations can segregate to homoplasmic, but the severe mutations, which are lethal in the homoplasmic state, are maintained within

TABLE 2. *Proposed characteristics for the three primary classes of OXPHOS disease*

Character	mtDNA point mutation	mtDNA del-ins mutation	nDNA mutation
Mutation site	Germ line	Somatic	Germ line
Cells with mutation	All	Tissue lineage	All
Inheritance	Maternal	Spontaneous	Mendelian
Enzyme level	Homoplasmic (constant level) Heteroplasmic (continuous variation)	Heteroplasmic (continuous variation)	Present or absent
Phenotype	Threshold expression	Threshold expression	Affected or unaffected
Developmental course	Progressive	Progressive	Stage and tissue specific

del-ins, deletion-insertion mutations.

the pedigrees by heteroplasmy. Because of the large number of mtDNA copies, the severity of the OXPHOS defect varies among the heteroplasmic maternal relatives depending on their proportion of mutant mtDNAs. The varying energy defects result in different phenotypes depending on the organ-specific thresholds that were traversed by the enzymatic defect. Finally, these diseases frequently progress in affected individuals, although the mechanism for this progression is unknown. One possibility is that the partial energy deficiency caused by the mtDNA mutation is exacerbated by an age-related decline in OXPHOS levels. OXPHOS has been shown to decline with age in both normal muscle (43) and in mildly affected MERRF patient muscle (37). By this hypothesis, the energetic levels of normal individuals are high enough at birth such that the subsequent decline in OXPHOS never falls below organ-specific energetic thresholds. However, the energetic levels of patients start much lower and with further OXPHOS decline soon traverse critical organ-specific thresholds causing disease. A second possibility is that over the life span of the individual, the mtDNAs in the nondividing muscle and nervous tissues continue to replicate and segregate. Ultimately, regions of these long cells accumulate only respiratory-deficient mtDNAs leading to local energetic failure and cell death. Clearly, this second hypothesis is not adequate for LHON since many essentially homoplasmic patients have been observed and these individuals still go blind in middle age.

The second major class of OXPHOS mutations are mtDNA insertion and deletions. Since these mutations destroy one or more mtDNA genes, they would be lethal in the homoplasmic state and consequently are always heteroplasmic. Most reported cases with insertion-deletion mutations have been isolated cases. Since the insertions always duplicate the mtDNA origins (28) and the deletions make the mtDNAs smaller (48), these mutations may impart a replicative advantage and rapidly segregate to homoplasmy eliminating their maternal lineages.

Many individuals with mtDNA deletions are mosaic. This suggests that some of the deletions may occur during somatic development and that one cause of phenotypic variability of the ocular myopathies is the time in development that the deletions occurred. Of the organs that harbor mtDNA deletions, heteroplasmic replicative segregation will lead to variation in the OXPHOS defect. Combined with organ-specific thresholds, this adds further phenotypic variability to the mtDNA insertion-deletion syndromes.

As with the mtDNA point mutations, the mtDNA insertion-deletion cases progress. One possibility is that these molecules have a replicative advantage and become progressively enriched by mtDNA turnover in the nondividing muscle and nerve cells. This hypothesis might explain why muscle fibers of ophthalmoplegia patients can have alternating regions that are cytochrome c oxidase negative and positive. Possibly these are regions of cells with high and low proportions of deleted mtDNAs (19).

The third major class of OXPHOS diseases are the nDNA mutations. These are inherited through the germ line in a mendelian fashion. The nuclear OXPHOS genes are present in only two copies. Hence, when the deleterious nDNA mutation occurs in the homozygous state virtually all of the OXPHOS activity will be lost. Since mutations that eliminate the function of single-copy OXPHOS genes like ATPsynβ are likely to be lethal early in development, it seems likely that most of the commonly observed nDNA OXPHOS mutations will be in tissue-specific isoform genes such as ANT1. This might account for the predilection of these diseases to affect selected tissues (i.e., heart and muscle) and to appear at specific developmental stages (i.e., shortly after birth when the neonate is rapidly acquiring an oxidative metabolism).

In addition to these three primary classes of OXPHOS genetic disease, a variety of combinations of two or more classes probably also occur. Already, an autosomal dominant ocular myopathy has been reported in which each patient harbors multiple different mtDNA deletions. Presumably, the nuclear mutation affects mtDNA replication, which predisposes the mtDNAs to deletion (57). Other possibilities could be mtDNA point mutations in replication origins that increase deletion rates, nuclear mutations that increase mtDNA point mutation rates, or simply the chance association of incompatible nuclear and cytoplasmic OXPHOS alleles. Two possible instances of this latter phenomenon have been observed in relation to the mtDNA ND3 protein polymorphism MV-1/MV-2 (27,52,56). In rare mtDNAs of African origin, the tenth amino acid of the ND3 gene is changed from an asparagine to an aspartic acid residue. This mutation places a charged group in the middle of a hydrophobic membrane-spanning domain altering mobility of the protein on SDS gels (26). This mutation has been reported in one family of healthy consanguineous parents with seven affected male children: two who died shortly after birth, four who had lactic acidosis and cardiomyopathy, and one who had cardiomyopathy (3). We have observed this polymorphism in an independent child who died shortly after birth with severe lactic acidosis (38).

In conclusion a number of neurological and neuromuscular diseases have been found to be associated with mutations in mitochondrial OXPHOS genes. The unique nature and complexity of the genetics of these genes have until recently been a major impediment to associating neurological disease and energy metabolism. However, it seems likely that a variety of neurological and psychological disorders will soon be found to be associated with OXPHOS defects. The identification of the biochemical and molecular basis of these diseases will provide powerful new methods for diagnosis of these neurological diseases and suggest new strategies for their metabolic therapies.

ACKNOWLEDGMENTS

The author would like to thank Mr. Kang Li, Ms. Marie Lott, Dr. John Shoffner, and Ms. Xian Xian Zheng for their assistance in preparation of the figures. This work was supported by National Institutes of Health grants NS21328 and GM33022 and a Muscular Dystrophy clinical research grant.

GLOSSARY

Adenosine triphosphate (ATP) A nucleoside triphosphate that is a high-energy intermediate in energy-transferring metabolism and one of the precursors for RNA synthesis.

Adenosine triphosphate synthase (ATPsyn) The enzyme that hydrolyzes ATP to form ADP and inorganic phosphate and catalyzes the reverse reaction of ATP formation.

Amino acid The precursors of proteins having the structure NH_2-C(R)-COOH. There are 20 amino acids that are linked end to end to form a polypeptide.

Base pair (bp) In nucleic acids, adenine must always pair with thymine (or, in RNA, with uracil) and guanine with cytosine. The specificity of base pairing is fundamental to DNA replication and to its transcription into RNA.

CAT box A DNA sequence that regulates transcription of eukaryotic genes, frequently with some tissue specificity. It is located about 70 to 80 bases upstream from the start of transcription.

cDNA Complementary DNA, synthetic DNA transcribed from a specific RNA through the action of the enzyme reverse transcriptase.

Codon A triplet of three bases in a DNA or RNA molecule, specifying a single amino acid.

Complex I NADH dehydrogenase or NADH: ubiquinone oxidoreductase.

Complex II Succinate dehydrogenase or succinate: ubiquinone oxidoreductase.

Complex III The bc_1 complex or ubiquinol: cytochrome c oxidoreductase.

Complex IV Cytochrome c oxidase.

Complex V ATP synthase.

Cytochromes Electron-transport proteins containing heme or related prosthetic group components that transport electrons via valence changes of the iron atom. Examples cytochrome b (cytb), cytochrome c, cytochrome c_1, cytochrome $a+a_3$.

Deletion Loss of part of a DNA molecule.
Deoxyribonucleic acid (DNA) The genetic material.
D-loop synthesis The mode of DNA replication in mitochondria in which staggered copying of the parental strands produces a displacement (D) loop.
Duplication An extra copy of one or more genes in the DNA.
Electron transport chain A group of enzyme complexes that contain electron carriers such as flavins, cytochromes, and iron-sulfur centers. Electrons are donated from $NADH_2$ or $FADH_2$ and traverse the chain from Complex I to C_0O to Complex III to cytochrome c to Complex IV to oxygen. As electrons are transferred from donor to acceptor, energy is released and used to synthesize ATP.
Genotype The genetic constitution of a cell.
Heteroplasmy A cell that contains two or more mitochondrial DNAs. The mitochondrial DNAs could differ by a single nucleotide, insertion, deletion, or rearrangement.
Homoplasmy A cell that contains only one type of mitochondrial DNA.
Hybridization Formation of a double-stranded structure, DNA-DNA, DNA-RNA by hydrogen-bonding of complementary single-stranded molecules or parts of molecules.
Kb (kilobase) A unit of 1,000 bases in DNA or RNA.
Messenger RNA (mRNA) RNA molecules that carry information for a particular polypeptide from the gene in the nucleus to the cytoplasm. In the cytoplasm, they combine with the ribosomes and tRNAs to direct the synthesis of protein molecules.
Mitochondrial DNA (mtDNA) The circular DNA within the mitochondrion that codes for large and small rRNA, a complete set of tRNAs, and 13 OXPHOS proteins. Each cell contains 100s to 1,000s of mtDNAs.
Mitochondrion The double-membrane cytoplasmic organelle in eukaryotic cells characterized by inner membrane infolds called cristae; in this organelle, fatty acids and organic acids are oxidized to generate energy in the form of ATP plus CO_2 and H_2O.
Oxidative phosphorylation (OXPHOS) The pathway by which mitochondria generate energy in the form of ATP by oxidation of $NADH + H^+$ or $FADH_2$ generated from organic acids with oxygen. OXPHOS is composed of the electron transport chain (Complexes I, II, III, and IV) and the ATP synthase (Complex V).
Phenotype The observable physical, biochemical, and physiological characteristics of an individual.
Polymorphism The occurrence together in a population of two or more different gene structures. In molecular genetics, a restriction fragment length polymorphism is a polymorphism in DNA sequence that can be detected on the basis of differences in the length of DNA fragments produced by digestion with a specific restriction enzyme.
Promoter A specific nucleotide sequence upstream (5') to a gene to which RNA polymerase binds and initiates transcription.
Replicative segregation The separation of heteroplasmic mtDNAs in a progenitor cell toward homoplasmic mtDNA in descendant cells during mitotic or meiotic cell replications.

Replication fork A site within a replicating duplex DNA molecule at which synthesis of complementary strands is occurring.

Respiration The principal energy-yielding reactions of aerobic cells, involving the transfer of electrons from organic fuel molecules to O_2 via the OXPHOS pathway.

Ribosomal RNA (rRNA) RNAs that are part of the ribosome structure and function in protein synthesis. All ribosomes have at least two rRNAs, a small and a large. The mitochondrial ribosomes have rRNAs of the relative sizes of 12S and 16S.

Ribosome A complex structure composed of RNA and protein, which is the site of protein synthesis.

TATA box A conserved DNA sequence about 25 bp upstream from the startpoint of the coding region of genes, involved in the initiation of transcription.

Transfer RNA (tRNA) RNAs that associate specific three base, codon, sequences in the mRNA with their cognate amino acids during protein synthesis.

REFERENCES

1. Anderson, S., Bankier, A. T., Barrell, B. G., et al. (1981): Sequence and organization of the human mitochondrial genome. *Nature*, 290:457–465.
2. Battini, R., Ferrari, S., Kaczmarek, L., Calabretta, B., Chen, S., and Baserga, R. (1987): Molecular cloning of a cDNA for a human ADP/ATP carrier which is growth regulated. *J. Biol. Chem.*, 262:4355–4359.
3. Bolhuis, P. A., Barth, P. G., Wijburg, F. A., Sinjorgo, K. M. C., and Ruttenbeek, W., (1988): Molecular basis of mitochondrial myopathies. *Lancet*, 1:884.
4. Capaldi, R. A. (1988): Mitochondrial myopathies and respiratory chain proteins. *TIBS*, 12:144–148.
5. Case, J. T., and Wallace, D. C. (1981): Maternal inheritance of mitochondrial DNA polymorphisms in cultured human fibroblasts. *Somatic Cell Mol. Genet.*, 7:103–108.
6. Cozens, A. L., Runswick, M. J., and Walker, J. E. (1989): DNA sequences of two expressed nuclear genes for human mitochondrial ADP/ATP translocase. *J. Mol. Biol.*, 206:261–280.
7. Fabrizi, G. M., Rizzuto, R., Nakase, H., Mita, S., Kadenbach, B., and Schon, E. A. (1989): Sequence of a xcDNA specifying subunit VIa of human cytochrome c oxidase. *Nucleic Acids Res.*, 17:6409.
8. Giles, R. E., Blanc, H., Cann, H. M., and Wallace, D. C. (1980): Maternal inheritance of human mitochondrial DNA. *Proc. Natl. Acad. Sci. USA*, 77:6715–6719.
9. Holt, I. J., Harding, A. E., and Morgan-Hughes, J. A. (1988): Deletions of muscle mitochondrial DNA in patients with mitochondrial myopathies. *Nature*, 331:717–719.
10. Holt, I. J., Harding, A. E., and Morgan-Hughes, J. A. (1989): Deletions of muscle mitochondrial DNA in mitochondrial myopathies: sequence analysis and possible mechanisms. *Nucleic Acids Res.*, 17:4465–4469.
11. Holt, I. J., Harding, A. E., Petty, R. K. H., and Morgan-Hughes, J. A. (1990): A new mitochondrial disease associated with mitochondrial DNA heteroplasmy. *Am. J. Hum. Genet.*, 46:428–433.
12. Holt, I. J., Miller, D. H., and Harding, A. E. (1989): Genetic heterogeneity and mitochondrial DNA heteroplasmy in Leber's hereditary optic neuropathy. *J. Med. Genet.*, 26:739–743.
13. Houldsworth, J., and Attardi, G. (1988): Two distinct genes for ADP/ATP translocase are expressed at the mRNA level in adult and human liver. *Proc. Natl. Acad. Sci. USA*, 85:377–381.
14. Johns, D. R., Rutledge, S. L., Stine, O. C., and Hurko, O. (1989): Directly repeated sequences associated with pathogenic mitochondrial DNA deletions. *Proc. Natl. Acad. Sci. USA*, 86:8059–8062.

15. Lestienne, P., and Ponsot, G. (1988): Kearns-Sayre syndrome with muscle mitochondrial DNA deletion. *Lancet*, 1:885.
16. Li, K., Warner, C. K., Hodge, J., et al. (1989): A human muscle adenine nucleotide translocator gene has four exons, is located on chromosome 4, and is differentially expressed. *J. Biol. Chem.*, 264:13998–14004.
17. Lott, M., Voljavec, A. S., and Wallace, D. C. (1990): Variable genotype of Leber's hereditary optic neuropathy. *Am. J. Ophthal.*, 109:625–631.
18. Mita, S., Rizzuto, R., Moraes, C. T., et al. (1990): Recombination via flanking direct repeats is a major cause of large-scale deletions of human mitochondrial DNA. *Nucleic Acids Res.*, 18:561–567.
19. Mita, S., Schmidt, B., Schon, E. A., DiMauro, S., and Bonilla, E. (1989): Detection of "deleted" mitochondrial genomes in cytochrome-c oxidase-deficient muscle fibers of a patient with Kearns-Sayre syndrome. *Proc. Natl. Acad. Sci. USA*, 86:9509–9513.
20. Moraes, C. T., DiMauro, S., Zeviani, M., et al. (1989): Mitochondrial DNA deletions in progressive external ophthalmoplegia and Kearns-Sayre syndrome. *N. Engl. J. Med.*, 320:1293–1299.
21. Neckelmann, N., Li, K., Wade, R. P., Shuster, R., and Wallace, D. C. (1987): cDNA sequence of a human skeletal muscle ADP/ATP translocator: lack of a leader peptide, divergence from a fibroblast translocator cDNA, and coevolution with mitochondrial DNA genes. *Proc. Natl. Acad. Sci. USA*, 84:7580–7584.
22. Neckelmann, N., Warner, C., Chung, A., et al. (1989): The human ATP synthase β subunit gene: sequence analysis, chromosome assignment, and differential expression. *Genomics*, 5:829–843.
23. Nelson, I., d'Auriol, L., Galibert, F., Ponsot, G., and Lestienne, P. (1989): Identification nucléotidique et modéle cinétique d'une délétion hétéroplasmique de 4666 paires de bases de l'ADN mitochondrial dans le syndrome de Kearns-Sayre. *C. R. Acad. Sci. [III]*, 309:403–407.
24. Nelson, I., Degoul, F., Obermaier-Kusser, B., et al. (1989): Mapping of heteroplasmic mitochondrial DNA deletions in Kearns-Sayre syndrome. *Nucleic Acids Res.*, 17:8117–8124.
25. Ohta, S., Tomura, H., Matsuda, K., and Kagawa, Y. (1988): Gene structure of the human mitochondrial adenosine triphosphate synthase β subunit. *J. Biol. Chem.*, 263:11257–11262.
26. Oliver, N. A., Greenberg, B. D., and Wallace, D. C. (1983): Assignment of a polymorphic polypeptide to the human mitochondrial DNA unidentified reading frame 3 gene by a new peptide mapping strategy. *J. Biol. Chem.*, 9:5834–5839.
27. Oliver, N. A., and Wallace, D. C. (1982): Assignment of two mitochondrially synthesized polypeptides to human mitochondrial DNA and their use in the study of intracellular mitochondrial interaction. *Mol. Cell. Biol.*, 2:30–41.
28. Poulton, J., Deadman, M. E., and Gardiner, R. M. (1989): Duplications of mitochondrial DNA in mitochondrial myopathy. *Lancet*, 1:236.
29. Powell, S. J., Medd, S. M., Runswick, M. J., and Walker, J. E. (1989): Two bovine genes for mitochondrial ADP/ATP translocase expressed differently in various tissues. *Biochemistry*, 28:866–873.
30. Rizzuto, R., Nakase, H., Darras, B., et al. (1989): A gene specifying subunit VIII of human cytochrome c oxidase is localized on chromosome 11 and is expressed in both muscle and non-muscle tissues. *J. Biol. Chem.*, 264:10595–1060.
31. Rosing H. S., Hopkins, L. C., Wallace, D. C., Epstein, C. M., and Weidenheim, K. (1985): Maternally inherited mitochondrial myopathy and myoclonic epilepsy. *Ann. Neurol.*, 17:228–237.
32. Rotig, A., Colonna, M., Blanche, S., et al. (1989): Mitochondrial DNA deletions in Pearson's marrow/pancreas syndrome. *Lancet*, 1:902–903.
33. Schlerf, A., Droste, M., Winter, M., and Kadenbach, B. (1988): Characterization of two different genes (cDNA) for cytochrome c oxidase subunit VIa from heart and liver of the rat. *EMBO J.*, 7:2387–2391.
34. Schon, E. A., Rizzuto, R., Moraes, C. T., Nakase, H., Zeviani, M., and DiMauro, S. (1989): A direct repeat is a hotspot for large-scale deletion of human mitochondrial DNA. *Science*, 244:346–349.
35. Seelan, R. S., Scheuner, D., Lomax, M. I., and Grossman, L. I. (1989): Nucleotide sequence of the cDNA for bovine cytochrome c oxidase subunit VIIa. *Nucleic Acids Res.*, 17:6410.
36. Shanske, S., Moraes, C. T., Lombes, A., et al. (1990): Widespread tissue distribution of mitochondrial DNA deletions in Kearns-Sayre syndrome. *Neurology*, 40:24–28.
37. Shoffner, J. M., Lott, M. T., Lezza, A. M. S., Seibel, P., Ballinger, S. W., and Wallace, D. C. (1990): Myoclonic epilepsy and ragged-red fiber disease (MERRF) is associated with a mitochondrial DNA tRNA^{Lys} mutation. *Cell*, 61:931–937.

38. Shoffner, J. M., and Wallace, D. C. (1990): Oxidative phosphorylation diseases: disorders of two genomes. *Adv. Hum. Genet.*, 19:267–330.
39. Schoffner, J. M., Lott, M. T., Voljavec, A. S., Soueidan, S. A., Costigan, D. A., and Wallace, D. C. (1989): Spontaneous Kearns-Sayre/chronic external ophthalmoplegia plus syndrome associated with a mtDNA deletion: a slip-replication model and metabolic therapy. *Proc. Natl. Acad. Sci. USA*, 86:7952–7956.
40. Shuster, R. C., Rubenstein, A. J., and Wallace, D. C. (1988): Mitochondrial DNA in anucleate human blood cells. *Biochem. Biophys. Res. Commun.*, 155:1360–1365.
41. Singh, G., Lott, M. T., and Wallace, D. C. (1989): A mitochondrial DNA mutation as a cause of Leber's hereditary optic neuropathy. *N. Engl. J. Med.*, 320:1300–1305.
42. Suske, G., Mengel, T., Cordingley, M., and Kadenbach, B. (1987): Molecular cloning and further characterization of cDNAs for rat nuclear-encoded cytochrome c oxidase subunits VIc and VIII. *Eur. J. Biochem.*, 168:233–237.
43. Trounce, I., Byrne, E., and Marzuki, S. (1989): Decline in skeletal muscle mitochondrial respiratory chain function: possible factor in ageing. *Lancet*, 1:637–639.
44. Van Kuilenburg, A. B. P., Muijsers, A. O., Demol, H., Dekker, H. L., and Beeumen, J. J. V. (1988): Human heart cytochrome c oxidase subunit VIII. Purification and determination of the complete amino acid sequence. *FEB*, 240:127–132.
45. Wallace, D. C. (1986): Mitochondrial genes and disease. *Hosp. Pract.*, 21:77–92.
46. Wallace, D. C. (1986): Mitotic segregation of mitochondrial DNAs in human cell hybrids and expression of chloramphenicol resistance. *Somatic Cell Mol. Genet.*, 12:41–49.
47. Wallace, D. C. (1987): Maternal genes: mitochondrial diseases. In: *Medical and Experimental Mammalian Genetics: A Perspective*, edited by V. A. McKusick, T. H. Roderick, J. Mori, and N. W. Paul (*Birth Defects*, vol. 23) pp. 137–190. A. R. Liss, New York.
48. Wallace, D. C. (1989): Mitochondrial DNA mutations and neuromuscular disease. *Trends in Genetics*, 5:9–13.
49. Wallace, D. C., Lott, M. T., Lezza, A. M. S., Seibel, P., and Shoffner, J. M. Mitochondrial DNA mutations associated with neuromuscular diseases: analysis and diagnosis using the polymerase chain reaction. *Pediatr. Res. (in press).*
50. Wallace, D. C., Singh, G., Hopkins, L. C., and Novotny, E. J., Jr. (1986): Maternally inherited diseases of man. In: *Achievements and Perspectives of Mitochondrial Research*, vol. 2, edited by E. Quagliariello, E. C. Slater, F. Palmieri, C. Saccone, C., and A. M. Kroon, pp. 427–436. Elsevier Science, Amsterdam.
51. Wallace, D. C., Singh, G., Lott, M. T., et al. (1988): Mitochondrial DNA mutation associated with Leber's hereditary optic neuropathy. *Science*, 242:1427–1430.
52. Wallace, D. C., Yang, J., Ye, J., Lott, M. T., Oliver, N. A., and McCarthy, J. (1986): Computer prediction of peptide maps: assignment of polypeptides to human and mouse mitochondrial DNA genes by analysis of two-dimensional-proteolytic digest gels. *Am. J. Hum. Genet.*, 38:461–481.
53. Wallace, D. C., Ye, J., Neckelmann, N., Singh, G., Webster, K. A., and Greenberg, B. D. (1987): Sequence analysis of cDNAs for the human and bovine ATP synthase β subunit: mitochondrial DNA genes sustain seventeen times more mutations. *Curr. Genet.*, 12:81–90.
54. Wallace, D. C., Zheng, X., Lott, M. T., et al. (1988): Familial mitochondrial encephalomyopathy (MERRF): genetic, pathophysiological, and biochemical characterization of a mitochondrial DNA disease. *Cell*, 55:601–610.
55. Webster, K. A., Gunning, P., Hardeman, E., Wallace, D. C., and Kedes, L. (1990): Coordinate reciprocal trends in glycolytic and mitochondrial transcript accumulations during the in vitro differentiation of human myoblasts. *J. Cell. Physiol.*, 142:566–573.
56. Yatscoff, R. W., Goldstein, S., and Freeman, K. B. (1978): Conservation of genes coding for proteins synthesized in human mitochondria. *Somatic Cell Mol. Genet.*, 4:633–645.
57. Zeviani, M., Servidei, S., Gellera, C., Bertini, E., DiMauro, S., and DiDonato, S. (1989): An autosomal dominant disorder with multiple deletions of mitochondrial DNA starting at the D-loop region. *Nature*, 339:309–311.
58. Zheng, X., Shoffner, J. M., Lott, M. T. (1989): Evidence in a lethal infantile mitochondrial disease for a nuclear mutation affecting respiratory complexes I and IV. *Neurology*, 39:1203–1209.

Genes, Brain, and Behavior, edited by
P. R. McHugh and V. A. McKusick.
Raven Press, Ltd., New York © 1991.

Muscular Dystrophy Research: What Have We Learned and Where Do We Go from Here?

*Frederick M. Boyce, *†‡Alan H. Beggs, and *†‡Louis M. Kunkel

Division of Genetics and Mental Retardation Center, The Children's Hospital, †Department of Pediatrics, Harvard Medical School, and ‡Howard Hughes Medical Institute, Boston, Massachusetts 02115

Research into the muscular dystrophies has progressed rapidly since the application of molecular genetics to the problem. The gene responsible for Duchenne muscular dystrophy (DMD) has been isolated and the protein product, dystrophin, partly characterized (reviewed in [11]). Analysis of dystrophin in patient biopsy samples has led to improved diagnosis of this disorder (10), and molecular genetic approaches have enabled accurate genotypic prediction of at-risk individuals (3). Our knowledge of dystrophin and its gene has suggested potential approaches to alter the course of the disease in affected individuals and has led to the design of experiments aimed at treating this devastating disease (19). The purpose of this chapter is to highlight some current knowledge and to outline how one can use this information to begin the characterization of other disorders of muscle and nerve. Our premise is that dystrophin, as part of the membrane cytoskeleton of both muscle and nerve, interacts with other proteins heretofore uncharacterized and that these other proteins are prime candidates to be disrupted in other neuromuscular disorders.

DMD and its milder allelic form, Becker muscular dystrophy (BMD), are muscle-wasting diseases of children and young adults (1). They are inherited as X-linked recessive disorders and are distinguished from other neuromuscular diseases by both their severity and inheritance patterns. There are, however, many other neuromuscular disorders that present with overlapping clinical features as DMD/BMD (1,22). Our knowledge of the molecular basis for these other diseases is in the same state of ignorance as was our understanding of DMD/BMD in the early 1980s. There is a reasonable set of clinical information on each disorder, yet despite extensive research, there is little known about the underlying biochemical defect. One fact remains certain, namely, that these disorders are inherited and, hence, there must be a gene that is disrupted by mutation to yield the observed phenotype. A molecular genetic approach to these disorders seems warranted given the success with DMD/BMD. Our work for the past year has been to start this analysis using our knowledge of dystrophin and our store of patient specimens from disorders other than DMD/BMD.

THE DYSTROPHIN GENE AND PROTEIN

The cloning of the dystrophin gene yielded the unexpected finding that the high incidence of DMD was the result of an extremely large gene (2,13,20). Studies have demonstrated that the more than 70 exons of the gene are spaced over 2.5 million base pairs of the human X chromosome making this locus nearly 10 times larger than any other characterized gene. The unprecedented size made this locus highly susceptible to mutations with nearly two-thirds being intragenic deletions (6,13). Deletions were found in both DMD and the more mild BMD patients, leading to the hypothesis that various deletions had different effects on the translational reading frame of the mature protein (18). The prediction was that Duchenne patients had deletions that removed exons of the gene containing an uneven number of triplet codons, thus causing a shift of the translational reading frame and leading to premature termination. In contrast, Becker patients would remove exons that would not affect the translational reading frame. Correlation of many deletions with clinical severity indicated that more than 90% of patients had deletions that fit the reading frame hypothesis (15). Many of the remaining patients had deletions in one region of the N terminus where alternative mRNA splicing may correct the frame shift. In the remainder, the reasons that the molecular results do not fit with the observed clinical results are unknown. These findings with DNA analysis have ramifications at the protein level and have important diagnostic and prognostic implications.

The fact that more than 65% of patients had deletion mutations as the cause of their disease has led to rapid means of genotype detection. Through the use of DNA-based diagnosis the exact mutations can be determined and those family members who have inherited the deletion detected. Now a female family member at risk can be counseled accurately and her offspring genotyped *in utero*. Birth choices can be made in an informed way and family planning can result in a drop in the incidence of DMD in families with a history of the disease. The ability to confidently predict normal offspring from such carriers and to determine which at-risk family members are not carriers has led to the birth of many normal males that otherwise would have been terminated due to risk for DMD.

Knowledge of the gene rapidly led to information on the encoded protein, dystrophin (8). The sequence of the RNA transcript (as cDNA) predicted a 3685 amino acid protein that exhibited sequence similarity to the cytoskeletal α-actinin and spectrin proteins (4,7,14). From this similarity, dystrophin was predicted to be composed of four domains (14). The N-terminal domain of 200 amino acids is highly similar to the same region of α-actinin that has been shown to bind actin. This domain is followed by 24 repeating groups of 109 amino acids that are similar to the repeats found in the spectrins. A cysteine-rich domain similar to that found in α-actinin is followed by a fourth domain that is highly conserved among mammals and birds and has been shown to be altered by RNA splicing to yield different isoforms that appear to show some tissue specificity (5). This last domain has been hypothesized to confer binding specificity to the protein for each of the tissues that express reasonable levels of dystrophin (11).

Portions of dystrophin have been expressed in bacteria as fusion proteins and these proteins used to immunize rabbits and sheep (8). The resulting antisera detect a large molecular weight protein (dystrophin) that is present in all muscle types (skeletal, cardiac, and smooth) as well as in brain. By biochemical fractionation, dystrophin has been detected in membrane fractions (9), and by immunohistochemistry the protein is localized on the inner face of the plasma membrane of all muscle fibers (21,23). Localization in the brain has been hampered by its low abundance and by cross-reaction of dystrophin antisera with other more abundant brain-specific proteins. The association of dystrophin with the membrane appears to be mediated by interactions with other proteins because there is no evidence from sequence analysis that dystrophin itself spans the membrane (14). Our current best guess about dystrophin's function comes from the similarity with other proteins (16). Dystrophin is thought to confer flexibility and strength to the membrane during contraction and relaxation. Dystrophin might also anchor proteins of the membrane to specific locations; the exact molecular basis of dystrophin's function must await further experimentation.

IMPROVED DIAGNOSIS OF THE MUSCULAR DYSTROPHIES

From deletion analysis it was predicted that Duchenne patients would produce a severely truncated and potentially unstable protein. Protein analysis using antisera directed against dystrophin established that indeed there was little or no detectable dystrophin in the muscle biopsies of Duchenne patients (10). In contrast, most muscle biopsies from BMD patients were found to contain an altered-size protein of near normal abundance. These observations allow routine testing of muscle biopsies from patients with neuromuscular disorders to discriminate between DMD, BMD, or unrelated disorders. Taken together with other clinical and pathological results, the diagnosis and prognosis for a patient with muscular dystrophy is now extremely accurate. One benefit of these studies has been the clear demarcation of those disorders that overlap with DMD/BMD clinically but are the result of mutations at other loci.

APPROACHES TO OTHER NEUROMUSCULAR DISORDERS

Dystrophin is known to be associated with the membrane cytoskeleton of both muscle and nerve cells (reviewed in [11]). Like the well-characterized erythroid-membrane cytoskeleton, it is likely that there are also many proteins involved in the muscle/nerve cell cytoskeletons. These are important proteins to characterize because their study will also address the function of dystrophin in this complex. Furthermore, these are novel proteins that are important for normal function of muscle and nerve, and their dysfunction may well cause other neuromuscular diseases. One goal of our laboratory is to identify these proteins and then to clone their cDNAs. These can then be sequenced and the corresponding protein sequence predicted. As was done with dystrophin, fusion proteins can be produced in bacteria and used to raise antisera to these novel cytoskeletal elements. Thus, the cDNA can be used as a molecular probe for the gene locus and the antibodies as probes for the protein product. These two complementary approaches can then be used to study patient materials derived from the numerous samples sent to us as part of our dystrophin studies. We now have nearly 200 samples from patients who do not have dystrophin deficiency yet have various neuromuscular diseases.

DYSTROPHIN-BINDING PROTEINS

Our laboratory is currently developing protocols to detect proteins that may bind to dystrophin. Both ends of the dystrophin protein have been expressed as fusion proteins and antibodies developed to specifically detect these two domains. Total proteins of muscle or nerve are solubilized and separated by electrophoresis. Following transfer of the separated proteins to nitrocellulose, the membrane is placed in a buffer that allows partial renaturation of the immobilized proteins. The filter is then incubated with a specific fusion protein of dystrophin and the peptide allowed to bind to proteins on the filter. The binding of the peptide is visualized by using antisera directed against that peptide. Specificity of the binding is controlled by use of different peptides, different tissues, and different antisera. To date, several proteins have been detected in skeletal muscle and smooth muscle. These proteins are associated with membrane fractions and presumably represent dystrophin-binding proteins. Each is currently being cloned from expression cDNA libraries and their sequence determined. The ability to detect these proteins in muscle from normal individuals would indicate that they should be testable in patient biopsy materials. If one is found to be missing or abnormal, then it would become a candidate protein product to be disrupted in that disorder. As more of these proteins are identified, more information should emerge concerning their function in the cytoskeletal complex of dystrophin underlying the plasma membrane.

PROTEINS WITH SIMILAR DOMAIN STRUCTURE TO DYSTROPHIN

Dystrophin is a member of an ever-expanding family of related cytoskeletal proteins that includes the α-actinins and spectrins. A new member of this family (named B3) has recently been identified by hybridization using dystrophin cDNA clones as probes. This protein, although not completely cloned, appears to have size and sequence characteristics that make it very similar to dystrophin (17). The locus for this protein is chromosome 6, and we as well as others are currently trying to determine whether there might be a disorder in which this protein is either absent or abnormal. A potentially more direct way to identify additional proteins in the family would be to take advantage of the fact that many of the polyclonal antibodies directed against dystrophin also detect other antigenically related proteins. Using these dystrophin antibodies, we have identified at least two new uncharacterized proteins. One of these is not muscle specific and appears to be expressed in many different tissues (12). A second relative of dystrophin is detected only with our C-terminal most antisera. This protein is detectable only in the brain and specifically at the glial cell end processes contiguous with the vasculature and periphery of the brain. Thus, this protein may play a role in the maintenance of the blood-brain barrier.

As with the dystrophin-binding proteins, each of these relatives can be cloned from an expression cDNA library and characterized as above. Thus, with both DNA and protein based assays, it should be possible to elucidate the molecular basis of many heretofore uncharacterized neuromuscular diseases.

ACKNOWLEDGMENTS

This work was supported by the Muscular Dystrophy Association and the National Institutes of Health (NS23740 and HD18658). We thank Eric Hoffman for advice. L. M. Kunkel is an associate investigator of the Howard Hughes Medical Institute.

GENETIC TERMS

Affinity purification A procedure used to prepare antibodies that are directed against a specific protein. Usually crude serum from an inoculated animal contains many different antibodies. One can bind the protein used in the immunization to a column support and pass the crude serum over the column. The antibodies directed against the specific protein will bind to the column and the unbound antibodies washed through. The specific antibodies are removed from the column under conditions that reverse binding. These antibodies are considered affinity purified by the fact that they had affinity for the protein on the column.

cDNA Complementary DNA produced by reverse transcriptase of RNA; the *in vitro* process is used to make a stable copy of RNA as DNA. The procedure is one of the steps leading to a cDNA library.

cDNA library The DNA complement of all RNA of a cell or tissue type is modified so that it is compatible with cloning in a plasmid or phage vector. Hundreds of thousands of clones are produced, each containing a single independent DNA molecule. One thus has a library of the RNA represented as cloned individual molecules.

Codon Refers to the triple set of nucleotides that encode a specific amino acid according to the genetic code.

Cytoskeleton Refers to the complex of proteins that make up the scaffolding of a cell. They may be used for motility of the cell or internal molecules. There is also a strong structural role in the stability of the cell.

Deletion Type of mutation that refers to the loss of DNA. Detectable as absence of particular sequences.

Dystrophin The name given to the Duchenne/Becker gene protein product.

Exon/intron Terms given to regions of DNA that are represented as part of a mature mRNA (exon) and those regions that are between coding sequences of a gene (intron).

Fusion peptide An artificially constructed protein containing part of a bacterial protein and part of the protein that has been cloned and that you are trying to produce in bacteria. The construct is made by joining a desired cloned segment with a cloned bacterial gene.

Immunofluorescence Tissue sections are mounted on a slide and incubated with antibodies directed against a specific protein. The binding of the antibody is detected by use of fluorescent antibodies directed against the first antibody. The fluorescent dye attached to the antibody is excited by light of a specific wavelength, and the dye emission is visualized by a microscope. By this means, the location of the protein desired to be detected can be observed.

Locus This genetic term refers to the region of DNA that contains the entire set of information to express the protein product encoded by the DNA.

Myoblast Term given to the cell type that will divide and form new muscle. Muscle is formed by fusion of multiple myoblasts into a single multinucleate cell termed a myofiber.

Polymerase chain reaction (PCR) A technique that allows one to use enzymes that synthesize DNA to specifically produce large amounts of DNA from a specific region defined by oligonucleotide sequence.

Reading frame Proteins are translated from an RNA template that encodes the specific amino acid by a set of three nucleotides. The translation process starts at a specific triplet and continues in sets of three nucleotides. This is called the reading frame of the protein, and any mutation that removes nucleotides in sets other than three would be termed to cause a frame shift.

Southern blot A technique first developed by Ed Southern that allows one to observe a rare DNA molecule among many others. DNA is normally cleaved at specific nucleotide sites defined by a restriction enzyme. The many different cleavage products are separated by molecular weight in an electric field. The separated molecules are transferred to a solid-membrane support as an image of the electrophoretic separation. The membrane is incubated with a tagged molecule that has a single copy within the original mixture. The tagged molecule will bind to its corresponding sequence and is visualized by means of the tag that is usually radioactive and seen on common X-ray film.

Western blot The procedure is in principle the same as a Southern blot except that the electrophoretically separated molecules are proteins, and a specific protein is visualized by a tagged antibody directed against the protein of interest.

REFERENCES

1. Brooke, M. (1986): *A Clinician's View of Neuromuscular Diseases.* Williams and Wilkins, Baltimore.
2. Burmeister, M., Monaco, A. P., Gillard, E. F., et al. (1988): A 10-megabase physical map of human Xp21, including the Duchenne muscular dystrophy gene. *Genomics*, 2:189–202.
3. Darras, B. T., Koenig, M., Kunkel, L. M., and Francke, U. (1988): Direct method for prenatal diagnosis and carrier detection in Duchenne/Becker muscular dystrophy using the entire dystrophin cDNA. *Am. J. Med. Genet.*, 29:713–726.
4. Davison, M. D., and Critchley, D. R. (1988): α-Actinins and the DMD protein contain spectrin-like repeats. *Cell*, 52:159–160.
5. Feener, C. A., Koenig, M., and Kunkel, L. M. (1989): Alternative splicing of human dystrophin mRNA generates isoforms at the carboxy terminus. *Nature*, 338:509–511.
6. Forrest, S. M., Cross, G. S., Speer, A., Gardner-Medwin, D., Burn, J., and Davies, K. E. (1987): Preferential deletion of exons in Duchenne and Becker muscular dystrophies. *Nature*, 329:638–640.
7. Hammond, R. G., Jr. (1987): Protein sequence of DMD gene is related to actin-binding domain of α-actinin. *Cell*, 51:1.
8. Hoffman, E. P., and Kunkel, L. M. (1987): Dystrophin: the protein product of the Duchenne muscular dystrophy locus. *Cell*, 51:919–928.
9. Hoffman, E. P., Knudson, C. M., Campbell, K. P., and Kunkel, L. M. (1987): Subcellular fractionation of dystrophin to triads of skeletal muscle. *Nature*, 330:754–758.
10. Hoffman, E. P., Fischbeck, K., Brown, R. H., et al. (1988): Dystrophin characterization in muscle biopsies from Duchenne and Becker muscular dystrophy patients. *N. Engl. J. Med.*, 318:1363–1368.
11. Hoffman, E. P., and Kunkel, L. M. (1989): Dystrophin abnormalities in Duchenne/Becker muscular dystrophy. *Neuron*, 2:1019–1029.
12. Hoffman, E. P., Beggs, A. H., Koenig, M., Kunkel, L. M., and Angelini, C. Cross-reactive protein in Duchenne muscle. *Lancet (in press)*.
13. Koenig, M., Hoffman, E. P., Bertelson, C. J., Monaco, A. P., Feener, C., and Kunkel, L. M. (1987): Complete cloning of the Duchenne muscular dystrophy (DMD) cDNA and preliminary genomic organization of the DMD gene in normal and affected individuals. *Cell*, 50:509–517.
14. Koenig, M., Monaco, A. P., and Kunkel, L. M. (1988): The complete sequence of dystrophin predicts a rod-shaped cytoskeletal protein. *Cell*, 53:219–228.
15. Koenig, M., Beggs, A. H., Moyer, M., et al. (1989): The molecular basis for Duchenne versus Becker muscular dystrophy: correlation of severity with type of deletion. *Am. J. Hum. Genet.*, 45:498–506.
16. Koenig, M., and Kunkel, L. M. Detailed analysis of the repeat domain of dystrophin reveals 4 potential hinge segments that may confer flexibility. *J. Biol. Chem. (in press)*.
17. Love, D. R., Hill, D. F., Dickson, G., et al. (1989): An autosomal transcript in skeletal muscle with homology to dystrophin. *Nature*, 339:55–58.
18. Monaco, A. P., Bertelson, C. J., Liechti-Gallati, S., Moser, H., and Kunkel, L. M. (1988): An explanation for the phenotypic differences between patients bearing partial deletions of the DMD locus. *Genomics*, 2:90–95.
19. Partridge, T. A., Morgan, J. E., Coulton, G. R., Hoffman, E. P., and Kunkel, L. M. (1989): Conversion of mdx myofibres from dystrophin-negative to dystrophin-positive by injection at normal myoblasts. *Nature*, 337:176–179.
20. van Ommen, G. J. B. Verkerk, J. M. H., Hofker, M. H., et al. (1986): A physical map of 4 million bp around the Duchenne muscular dystrophy gene on the human X-chromosome. *Cell*, 47:499–504.
21. Watkins, S. C., Hoffman, E. P., Slayer, H. S., and Kunkel, L. M. (1988): Immunoelectron microscopic localization of dystrophin in myofibres. *Nature*, 333:863–866.
22. Zatz, M., Passos-Buenos, M. R., and Rapaport, D. (1989): Estimate of the proportion of Duchenne muscular dystrophy with autosomal recessive inheritance. *Am. J. Med. Genet.*, 32:407–410.
23. Zubrzycka-Gaarn, E. E., Bulman, D. E., Karpati, G., et al. (1988): The Duchenne muscular dystrophy gene product is localized in the sarcolemma of human skeletal muscle fibres. *Nature*, 333:466–469.

Genetics of Alzheimer's Disease

Marshal F. Folstein and Andrew Warren

Department of Psychiatry, The Johns Hopkins Hospital, Baltimore, Maryland 21205

Alzheimer's case report appeared in the decade of Mendel's rediscovery. But if Alzheimer was aware of mendelism, it is unlikely that he would study the genetics of Alzheimer's disease because people did not live long enough to express the disease in recognizable patterns and because dementia was considered a consequence of aging rather than a disease that environment and genes might cause.

The rationale for using the genetic approach in Alzheimer's disease depends in part on the concept that Alzheimer's disease is a disease category and not an inevitable consequence of aging. Epidemiological studies support the idea that Alzheimer's disease is a disease entity because *the risk is not homogeneous*. Alzheimer's disease affects certain people at certain times more than others, as is the case with any disease. Our studies of the epidemiology of Alzheimer's disease in Baltimore indicate that Alzheimer's disease strictly defined is present in 2% of the over 65 population but at least 8% of the over 85 population (see Table 1) (12).

Of the over 85 age group 29% suffer from a dementia of some type (10). Since it is currently impossible to diagnose Alzheimer's disease when it occurs in the presence of another neurological disorder such as stroke, the true prevalence of Alzheimer's disease at age 85 is between 8% and 29%, perhaps 18%, a rate similar to many others in the world literature (10) (see Table 2).

Other evidence of the heterogeneity of risk of Alzheimer's disease comes from genetic studies. Alzheimer's disease runs in families (11) and monozygotic twins are often concordant for the disorder (8,29). Trisomy 21 causes Alzheimer's disease, and early onset cases have been linked to chromosome 21 (Gusella, *this volume*).

Genetic studies of Alzheimer's disease and other geriatric genetic diseases are limited by the special attributes imposed by the onset of disease in the geriatric period. The onset of symptoms after reproduction age will diminish the selection pressure resulting in higher gene frequencies and thus higher prevalence rates than diseases with onset before the age of reproduction. But the incidence rate of any disease in the geriatric period is lower than expected by estimate of the gene frequency because of competing causes of death. Many gene carriers of geriatric diseases will not express symptoms because the carrier will not survive to the age of onset. This phenomenon will confound traditional segregation analyses and modern linkage analysis, which depend on counting cases of those who are affected or who

TABLE 1. *Alzheimer's disease prevalence in 85 year olds: Baltimore 1981*

All neuropsychiatric disorders	39%
All dementia	29%
Alzheimer's disease	8%

have lived through the age at risk. Also, confounded will be estimates of the gene frequency based on prevalence since the genotype of geriatric genetic diseases will be more frequent than the phenotype. To the clinician's eye most cases will appear to be sporadic because most relatives who are carriers will not express the disease (3,4).

In our studies of the genetics of Alzheimer's disease we considered the *phenotype*, the *risk* to relatives, and the *prevalence* of the nongenetic forms. In order to clarify the question we made a conjecture in 1981 that has guided our work ever since. Conjecture making is something more than prophecy. It has the virtue of reducing confusion by increasing the possibility of error and error is better than confusion according to Bacon. Here is the conjecture. *If Alzheimer's disease is classically defined, then the trait is transmitted as a fully penetrant, but age-dependent autosomal dominant and is the most prevalent dementia.* The implications of this conjecture are that an Alzheimer's disease gene exists and will be expressed in approximately 50% of the parents, sibs, and children of properly identified probands if they live to a sufficient age and, furthermore, that the genetic form of Alzheimer's disease is frequent (5,13–15).

In order to test this idea, we specified a phenotype similar but not identical to one of Alzheimer's cases. Alzheimer described a patient who was 51 years old and suffered from morbid jealousy and an intellectual deterioration, which was characterized eventually by amnesia, a language disorder, and a disorder of recognition. She died after 4½ years of illness (1). In modern studies, the clinical symptoms on average progress with a loss of 4 Mini-Mental points per year until death an average of 7 years after onset (16), but in addition to increasing severity of intellectual deficits along a single dimension such as MMSE score, a changing pattern of deficits emerges that was described earlier by Sjogren et al. (29). Thus, we expect to see amnesia and other behavioral changes in the first 3 years followed by amnesia, aphasia, apraxia, and agnosia in years 3 to 5, the four A's of Alzheimer's disease. Abnormal gait and other motor signs appear in the disorder after the cognitive impairment is severe. Another aspect of the phenotype is the neuropathology. Alz-

TABLE 2. *Alzheimer's disease prevalence in 85 year olds (26)*

Kaneko	17%
Sulkava	15%
Hagnell	13%
Larsson estimate	12%

heimer described the characteristic silver-staining neurofibrillary tangles and noted the amyloid plaques that had been described earlier. Amyloid is also deposited in the blood vessels in the brain in Alzheimer's disease victims. Amyloid is a pleated sheet of precipitated preprotein that is coded on chromosome 21 but is not closely linked to the Alzheimer's disease locus. There is not a consensus as to the primacy of the plaques or tangles in relation to cell loss or of the specificity of plaques and tangles as pathognomonic sign of disease. These structures might be markers for the causative toxins or markers of secondary attempts at repair of cell damage (34).

The specified phenotype we used for genetic study differed from that of Alzheimer in that we included cases of any age of onset. In recent years, it has become clear that this clinical picture is a reasonably accurate predictor of neuropathology (30). Furthermore, the distribution of the major neuropathology in the temporal parietal regions is consistent with the clinical description of the four As: amnesia, aphasia, apraxia, and agnosia (6,10,20,21).

With the confidence that we could identify a phenotype during life, we conducted a genetic study using the family history method. We asked whether the relatives of classically symptomatic cases of dementia would more often be demented than the relatives of controls.

From a geographically defined nursing home population of 3,000, John Breitner selected probands likely to be suffering from typical Alzheimer's disease (5). They were clinically demented and agraphic. There was no clinical evidence of stroke, diabetes, or hypertension. Their relatives were compared to the relatives of several *control* groups including individuals who were demented but not agraphic, individuals not demented, and to relatives of spouses.

The probands and controls were Caucasian women aged 84 who had been ill for many years. Thus, the cases had developed amnesia, apraxia, aphasia, and agnosia and the controls had been ill long enough to have developed amnesia, apraxia, aphasia, and agnosia if they were ever going to.

Interviewers blind to whether the proband was a case or control interviewed many relatives in each family using a structured questionnaire developed for the study and subsequently shown to be reliable (2). The relatives' descriptions of the mental state of probands agreed with our examinations and thus we assumed some degree of validity of the relatives' descriptions of other affected relatives.

Life table methods were used to determine the risk of relatives at each age. These methods were necessary because the number of individuals exposed at each age group is changed by death from competing causes. Thus crude prevalence rates of numbers affected do not represent the true risk (7).

We found that by age 85 the risk of becoming demented was very high in the first-degree relatives of nursing home cases compared to the relatives of controls. The rate was consistent with the expected rate of 50% found in the relatives of a proband transmitting an autosomal dominant trait.

This study was then replicated in the Hopkins Dementia Research Clinic. Because the nursing home probands were not consistently examined with laboratory tests we repeated the study in a group of clinic patients who had been thoroughly

TABLE 3. *Risk of dementia in relatives by age 85: proband sample*

NH	55%
Clinic	48%
Autopsy	50%
Others	Variable
Controls	12%
Controls	8%
Controls	0%

evaluated and met NINCDS criteria for probable Alzheimer's disease. The risk to the first-degree relatives was 48%. We repeated the study a third time in relatives of a group of patients who had autopsy-proven Alzheimer's disease. We found the same rate.

Similar results have been obtained by many other groups as shown in Table 3 (10,17,19,23), but some have found lower rates in the relatives (9,18).

To further test the conjecture we determined whether Alzheimer's disease shared characteristics with other known autosomal dominant disorders. If this disorder were an autosomal dominant disorder, we might expect to see a paternal age effect. It is well-known that advanced maternal age, as in Down's syndrome, is associated with aneuploidy. It is less well-known that in autosomal dominant diseases like Marfan's syndrome advanced paternal age is related to new mutations (Pyeritz, *this volume*).

Diane Powell investigated the age of a potential founding father of an Alzheimer's disease line and compared that person to controls from the 1919 census. The first individual in the line of sufficient age yet unaffected was significantly older at the birth of Alzheimer cases than controls (25). Replication of this study will be feasible after the genes have been discovered.

Several attempts have been made to determine whether the parents of Alzheimer's disease patients are older than controls (31). However, the advanced age is expected in parents of founders not in gene carriers who are offspring of the founder.

Parental age effect (see Table 4) is to be distinguished from parental transmission effect. In Huntington's disease (22) and other conditions, the age of onset and severity of a dominant condition are dependent on the sex of the transmitting parent. Affected children of Huntington's disease mothers have a later age of onset than affected children of Huntington's disease fathers (24). In our Alzheimer's disease

TABLE 4. *Parental age effect*

	Mean age	
	Paternal	Maternal
FAD	45(12)	31(6)
1919 Population	33(8)	28(7)

families we found no difference in the age of onset in cases with either parent affected.

If Alzheimer's disease were transmitted as a dominant, then we would expect to find both genetic and environmental forms, and within the genetic forms we would expect to find more than one mutation to be causing the same phenotype (Pyeritz, *this volume*). There is increasing evidence of etiological heterogeneity in Alzheimer's disease (10,16). In addition there certainly are genocopies in that Down's syndrome due to trisomy 21 is not the cause of most cases of Alzheimer's disease. The recent linkage work suggesting that some of the families of older age of onset including the Volga German families do not link to the 21 locus supports the idea of genetic heterogeneity (27,28; Gusella, *this volume*).

In genetic disease such as Marfan's syndrome and homocystinuria, clinical features suggest genetic subtypes. Clinical features also suggest subtypes of Alzheimer's disease. A subgroup of patients of the earlier onset form have an abnormality in their platelet membranes (32). Age of onset of the disorder varies between families. Figure 1 shows the age of onset between probands and relatives. When the disease tends to occur early in the proband, it tends to occur early in the relative and when it occurs late in the proband, it occurs late in the relative, suggesting that age of onset might be inherited. Possibly the gene causing the early-onset form is different from the gene causing the late-onset form (16).

If Alzheimer's disease were an autosomal dominant trait, then we might expect to find similar clinical and pathological features to be caused by environmental factors. In our initial nursing home study there were patients with dementia but without parietal signs of agraphia whose family members were not at increased risk. Some of these cases are likely to be phenocopies or environmentally caused forms. Some are possibly new mutations. Similar but not identical clinical-pathological entities have been reported due to head trauma and possibly a slow virus.

The prevalence of familial cases gives an indication of the prevalence of the genetic forms and by inference of the phenocopies even though sporadic or single cases in a family are often but not always phenocopies. Many individuals carrying the Alzheimer's disease gene will die from competing causes of death before they express the disease, and therefore estimates of the prevalence of the familial form are likely to be underestimates (3). Nevertheless, even with these underestimates the prevalence is much higher than previously thought.

Table 5 lists studies of prevalence of familial disease. The number of cases with affected first-degree relatives ranges from 26% to 75% and is usually around 40%. If cases are counted who have parents that lived to be at least as old as the proband, then 75% of cases have an affected first-degree relative (25).

So, the 1981 conjecture has not yet been refuted. We now propose three genetic forms of Alzheimer's disease; Down's syndrome, the early onset autosomal form linked to chromosome 21, and the late onset form likely to be autosomal but as yet not linked to any chromosome. Although no compelling evidence of environmental risks is known, we expect to find phenocopies (16).

Given those conclusions, what do we tell our patients? There are certain princi-

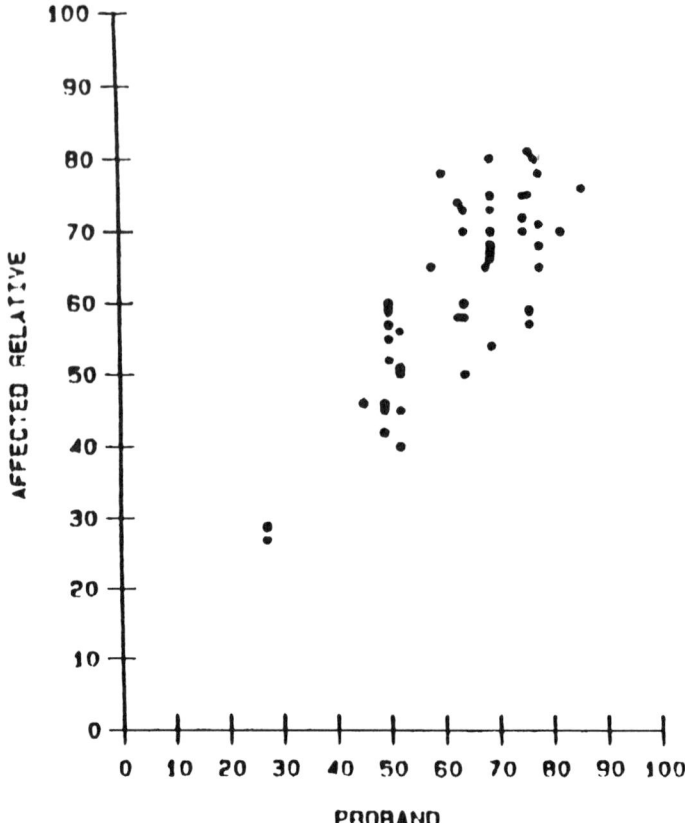

FIG. 1. Age of onset in probands and relatives.

ples that are the basis for counseling families regarding Alzheimer's disease (35). First, the actual risk of expressing an age-dependent disease is equal to the joint probability of the theoretical risk and the risk of surviving to that age from the current age. Theoretical risk depends on the individual pedigree, that is, in some cases it might be 50% and in other cases it might be unknown. Finally, the survival risk depends on individual time, place, and person. So, for example, for a 40-year-old male with an affected parent and grandparent we might assume a theoretical risk

TABLE 5. Prevalence of familial forms

Meggendorf	1927	26%
Heston	1981	40%
Breitner	1984	50%
Powell	1984	75%
Autopsy	1988	60%

of 50% by age 85. The risk of surviving to the age of maximal expression (85 years) of the disease would be 20%. The actual risk that individual would ever develop Alzheimer's disease is 0.5×0.2 or 0.1. In females the risk is higher because their survival is longer. Thus, a 40-year-old female would have a 40% chance of surviving to age 84 and if her risk were 50% because of her pedigree, then her risk of expressing Alzheimer's disease by age 85 would be 20%. These estimates are given to illustrate that even in a worse case scenario, the actual risk is close to the rates stated for the general population. Since the age of onset is correlated in families, the risk for very early onset families would be higher. Fortunately, these cases are rare in the general population.

These extreme age-dependent disorders then have implications for the future. First of all, as medical advances eliminate the competing causes of death, they will increase in prevalence. The better we are at preventing heart disease and cancer, the more Alzheimer's disease we will have.

But there is a hopeful side to the extreme age-dependent diseases. To delay their onset by only a few years will prevent their occurrence. In this disease and other old-age onset conditions, we are interested in finding not only the gene and gene product, but also those features of the environment and the genome that will lead to expression of symptoms late in life. If environmental interventions delayed the onset of the disease by only a few years, its prevalence could be radically reduced. Discovery of the genes causing Alzheimer's disease would greatly help us to find environmental triggers that could be modified to delay onset and thus prevent the disease.

REFERENCES

1. Alzheimer, A. (1907): Uber eine eigenartige Erkrankung der Hirnrinde. *Allg. Z. Psychiatrie Psychisch-Gerichtlich Med.*, 64:146–148.
2. Breitner, J., Murphy, E., Silverman, J., Mohs, R., and Davis, K. (1988): Age-dependent expression of familial risk in Alzheimer's disease. *Am. J. Epidemiol.*, 128:536–548.
3. Breitner, J., Folstein, M., and Murphy, E. (1986): Familial aggregation in Alzheimer dementia: I. A model for age-dependent expression of an autosomal dominant gene. *J. Psychiatr. Res.*, 20:31–43.
4. Breitner, J., Murphy, E., and Folstein, M. (1986): Familial aggregation in Alzheimer dementia: II. Clinical genetic implications of age-dependent onset. *J. Psychiatr. Res.*, 20:45–55.
5. Breitner, J., and Folstein, M. (1984): Familial Alzheimer dementia: a prevalent disorder with specific clinical features. *Psychol. Med.*, 14:63–80.
6. Constantinidis, J. (1978): Is Alzheimer's disease a major form of senile dementia? In: *Alzheimer's Disease: Senile Dementia and Related Disorders*, edited by R. Katzman, R. Terry, and K. L. Bick, pp. 15–25. Raven Press, New York.
7. Chase, G., Folstein, M., Breitner, J., Beaty, T., and Self, S. (1983): The use of life tables and survival analysis in testing genetic hypotheses with an application to Alzheimer's disease. *Am. J. Epidemiol.*, 117:590–597.
8. Creasey, H., Jorm, A., Longley, W., Broe, G. A., and Henderson, A. S. (1989): Monozygotic twins discordant for Alzheimer's disease. Department of Geriatric Medicine, University of Sydney, NSW, Australia. *Neurology*, 39:1474–1476.
9. Farrer, L. A., O'Sullivan, D. M., Cupples, L. A., Growdon, J. H., and Myers, R. H. (1989): Assessment of genetic risk for Alzheimer's disease among first degree relatives. Department of Neurology, Boston University School of Medicine. *Ann. Neurol.*, 25:485–493.

10. Farrer, L. A., Myers, R. H., Cupples, L. A. (1990): Transmission and age-at-onset patterns in familial Alzheimer's disease: evidence for heterogeneity. *Neurology*, 40:395–403.
11. Folstein, M. (1986): Genetics and Alzheimer's disease: promises and caveats. *Neurobiol. Aging*, 7: 482.
12. Folstein, M., Anthony, J., Parhad, I., Duffy, B., and Gruenberg, E. (1985): The meaning of cognitive impairment in the elderly. *J. Am. Geriatr. Soc.*, 33:228–235.
13. Folstein, M. F., and Breitner, J. (1981): Language disorder predicts familial Alzheimer's disease. *Johns Hopkins Med. J.*, 149:145–147.
14. Folstein, M. F., Powell, D., and Breitner, J. C. S. (1983): The cognitive pattern of familial Alzheimer disease (FAD). Banbury report 15: biological aspects of Alzheimer's disease, Banbury Center. Cold Spring Harbor Laboratory, New York, pp. 337–349.
15. Folstein, M., and Powell, D. (1984): Is Alzheimer's disease inherited? A methodologic review. *Integrative Psych.*, 2:163–170.
16. Folstein, M. F., Warren, A., and McHugh, P. R. (1988): Heterogeneity in Alzheimer disease: an exercise in the resolution of a phenotype. In: *Molecular Genetic Mechanism in Neurological Disorder*, edited by P. Brown and L. Bolis, pp. 85–89. FESN, Geneva.
17. Huff, F. J., Auerbach, J., Chakravarti, A., and Boller, F. (1988): Risk of dementia in relatives of patients with Alzheimer's disease. Department of Neurology, Graduate School of Public Health, University of Pittsburgh School of Medicine. *Neurology*, 38:786–790.
18. Knesevich, J., Toro, F., Morris, J., and LaBarge, E. (1985): Aphasia, family history, and the longitudinal course of senile dementia of the Alzheimer type. *Psychiatr. Res.*, 14:255–263.
19. Martin, R., Gerteis, G., and Gabrielle, W. (1988): A family-genetic study of dementia of Alzheimer's type. *Arch. Gen. Psychiatry*, 45:894–900.
20. McHugh, P. R., and Folstein, M. F. (1987): Organic mental disorders. In: *Psychiatry*, 2nd ed. J. B. Lippincott, Philadelphia.
21. McKhann, G., Drachman, D., Folstein, M. F., Katzman, R., Price, D., and Stadlan, E. (1984): Clinical diagnosis of Alzheimer's disease. *Neurology*, 34:939–944.
22. Myers, R., Madden, J., Teague, J., and Falck, A. (1982): Factors related to onset age of Huntington disease. *Am. J. Hum. Genet.*, 34:481–488.
23. Mohs, R., Breitner, J., Silverman, J., and Davis, K. (1987): Alzheimer's disease, morbid risk among first-degree relatives. *Arch. Gen. Psychiatry*, 44:405–408.
24. Myers, R., Sax, D., Schoenfeld, M., et al. (1985): Late onset of Huntington's disease. *J. Neurol. Neurosurg., Psychiatry*, 48:530–534.
25. Powell, D., and Folstein, M. (1984): Pedigree study of familial Alzheimer's disease. *J. Neurogenet.*, 1:189–197.
26. Rocca, W., Amaducci, L., and Schoenberg, B. (1986): Epidemiology of clinically diagnosed Alzheimer's disease. *Ann. Neurol.*, 19:415–424.
27. Roses, A., Pericak-Vance, M., Haynes, C., et al. (1988): Genetic linkage studies in Alzheimer's disease. *Neurology*, 38(Suppl. 1):173.
28. Schellenberg, A., Bird, T., Wijsman, E., et al. (1988): Absence of linkage of chromosome 21q21 markers to familial Alzheimer's disease. *Science*, 241:1507–1510.
29. Sjogren, T., Sjogren, H., and Lindgren, A. G. H. (1952): Morbus Alzheimer's and morbus pick: a genetic clinical and patho-anatomical study. *Acta Psychiatr. Neurol. Scand.*, 82:1–152.
30. Wade, J., Mirsen, T., Hachinski, V., Fisman, M., Lau, C., and Merskey, H. (1987): The clinical diagnosis of Alzheimer's disease. *Arch. Neurol.*, 44:24–29.
31. White, J., McGue, M., and Heston, L. (1986): Fertility and parental age in Alzheimer disease. *J. Gerontol.*, 41:40–43.
32. Zubenko, G., Wusylko, M., Cohen, B., Boller, F., and Teply, I. (1987): Family study of platelet membrane fluidity in Alzheimer's disease. *Science*, 238:539–542.
33. Zubenko, G. S., and Ferrell, R. E. (1988): Monozygotic twins concordant for probable Alzheimer disease and increased platelet membrane fluidity. Department of Psychiatry, University of Pittsburgh School of Medicine, Pennsylvania. *Am. J. Med. Genet.*, 29:431–436.
34. Reisberg, B. (1983): Alzheimer's disease. *Standard Reference*, pp. 37–47.
35. Chase, G. A. (1986): Genetic counselling in Alzheimer's disease. *Neurobiol. Aging*, 7:483–485.

Genes, Brain, and Behavior, edited by
P. R. McHugh and V. A. McKusick.
Raven Press, Ltd., New York © 1991.

The Current Status of Linkage Studies in Schizophrenia

*Joel Gelernter and *†Kenneth K. Kidd

*Departments of *Psychiatry and †Human Genetics, Yale University School of Medicine, New Haven, Connecticut 06510*

Schizophrenia is a disorder with a long recognized genetic contribution. With the development of molecular genetic methods of linkage analysis, especially restriction fragment length polymorphisms (RFLPs), increasing research activity is being directed toward discovering genetic linkage between schizophrenia and some marker locus. Identification of such a linkage would imply localization of a gene that can cause schizophrenia. Recent linkage studies in schizophrenia have disagreed about the possible presence of a susceptibility locus on the proximal long arm of chromosome 5. Here we review the background of those papers and discuss other current approaches to linkage studies in schizophrenia.

The genetic contribution to the development of schizophrenia, although widely recognized for decades, has been under special scrutiny of late since the development of new molecular techniques of genetic mapping. These mapping methods carry the promise of aiding our eventual identification of a gene that may have an important predisposing effect toward the development of schizophrenia. Were such a gene located and described, deducing the structure of the protein it specifies could help elucidate basic steps in the etiology of the disorder. This could lead to treatments specifically directed to the cause of the disorder. Knowledge of the abnormality could correspondingly be expected to enrich our knowledge of normal behavior.

Linkage studies are fundamental to this progress. In a linkage study, genetic markers are used to identify specific segments of chromosomes, so that their inheritance may be followed across generations. A genetic marker is a genetic locus with heritable normal variation that can be assessed phenotypically to determine something about an individual's genetic makeup. Such a marker can be something of relevance in clinical contexts, such as color blindness or blood type, or it can be a clinically irrelevant trait detectable only by special assays or on the molecular level. Markers are useful because each is tied to a specific physical location on one of the chromosomes; when a given allelic form is passed down from parent to child, it takes with it a contiguous segment of DNA and the specific alleles at the loci in that segment. The boundaries of this continuous segment of DNA are either places where recombination events have occurred or chromosomal telomeres. Alleles at a marker locus are more likely to be inherited along with the alleles at close pieces of DNA than with alleles at more distant pieces, because of the possibility of recombination; if recombination occurs between two markers, the alleles at the two loci are physically separated and put together in a different combination (with whatever alleles happen to be on the chromosome inherited from the other parent). (If two markers are on different chromosomes, their inheritance is completely independent (as predicted by Mendel's Second Law).) If a trait of interest is inherited more often than would be expected on the basis of chance along with a genetic marker, then the marker and the trait are said to be "linked" and, by inference, if the location of the marker is known, the general location of the gene that predisposes to development of the trait is known too (because it must be close to the marker). Discovery of linkage therefore allows localization of a disease susceptibility locus. (This may still be many steps removed from identifying the gene predisposing to disease itself.)

It is clear that there is an important genetic contribution toward development of schizophrenia, as demonstrated by adoption studies (17,24), family studies (12,19), and twin studies (14). These findings are consistent. However, schizophrenia is a difficult disease to study genetically because even after decades of research (a) we do not know what causes it, (b) we have found few abnormalities consistently shared by patients, and (c) we do not know of any consistently distinguishable diagnostic subtypes based on biochemical differences between patients. Therefore, although the disease may be genetically heterogeneous, such heterogeneity is not established; we do not yet understand the biological basis for any heterogeneity, so we are not in a position to group "like" types of familial schizophrenia with each other for the purpose of genetic analyses. Linkage is reasonably promoted as a method that might eventually allow a clarification of the diagnostic spectrum. Once a linkage is established, it will be possible to review psychiatric histories for all members of a kindred in which the linkage has been demonstrated and compare clinical findings for relatives with and without the illness-associated allele at the susceptibility locus (10,25,28). Those illnesses (or symptom clusters) that are found in excess in nonschizophrenic people with the illness-associated allele at the schizophrenia susceptibility locus will be classifiable as genetically related to schizophrenia, and those illnesses found just as often in people without this disease susceptibility allele will be identifiable as genetically unrelated. This formulation will be applicable only when such a linkage is truly and irrefutably identified. A problem arises, however, when disease definition and linkage status are used to define *each other*, that is, when illness definition is varied in the search for the true parameters of linkage, and then those parameters are taken to be correct because a LOD score greater than 3 (traditionally considered the threshold for statistical significance) can be generated. Such a strategy is appropriate if exploratory, but the initial results must be validated in a separate, nonexploratory study designed to test that the specified clinical and genetic parameters really define a locus with linkage to the specific marker.

The problems of characterization of phenotype and identification of mode of inheritance (discussed below) are problems intimately related to the task of finding a major gene predisposing for schizophrenia. Linkage, although it has great possibilities, is also fraught with potential complication.

In searching for markers linked to schizophrenia, researchers have used two approaches to try to increase the odds of finding a susceptibility locus over simply testing markers at random. We will illustrate these with two examples. We will first discuss the situation on chromosome 5, where a linkage was announced in the wake of cytogenetic findings. Then we will discuss how we have applied a "candidate gene" strategy in the context of mapping.

CHROMOSOME 5 AND SCHIZOPHRENIA

For schizophrenia, recent attention has been focused on chromosome 5. The origin of this attention was a report by Bassett et al. (1), describing schizophrenia in an uncle/nephew pair who shared an unbalanced translocation involving a piece of chromosome 5 and were therefore trisomic for that small genetic region. That is, they had three copies instead of two of all of the genes located within the piece of the chromosome that was translocated. These two relatives had physical abnormalities as well, such as frontal bossing and hypertelorism. The sister/mother who "connected" these two schizophrenics carried the balanced translocation (and therefore was not trisomic for any genetic segment) and was physically and behaviorally normal. The implication was that the uncle and nephew might be schizophrenic because they received extra genetic material in that region and that therefore a gene for schizophrenia could lie somewhere in the trisomic region. (It has, however, been observed that this cannot be inferred as a statistically significant result from the translocation because too few family members were available for study, that is, the association between the translocation and schizophrenia may have been due to chance alone.)

Amplifying the interest in this region was the fact that the gene coding for glucocorticoid receptor, given the gene symbol GRL, was mapped to the translocation region, which corresponds to bands 5q11.1–5q13.3. Since steroid psychosis resembles schizophrenia in some ways, this made GRL a "candidate gene," and several groups started testing GRL and other chromosome 5 markers for linkage with schizophrenia.

There were thus two lines of evidence suggesting that genes in this region could have something to do with susceptibility to schizophrenia: the translocation and the presence of the "candidate gene" in the region. However, candidate gene support was eliminated in late 1988 when, in the course of their work, our group found that the location initially given for GRL (in 1987) was incorrect. GRL does not map to the translocation region at all but to the distal long arm of chromosome 5 (13) (Fig. 1). Such revisions are not at all uncommon at this early stage of mapping of the human genome. In this case, "moving" GRL weakened the reasoning in favor of potential linkage to markers in the translocation region.

In late 1988, the discovery of a schizophrenia susceptibility locus was announced

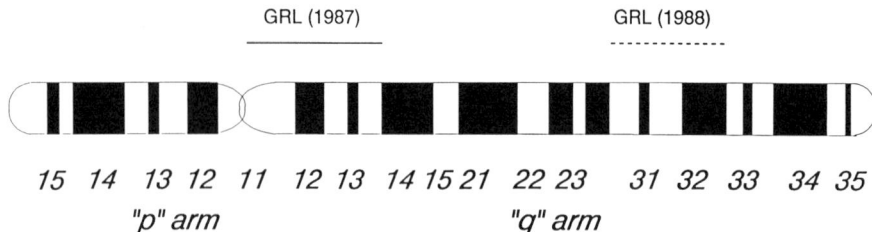

FIG. 1. Chromosome 5, with past and present locations of glucocorticoid receptor (GRL).

by Dr. Hugh Gurling's group, a result that generated considerable interest in the scientific community (39). Sherrington et al. studied a series of British and Icelandic pedigrees and reported a LOD score greater than 6 for linkage of schizophrenia (broadly defined) to two chromosome 5 markers that mapped within the translocation region. Several aspects of the analyses deserve comment; first we will consider the diagnostic criteria used to determine who should be considered "ill" in the linkage analysis. The highest LOD score (6.49) was obtained when the diagnostic spectrum of schizophrenia was broadened to accommodate "fringe" diagnoses such as phobia and alcoholism, a decision not well supported by available family study data. The procedure used, of employing various diagnostic schemata to maximize the LOD score, amounts to testing the diagnostic spectra to be used on the basis of genotype in the families involved. Considering a more restricted, and better supported, diagnostic spectrum (schizophrenia and schizophrenia spectrum considered as affected), the maximum LOD score drops to 4.33.

When a linkage is first proposed and the LOD scores are not yet absolutely convincing, defining the diagnosis in this way may be questioned if the diagnostic spectra involved are not well supported by other data. Treatment of diagnosis as a parameter may be expected to raise the LOD score required to demonstrate statistically significant linkage because of the increased number of tests performed. As discussed above, the criterion for acceptance of linkage is generally taken as a LOD score over 3; however, it has been suggested that a higher figure may be more appropriate (8,26,30,38).

The selection by Sherrington et al. (39) of a penetrance value for the putative schizophrenia susceptibility locus (which was 0.86 and which maximized the LOD score) could also have been better supported. A lower value might have provided a more realistic penetrance estimate, for example, 0.72 is a more realistic value for the Swedish kindred (discussed below), as determined from an analysis by Giuffra et al. (23). Spuriously high penetrance figures are expected to increase the absolute value of the LOD scores calculated.

The same issue of *Nature* carried a report by Kennedy et al. (23) ruling out presence of a schizophrenia susceptibility locus mapping to the same area based on analyses of the Swedish kindred studied by Böök (3) and Wetterberg (41–43). Kennedy et al. used data from five markers, D5S21, D5S76, D5S39, HEXB, and D5S78 (probes pJ0110HC, p105–599Ha, p105–153Ra, pHexX, and p105–798Rb, respectively). The map positions of these markers were known and the region of chromosome 5 excluded from harboring a schizophrenia susceptibility locus spanned about 40 centimorgans. The two markers used by Sherrington et al. (D5S76 and D5S39) were flanked by the others. A penetrance value of 0.72 was used; all patients considered "ill" in the analyses had schizophrenia.

(The Swedish kindred is an excellent resource for attempting to map a susceptibility locus for schizophrenia because it represents a geographically isolated sample [with some features in common with a genetic isolate] and therefore everyone in the kindred is likely to have the same genetic form of schizophrenia. This minimizes the problem of within-study genetic heterogeneity, a problem that could frustrate the search for linkage if some pedigrees in a series truly manifested linkage with a marker and others did not. However, by virtue of its being a single large kindred, there is the possibility that a linkage discovered in this kindred might not apply to any others. This does not deter us because to delineate the genetic basis of schizophrenia in even a single kindred could immeasurably improve understanding of the etiology of the disorder and could provide pathophysiological clues to other loci that may show linkage in other kindreds.)

Since the original two papers, several others have appeared, all consistent with no linkage of schizophrenia to the translocation region of chromosome 5. St. Clair et al. (40) studied 15 pedigrees with a series of diagnostic schemes employing different penetrance assumptions derived from their data set. The first of their models considered schizophrenia, schizoaffective disorder, bipolar affective disorder, and unspecified functional psychosis to be the disease spectrum, with penetrance 0.66. Two other models added major depression (penetrance 0.77) and all other RDC diagnoses as well (penetrance 0.94), respectively. They studied the loci D5S76, D5S39, and D5S78 for multipoint analyses. Linkage to the translocation region was excluded under all three models with highly significant LOD scores mostly in the range of -8 and below. An additional model applied penetrance of 0.44 to a disease model including only schizophrenia, schizoaffective disorder, and unspecified functional psychosis, but only with pairwise data from D5S76 (exclusion out to 5% recombination; LOD score -3.1). It has been proposed that inclusion of pedigrees with cases of bipolar affective disorder could account for the negative results (4). St. Clair et al. noted, however, that even with those pedigrees that included individuals with affective disorders excluded from the analyses, the negative LOD score still reached significance out to 10% recombination from D5S76. The same group recently performed additional analyses using only families with schizophrenia but no cases of affective disorder and obtained a strong negative result for 5q11–13 markers (2).

There have been three other negative reports regarding schizophrenia and chromosome 5 markers (6,7,18) and no other positive reports.

The situation may be summarized as follows. Linkage has been claimed by one group between schizophrenia and genetic markers on chromosome 5 (39) in a set of kindreds. Several other groups have studied genetic markers mapped to the same region on chromosome 5 and have found significant evidence against linkage, all studies using different sets of kindreds. Since in at least two cases (2,22,23) the analyses have been carried out under assumptions as conservative as those used by the group reporting linkage or more so, these results represent either a discrepancy, or genetic heterogeneity (meaning that some schizophrenia is chromosome 5 linked and some is not).

Before discussing which is more likely to be the case, we might reexamine the basic assumptions of linkage analysis (see also Robertson [38]). Specific requirements to carry out linkage studies have been identified (27). These may be summarized as follows:

1. adequate diagnosis and nosology,
2. availability of suitable family material,
3. sufficient genetic markers,
4. multipoint analytic methods.

The first requirement in this list is for adequate diagnosis and nosology. DSMIII and DSMIII-R have allowed for objective, reliable diagnoses for the core syndrome (that is, schizophrenia itself). Deciding what other diagnoses may be included for the purpose of genetic analyses poses a greater problem at present. The recurrence risk of schizophrenia in first-degree relatives of schizophrenics is only about 3.7% to 8.9% (reviewed in [20]); such a low rate of illness in relatives tends to provide an inadequate density of affected individuals to allow for significant results of analyses using the full schizophrenia syndrome alone as the disease definition. This problem has led many investigators to propose alternative disease definitions for the analyses, an approach that may be problematic if these definitions are not (a) decided on *a priori* and (b) consistent with family study data. It has resulted in disease definitions in various studies being inconsistent with each other. Matthysse et al. (33) have proposed one possible solution to this problem of low density of affected individuals (and understanding of the transmission of schizophrenia in general) with a "latent trait" model of schizophrenia, involving transmission not of schizophrenia itself but of a "latent trait" capable of causing either schizophrenia or some other abnormality (in this case, smooth pursuit eye tracking abnormalities).

The second requirement is availability of suitable family material. Kindreds like the North Swedish one are rare and few groups are able to study such isolates, decreasing their chances for discovering linkage. Kendler and associates (21) are collecting schizophrenia families from County Roscommon, Ireland; the resulting collection may be nearly ideal and may be quite analogous to the North Swedish kindred. Other groups have generally assembled collections of many moderate-sized kindreds from different genetic backgrounds, all segregating for schizophrenia. Therefore it is the rule that no two groups are working with really comparable kindred collections; inclusion and exclusion criteria naturally vary. It may be that the positive chromosome 5 results have not been replicated because groups besides the group reporting linkage have failed to systematically exclude schizophrenia pedigrees including individuals affected with bipolar affective disorder. St. Clair et al. (40) note, however, that they retain their exclusionary result even when they only include data from pedigrees without affective disorder. The Swedish kindred also is notable for its absence of affective disorder.

The third requirement, that of availability of sufficiently many genetic markers, is finally easy to meet in most circumstances. Nearly 2,000 polymorphic markers detected with DNA methods (mostly RFLPs) have been catalogued (29) and most are readily available to researchers for linkage studies. The fourth, availability of suitable multipoint methods of linkage analysis, is within the technical reach of most groups at this point since computer versions of such programs as LINKAGE (32) are widely distributed.

Discussion: Chromosome 5 and Schizophrenia

It has been argued (16,31) that genetic heterogeneity may explain the absence of chromosome 5 linkage with schizophrenia outside of the single sample for which it has been reported, but this argument was made before the failure to replicate became a common finding. There is doubt now about chromosome 5 linkage to schizophrenia, even in the original Icelandic and English sample; many investigators think that the finding may well have been spurious. This does not mean that the work itself was done wrong or that errors were made, simply that possibly a more stringent statistical test should have been applied before accepting linkage. It is also possible that a true linkage was discovered but that the locus mapped may determine a broad susceptibility to psychiatric abnormality rather than schizophrenia itself. We should not regard linkage of schizophrenia to chromosome 5 as verified until an independent replication of the finding satisfying stringent statistical criteria becomes available.

Mode of Inheritance—A Caveat for Linkage Studies

Although work on searching for a genetic marker linked to schizophrenia trait is proceeding, we may not really know how to set the parameters for our analyses, as schizophrenia is not a genetically simple disorder. All of the studies quoted have assumed dominant inheritance, which seems plausible in the kindreds studied; however, it is by no means established that this is the correct description in general. Certain facts, e.g., recurrence risk of schizophrenia in relatives, may be more consistent with oligogenic inheritance or some other kind of inheritance more complicated than single major locus autosomal dominant (37). If there truly is genetic heterogeneity, then the mode of inheritance may be different for different loci. In such a case, the correct model would have to be used for each family.

CANDIDATE GENE STUDIES IN SCHIZOPHRENIA

We will now discuss a candidate gene study in schizophrenia. This will illustrate a method possible only since the cloning of many genes of importance in the central nervous system. With a candidate gene linkage study, a cloned gene that may have some function in the pathophysiology of the illness under study is selected and tested for linkage with that illness. If there is no linkage, a mutation in that gene cannot cause the illness, but if there is linkage, a pathophysiological relationship is possible. Candidate gene studies of this sort illustrate another use of genetic linkage, testing of a pathophysiological hypothesis. In the case we will discuss, the candidate gene was a D_2 dopamine receptor, recognized by probe hD2G1. This gene, given the symbol DRD2, was cloned at the end of 1988 by Civelli's group (5). The dopamine hypothesis of schizophrenia is well known; clearly the dopamine system has some involvement in schizophrenic symptomatology. However, it had not been possible to test for a mutation in a gene coding for a D_2 receptor before, and it was an obvious step to try to do so.

A linkage study tests whether a disease susceptibility locus is coincident with the "candidate gene" by examining whether the disease trait and an allele at the locus of the candidate gene are inherited together or segregate independently. If they segregate independently, that is, if whether or not a person in the kindred is ill has nothing to do with whether or not he gets a certain allele at the candidate gene locus, then the disease susceptibility locus is not near the candidate gene. Consequently, the two loci cannot be the same, and, at least in the families studied, a mutation in the candidate gene cannot cause the disease. While such a negative finding demonstrates conclusively that the candidate gene does not cause *all* cases of the disorder, it can never exclude the possibility of the candidate gene causing *some* cases of the disorder.

In our approach to a candidate gene study, we first try to place the candidate gene in its genomic context (Fig. 2). This has several advantages. Studying segregation simultaneously at several genetic loci adjacent to and surrounding the candidate gene almost always leads to "stronger" results. The multiple markers allow extraction of segregation information about the chromosomal region containing the candidate gene from more of the meioses occurring in the kindred. Since we often have disease kindreds of only limited size, we need to obtain all the information we can

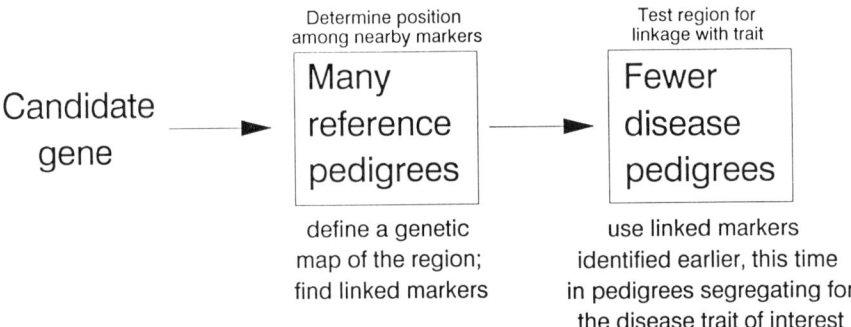

FIG. 2. Overall strategy for the use of candidate genes in the context of exclusion mapping.

from each of them. Studying nearby markers allows us to derive information about transmission of the region containing the candidate gene even when the polymorphism at the gene itself is entirely uninformative. Placing the candidate gene in context also serves the goal of exclusion mapping, so that at the end of the study there is a genomic region of some significance (that region which also contains the candidate gene) that is known not to contain a locus responsible for the trait of interest.

DRD2 was previously mapped by physical techniques to chromosome 11q23 (i.e., region q23 of chromosome 11) (15); however, its position in the genetic linkage map needed to be established. We used hD2G1, a probe for DRD2, and probes for other loci previously mapped to the same general area to phenotype several large reference families (families which bore no relationship to schizophrenia trait). The marker typings were used to construct the map shown in Fig. 3 (11). This map was based on data from 250 to 400 individuals for each marker, a sample large enough to give a reasonably accurate estimate of the frequency of crossovers between any two markers. One of the markers mapping close to DRD2 is PBGD, which is the gene for porphobilinogen deaminase. An abnormal allele at this locus is the actual "disease gene" that causes acute intermittent porphyria (AIP). AIP is an illness that sometimes presents with psychotic symptoms that can be confused with schizophrenia, so PBGD was also a candidate gene for schizophrenia causation. (AIP has also been proposed as a model for genetic transmission of schizophrenia [42].)

This map has been used as the basis for a multipoint linkage analysis, considering

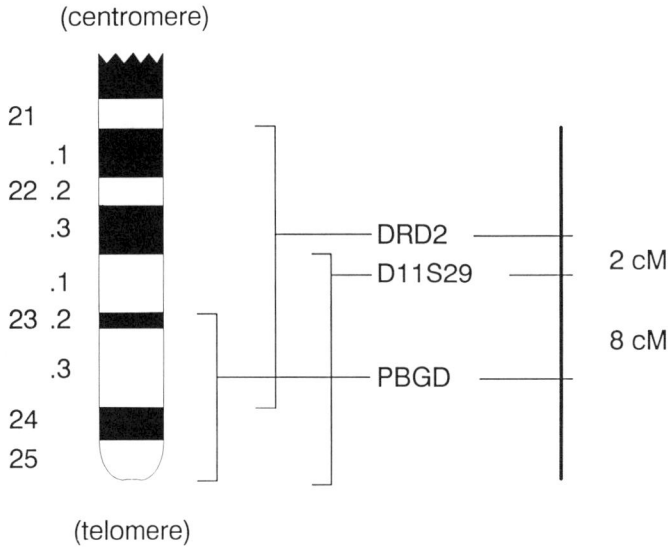

FIG. 3. Physical and linkage map for three markers on the long arm of chromosome 11 (i.e., 11q).

data from all of the markers simultaneously, of schizophrenia trait in the Swedish kindred and another family (34). For the Swedish kindred, we examined three sets of penetrance assumptions: penetrances of 0.85 (close to that used in Sherrington et al. [39]); 0.72, as in the Kennedy et al. (23) analyses of 5q markers (this is the value we feel is most likely to represent the correct one for the Swedish kindred); and 0.56, a lower bound for true penetrance in the Swedish kindred (discussed in [23]). A locus causing schizophrenia is excluded from the region containing the DRD2 and PBGD loci in the Swedish kindred under the less conservative penetrance assumptions, and, with penetrance of 0.56, at the DRD2 and PBGD loci themselves (Fig. 4; this is a subset of the data presented in [34]). Mutations in these genes therefore cannot be responsible for schizophrenia, if the assumptions about its mode of inheritance were correct. As predicted, higher penetrance parameters resulted in an apparently larger genomic area from which a susceptibility locus for schizophrenia trait could be excluded, a region of exclusion that we think is probably spuriously large when penetrance is set at 0.85.

Discussion: A Dopamine Receptor and Schizophrenia

One should draw only fairly cautious conclusions. For example, this D_2 receptor *molecule* could still be relevant because other DRD2-related defects could arise any

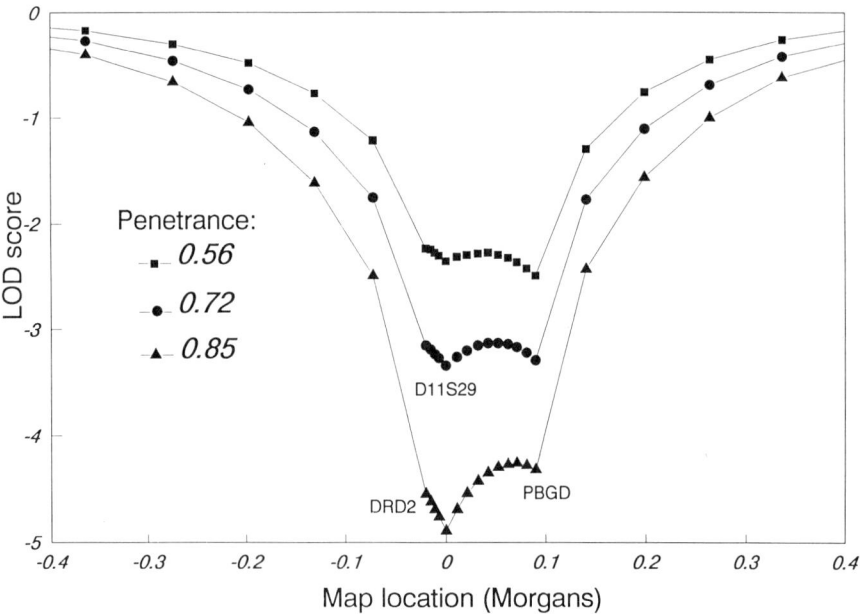

FIG. 4. LOD scores, schizophrenia trait, and three chromosome 11 markers; Swedish kindred.

time after transcription of the genetic message from this gene. In addition, we know now that there are other D_2 receptor genes also (35). This finding may actually strengthen arguments for any one of these genes causing psychiatric illness. If there were only one dopamine receptor gene, one might expect a mutation in it to cause even more pervasive physical and neurological abnormalities than those of schizophrenia, or even to be lethal. However, mutation in this D_2 receptor *gene* cannot be causative in the Swedish kindred and whatever gene is causative cannot map to this region of the genome. This narrows the range of pathophysiological hypotheses for causation of schizophrenia, because it is now clear that schizophrenia cannot be caused exclusively by a mutation in at least one D_2 dopamine receptor gene.

CONCLUSION

We have discussed some of the current state of affairs in the molecular genetics of schizophrenia, focusing on one area of chromosome 5 and on a recent candidate gene study. We conclude that the weight of evidence does not yet support the presence of a susceptibility locus for schizophrenia on chromosome 5 and that genetic heterogeneity is not needed as an explanation for nonreplication of this positive result. Also, it has been demonstrated that a mutation in D_2 dopamine receptor cannot be causative for schizophrenia in the Swedish kindred. Although the candidate gene approach has not resulted in a positive linkage finding, it has allowed refinement in ideas of pathophysiology of schizophrenia.

Schizophrenia may be more complicated genetically than the assumptions made in some previous studies (37). It now appears that many of the simplifying assumptions made to render schizophrenia suitable for linkage analysis may have been oversimplifications. We need to recognize this possibility and adjust our models and analyses appropriately. Ultimately, a better understanding of the genetic models which should be employed for schizophrenia should lead to clarification of corresponding linkage methods. It is not impossible to study linkage of a complex disorder (such as diabetes) if it is possible to make reasonably good guesses about the mode of inheritance. If specific alleles at several loci must work together to cause schizophrenia, then given adequate pedigree resources, it should be possible to find linkage with each locus; and if the statistical models do not generate results of the expected level of certainty, thresholds for claims of positive results can be adjusted (as has already been advocated by Kidd [30]). New methods can be devised to facilitate analysis (36). More realistic assumptions and stricter statistical tests may be expected to result in more enduring interpretations for the results of linkage studies.

ACKNOWLEDGMENT

This work was partially supported by grants MH30929 and MH39239 from the National Institute of Mental Health.

BASIC TERMS USED IN THE POPULATION GENETICS

Allele   One form of the genetic information at a gene locus. All individuals considered in this program package would be diploid, in other words have inherited one copy of every gene from the mother (female parent) and a second copy of every gene from the father (male parent). Each of those copies can be referred to as an allele because it is a different copy but more commonly *allele* also carries the connotation of different relevant information. For example, there are three possible alleles for the ABO blood type: A, B, and O. Every person has just two of those, resulting in four possible blood types: A, B, O, and AB (one A allele + one B allele). There are no AO and BO blood types because those genetic types (genotypes) are indistinguishable from AA and BB, respectively.

Fitness   In population genetics fitness is a measure of an individual's success in producing offspring. The concept has nothing to do with health per se, because a healthy individual who is completely sterile has a fitness of zero. Of course, if an individual dies before reaching reproductive age, the individual's fitness is also zero. Because we are interested in changes in the genetic composition of a population, not in its overall size, it is reasonable to consider only relative fitness and the convention usually adopted is that the most fit individual has a fitness of one and all others have lower fitnesses.

Gamete   A gamete (egg or sperm) contains exactly half of the genetic information from the parent; each gamete contributes exactly half of the genetic information to the offspring. At each gene locus, a gamete contains only one allele.

Genetic drift   Changes in allele frequency caused by the accumulated sampling error of alleles being transmitted from one generation to another is termed genetic drift. Founder effect, a term used for an extreme situation, is one form of genetic drift. Consider one heterozygous individual, AB, who has five offspring. It is impossible for that individual to transmit equal numbers of A alleles and B alleles to the next generation. Even if there were two offspring, one quarter of the time the two offspring would both receive the A allele and only half of the time would one offspring receive the A allele and the other offspring the B allele. In extremely large populations this sampling error would average out, but in small populations it does not.

Genotype   The genetic constitution, i.e., the combination of the two alleles at a genetic locus, is called a genotype. At the ABO locus AO is one genotype and AA is another genotype even though they both have the same phenotype (appearance), the blood type A. In this case the relationship between the two genotypes and the phenotype blood group A is called dominance since the heterozygote AO is identical in phenotype to the homozygote AA.

Hardy-Weinberg Principle   Hardy and Weinberg independently devised the simple algebraic relationship stating what genotype frequencies would be in a population given the allele frequencies in that population. The simple algebraic formula strictly applies given a large number of simplifying assumptions. The principle has been modified to allow for the possibility of inbreeding.

Heterozygote A genotype in which the two alleles at a given locus are of different types is called a heterozygote. At the ABO blood group system AO, BO, and AB are three different kinds of heterozygotes.

Homozygote An individual in which the two alleles at a locus are of the same type is termed a homozygote. At the ABO blood group system the genotypes AA, BB, and OO are the three possible homozygotes.

Inbreeding The general term for closely related individuals mating and having offspring is inbreeding. In population genetics it is quantified as the inbreeding coefficient, F, which can be defined as the probability that both copies of a gene in an individual will have arisen from a recent common ancestral gene and therefore be identical by descent. In a randomly mating population of large size the inbreeding coefficient would be zero; if brother-sister matings were carried out for many generations (as in a line of inbred mice) or a plant were self-pollinated for many generations (as is common in peas), the inbreeding coefficient would rapidly reach its maximum value of 1.0. In the randomly mating population there would still be many homozygotes but the alleles would be identical in type, not identical by descent. In the completely inbred population all individuals eventually become homozygous for one allele or the other and that homozygosity is for alleles not only identical in type but also identical by recent descent from a common ancestral allele.

Locus A locus is the segment of DNA in a chromosome containing the genetic information for one particular function, i.e., a gene. In molecular terms the precise boundary of a locus is difficult to define—how far into the 5′ flanking region do the controlling sequences extend and how much of the 3′ flanking is necessary for messenger RNA stability? In classical transmissional and population genetics, however, the locus can be considered a single discrete entity existing in different allelic forms recognized by their phenotypic consequences. Many traits, e.g., tall versus short pea plants, the ABO blood group system in humans, etc., are determined by different alleles at a single locus. Many other traits such as hair color in humans, comb type in domestic chickens, etc., are determined by interactions of different genotypes at two or more separate loci. Some traits, such as height in humans, are determined by allelic variation at multiple loci.

Phenotype As opposed to genotype, the phenotype is the appearance of an organism. A tall plant has phenotype "tall," for instance. In most situations the genotype is not directly observable and only the phenotype can be studied. As mentioned before, ABO blood group genotypes AO and AA have the same phenotype.

Sex linkage An exception to the rule that all individuals have two copies at every locus occurs for those genes that are on the sex chromosomes: individuals of the heterogametic sex (males in mammals, females in birds) have only one copy of the gene on the X chromosome. Considering only mammals, females have two X chromosomes and hence two copies of each gene but males contain only the single X chromosome and the male-determining Y chromosome, which does not have any of the functional X-chromosome genes. Thus, males have only one copy of each gene for sex-linked genes and transmission patterns of alleles on their X chromosome are completely correlated with sex of the offspring: A Y-bearing gamete does not contain those X-chromosome alleles from the father but does determine that the offspring will be a male; an X-bearing sperm contains all of the alleles from the male's single X chromosome (which he got from his mother) and determines a female offspring. Since males have only one allele at each locus, there is no dominance and "what you see is what you've got," i.e., phenotype is identical to genotype. Thus, if a boy inherits an abnormal allele on an X chromosome from his mother, he has no chance of having a normal functional allele to cover for it and will show the abnormality. This explains why color blindness and hemophilia are more common in males; those disorders are caused by abnormal alleles at loci on the human X chromosome.

Linkage When two loci are sufficiently close on a chromosome, the alleles (one from each locus) tend to occur in gametes in the same two combinations in which they were inherited from the parents; this violation of Mendel's second law (independent assortment) is called linkage.

Recombination Linkage is usually quantified using the recombination frequency (symbolized r or Θ), which is the frequency of gametes that are not of the parent types. Complete linkage is equivalent to zero recombination and independent assortment (no linkage) is equivalent to 50% recombination.

Linkage disequilibrium Linkage disequilibrium occurs between two loci on the same chromosome if the relative frequency of alleles occurring together in the same haplotype departs significantly from chance association.

REFERENCES

1. Bassett, A. S., McGillivray, B. C., Jones, B. D., and Pantzar, J. T. (1988): Partial trisomy chromosome 5 cosegregating with schizophrenia. *Lancet*, 1:799–801.
2. Blackwood, D. H. R., Muir, W. J., St. Clair, D. M., and Evans, H. J. (1989): Schizophrenia and chromosomes [letter]. *Lancet*, 2(8277):1459.
3. Böök, J. A. (1953): A genetic and neuropsychiatric investigation of a North-Swedish population with special regard to schizophrenia and mental deficiency. *Acta Genet.*, 4:1–100.
4. Byerly, W. F. (1989): Genetic linkage revisited. *Nature*, 340:340–341.
5. Bunzow, J. R., Van Tol, H. H. M., Grandy, D. K., et al. (1988): Cloning and expression of a rat D_2 dopamine receptor cDNA. *Nature*, 336:783–787.
6. Detera-Wadleigh, S. D., Goldin, L. R., Sherrington, R., et al. (1989): Exclusion of linkage to 5q11–13 in families with schizophrenia and other psychiatric disorders. *Nature*, 340:391–393.
7. Diehl, S., Su, Y., Aman, M., MacLean, C., et al. (1989): Linkage studies of schizophrenia in Irish pedigrees. First World Congress on Psychiatric Genetics, Cambridge, U. K., August 1989.
8. Edwards, J. H., and Watt, D. C. (1989): Caution in locating the gene(s) for affective disorder (editorial). *Psychol. Med.*, 19:273–275.
9. Egeland, J. A., Gerhard, D. L. Pauls, J. N., et al. (1987): Bipolar affective disorders linked to DNA markers on chromosome 11. *Nature*, 325:783–787.
10. Gelernter, J., and Gershon, E. S. (1989): Psychiatric diagnosis in the age of molecular genetics. In: *The Validity of Psychiatric Diagnosis*, edited by Robins and Barrett, pp. 143–161. Raven Press, New York.
11. Gelernter, J., Grandy, D. K., Bunzow, J., et al. (1989): D_2 dopamine receptor locus (probe hD2G1) maps close to D11S29 (probe L7) and is also linked to PBGD (probe PBGD0.9) and D11S84 (probe p2-7-ID6) on 11q. *Cytogenet. Cell Genet.*, 51:1002.

12. Gershon, E. S., DeLisi, L. E., Hamovit, J., et al. (1988): A controlled family study of chronic psychosis, schizophrenia and schizoaffective disorder. *Arch. Gen. Psychiatry*, 45:328–336.
13. Giuffra, L. A., Kennedy, J. L., Castiglione, C. M., Evans, R. M., Wasmuth, J. J., and Kidd, K. K. (1988): Glucocorticoid receptor maps to the distal long arm of chromosome 5. *Cytogenet. Cell Genet.*, 49:313–314.
14. Gottesman, I. I., and Shields, J. (1972): *Schizophrenia and Genetics: A Twin Vantage Point*. Academic Press, New York.
15. Grandy, D. K., Litt, M., Allen, L., et al. (1989): The human dopamine D_2 receptor gene is located in chromosome 11 at q22-q23 and identifies a Taq I polymorphism. *Am. J. Hum. Genet.*, 45:778–785.
16. Gurling, H. (1989): Genetics of schizophrenia (letter). *Lancet*, 1(8632):277.
17. Heston, L. L. (1966): Psychiatric disorders in foster home reared children of schizophrenic mothers. *Br. J. Psychiatry*, 112:819–825.
18. Kaufman, C. A., DeLisi, L. E., Lehner, T., and Gilliam, T. C. (1989): Physical mapping, linkage analysis of a putative schizophrenia locus on chromosome 5q. *Schizophr. Bull.*, 15:441–452.
19. Kendler, K. S., Gruenberg, A. M., and Tsuang, M. T. (1985): Psychiatric illness in first-degree relatives of schizophrenic and surgical control patients. *Arch. Gen. Psychiatry*, 42:770–779.
20. Kendler, K. S. (1988): The genetics of schizophrenia and related disorders: a review. In: *Relatives at risk for mental disorder*, edited by D. L. Dunner, E. S. Gershon, and J. E. Barrett, pp. 247–266. Raven Press, New York.
21. Kendler, K. S., Walsh, D., Su, Y., et al. (1989): The Roscommon family and linkage study of schizophrenia: preliminary report. American College of Neuropsychopharmacology, 28th annual meeting, Maui, Hawaii, December 1989.
22. Kennedy, J. L., Giuffra, L. A., Moises, H. W., et al. (1989): Molecular genetic studies in schizophrenia. *Schizophr. Bull.*, 15:383–391.
23. Kennedy, J. L., Giuffra, L. A., Moises, H. W., et al. (1988): Evidence against linkage of schizophrenia to markers on chromosome 5 in a northern Swedish pedigree. *Nature*, 336:167–170.
24. Kety, S. S., Rosenthal, D., Wender, P. H., and Schulsinger, F. (1967): The types and prevalence of mental illness in the biological and adoptive families of adopted schizophrenics. In: *The Transmission of Schizophrenia*, edited by D. Rosenthal and S. S. Kety, pp. 345–362. Pergamon Press, London.
25. Kidd, K. K., and Matthysse, S. (1978): Research designs for the study of gene-environment interactions in psychiatric disorders. *Arch. Gen. Psychiatry*, 35:925–932.
26. Kidd, K. K., and Ott, J. (1984): Power and sample size in linkage studies. Human Gene Mapping 7. *Cytogenet. Cell Genet.*, 37:510–511.
27. Kidd, K. K. (1987): Research design considerations for linkage studies of affective disorders using recombinant DNA markers. *J. Psychiatr. Res.*, 21:551–557.
28. Kidd, K. K. (1987): Genetic research on affective disorders: current problems and future directions. In: *Affective Disorders: Recent Research and Related Developments. Proceedings of an Indo-U.S. Symposium.* Edited by S. M. Channabasavanna and S. A. Shah, pp. 79–91. National Institute of Mental Health and Neuro Sciences, Bangalore, India.
29. Kidd, K. K., Bowcock, A. M., Schmidtke, R. K., et al. (1989): Report of the DNA committee and catalogs of cloned and mapped genes and DNA polymorphisms. *Cytogenet. Cell Genet.*, 51:622–947.
30. Kidd, K. K., Cavalli-Sforza, L. L., and Wetterberg, L. A genetic linkage study of schizophrenia. In: *Proceedings of the VIIIth World Congress of Psychiatry*, Athens, October 1989, edited by C. Stefanis, et al. Elsevier Science, Amsterdam (*in press*).
31. Lander, E. S. (1988): Splitting schizophrenia. *Nature*, 336:105–106.
32. Lathrop, G. M., Lalouel, J. M., Julier, C., and Ott, J. (1985): Multilocus linkage analysis in humans: detection of linkage and estimation of recombination. *Am. J. Hum. Genet.*, 37:482–498.
33. Matthysse, S., Holzman, P. S., and Lange, K. (1986): The genetic transmission of schizophrenia: application of Mendelian latent structure analysis to eye tracking dysfunctions in schizophrenia and affective disorder. *J. Psychiatr. Res.*, 20:57–76.
34. Moises, H. W., Gelernter, J., Grandy, D. K., et al. No linkage between a D2-dopamine receptor gene and schizophrenia. *Arch. Gen. Psychiatry* (*in press*).
35. O'Malley, K. L., Stone, K. R., and Todd, R. D. (1989): Identification of a D_2 receptor subtype which elevates intracellular calcium. *Soc. Neurosci. Abstr.*, 15:424.
36. Ott, J. (1990): Invited editorial: Cutting a Gordian knot in the linkage analysis of complex human traits. *Am. J. Hum. Genet.*, 46:219–221.

37. Risch, N. (1990): Linkage strategies for genetically complex traits. I. Multilocus models. *Am. J. Hum. Genet.*, 46:222–228.
38. Robertson, M. (1989): False start on manic depression. *Nature*, 342:222.
39. Sherrington, R., Brynjolfsson, J., Petursson, H., et al. (1988): Localization of a susceptibility locus for schizophrenia on chromosome 5. *Nature*, 336:164–167.
40. St. Clair, D., Blackwood, D., Muir, W., et al. (1989): No linkage of chromosome 5q11-q13 markers to schizophrenia in Scottish families. *Nature*, 339:305–309.
41. Wetterberg, L. (1982): The genetic control of catecholamines and its possible implication in schizophrenia. In: *Biological Aspects of Schizophrenia and Addiction*, edited by G. Hemmings. John Wiley, New York.
42. Wetterberg, L. (1979): Clinical and biochemical manifestations of acute intermittent porphyria; a working model for schizophrenia as an inborn error of metabolism. In: *The Biological Basis of Schizophrenia*, edited by G. Hemmings, pp. 139–146. The Schizophrenia Association of Great Britain, MTP Press Ltd., Lancaster, England.
43. Wetterberg, L. Diagnosis of schizophrenia and affective disorders: a Swedish example. In: *Proceedings of the VIIIth World Congress of Psychiatry*, Athens, October 1989, edited by C. Stefanis, et al. Elsevier Science, Amsterdam (*in press*).

Genes, Brain, and Behavior, edited by
P. R. McHugh and V. A. McKusick.
Raven Press, Ltd., New York © 1991.

Genetics of Manic Depressive Illness: Current Status and Evolving Concepts

Miron Baron

Department of Psychiatry, Columbia University College of Physicians and Surgeons, New York State Psychiatric Institute, New York, New York 10032

Manic depressive illness, also known as bipolar affective disorder, is characterized by recurrent manic and depressive episodes, variable age of onset, and population prevalence of 0.5% to 1.0%. Genetic factors have long been implicated in the etiology of manic depression. However, progress in this field has been hampered by uncertainties concerning the mode of genetic transmission, the specific genes involved, etiologic heterogeneity, and phenotypic variation. Molecular biology techniques coupled with genetic marker studies will likely have a key role in resolving some of these issues. The implications of these advances for unraveling the biology of manic depression are discussed in the light of recent reports on linkage between the illness and marker loci mapped to specific genomic locations. The linkages hitherto reported may point to different hereditary forms of manic depression. As a possible first step in the elucidation of molecular pathology, these findings could shed light on the etiology, nosology, pathophysiology, and, possibly, prevention and treatment of affective disorders.

EVIDENCE OF GENETIC TRANSMISSION

Traditional approaches to behavioral genetics focus on family, twin, and adoption studies. Family studies have consistently shown that bipolar affective illness runs in families. In the recent well-designed studies, the morbidity risk (age-adjusted familial rate) for bipolar disorder among the first-degree relatives of bipolar probands is 4% to 9% as compared with 0.2% to 0.5% in the relatives of normals (1,19,41). The relative risk (the ratio of the risk to patients' relatives to the risk to relatives of normal controls) is 17 to 20, indicating significant familial clustering. When unipolar depression, a condition thought to be a milder clinical variant of bipolar illness, is included in the bipolar "spectrum," the corresponding figures are 13% to 35% versus 5% to 8%.

Twin and adoption studies show whether familial aggregation has a genetic component. Because monozygotic (identical) twins share all their genes whereas dizygotic (fraternal) twins share only 50% of their genetic constitution, a higher concordance rate in the former points to the role of genetic factors. The concordance rates for the bipolar spectrum are 80% versus 24% in monozygotic and dizygotic twins, respectively (a ratio of 3.3 to 1) (13). The heritability estimate (a measure of the genetic contribution to the overall familial resemblance) is 75%, suggesting a genetic component of large magnitude. However, since 20% of monozygotic twin pairs are discordant for the illness, nongenetic factors are clearly present. Using the adoptee's family method, which determines the risk for a disorder to the biologic and adoptive parents of adoptees versus controls, the risk for affective disorder in the biologic parents of bipolar adoptees was greater than that found in the biologic parents of normal adoptees; it was also greater than the risk to the adoptive parents, thus supporting the role of heredity in bipolar affective illness (28).

MODE OF INHERITANCE

Although the studies described in the previous section invoke a role for genetic factors in bipolar disorder, they do not offer insights into the underlying mode of genetic transmission. Mode of inheritance can be determined through the use of mathematical models that test the fit of specific genetic hypotheses to family data (for review, see [3,40]). Most efforts in this domain have focused on the single major locus (or gene) (SML) and multifactorial-polygenic (MFP) models.

According to the SML model, the familial transmission of the disorder can be explained solely by a single gene with two alleles. The same model can subsume dominant and recessive modes of inheritance, as well as contributions from the environment. When one dose of the abnormal allele may result in disease expression, the trait is dubbed dominant. When a double dose is required, the trait is said to be recessive. To account for deviations from classic mendelian inheritance, the concepts of reduced or incomplete penetrance (incomplete manifestation of the disorder in persons who have the abnormal genotype) and, conversely, phenocopies or sporadic ones (persons who do not have the abnormal genotype but who nevertheless exhibit the disorder) have been advanced. Both circumstances may be due to other genetic or nongenetic factors.

The MFP model stipulates multiple genes and random environmental effects, each making a small and additive contribution to phenotypic expression. When the genetic-environmental load exceeds a threshold, the clinical phenotype becomes manifest. Nongenetic factors, both those that are transmitted between generations as well as those that are not transmissible, can be accounted for in the model.

Both the SML and MFP models can be made more complex by incorporating other features, such as sex effect (assuming males have a different liability from females), severity-dependent thresholds (assuming different illness forms have different liability thresholds, for instance, bipolar disorder versus unipolar depression, the latter being considered a milder clinical variant), multiple alleles (SML model), more than one locus or gene (e.g., a two-locus model), graduated effects for the different genes involved (MFP model), and a "mixed" model combining SML and MFP formulations.

The application of statistical genetic techniques to family data on bipolar and related affective disorders has not resolved the underlying mode of inheritance (2,14,19,36). The failure to detect specific genetic mechanisms, particularly single genes, has been attributed primarily to diagnostic uncertainties and etiologic heterogeneity. It has become clear that additional genetic information, specifically biological and genetic marker data, is needed to complement and enrich the clinical diagnosis.

BIOLOGICAL MARKERS

Biological markers or endophenotypes (the exophenotype being the clinical condition) can be explored using diverse disciplines such as biochemistry (e.g., neurotransmitter enzymes, metabolites, and receptor proteins), endocrinology (e.g., hormones), and neurophysiology (e.g., electroencephalographic measures). To meet criteria for a vulnerability trait, the biological characteristic must distinguish affected persons from normal controls at the population level; it should be heritable and state independent (stable over time, regardless of clinical state), and it should segregate with the illness in families (37). Potential biological markers can be tested using standard statistical measures (37) or more involved methods, such as the statistical genetic models described earlier (9).

As reviewed (30), despite extensive efforts, no one biological trait has fulfilled all the aforementioned criteria. Biological characteristics that have been studied in this vein in bipolar illness include lithium transport in red blood cells, platelet imipramine binding, cholinergic rapid-eye-movement (REM) sleep induction, tyrosine excretion, plasma GABA, CSF 5-HIAA, lymphoblast beta receptors, platelet monoamine oxidase (MAO), and erythrocyte catechol-o-methyltransferase (COMT). Some characteristics, specifically lithium transport, cholinergic REM sleep induction, and plasma GABA, show some promise as potential biological markers but the available information, most notably family data, is incomplete.

GENETIC MARKERS

Definition and Principles

Arguably genetic marker strategies constitute the most definitive approach to disease-related genes. Genetic markers are inherited variations, or alleles, at specific chromosomal loci. The greater the variability among alleles (polymorphism), the greater the usefulness of the marker. The relation of genetic markers to a given disorder can be determined by linkage analysis. Linkage refers to the tendency of alleles at different loci to be co-inherited. The statistical measure of linkage is the lod score (the logarithm of the odds ratio between the probability of observing the data under the hypothesis of linkage and that of there being no linkage). A lod score greater than 3.0 (i.e., an odds ratio of 1,000:1 in favor of the linkage hypothesis) is considered sufficient evidence for linkage. A lod score smaller than -2.0 (odds ratio of 100:1 against the linkage hypothesis) speaks against a linkage being present. The distance between loci can be inferred from the recombination frequency (recombination is a rearrangement of alleles in the offspring generation due to exchange of material between homologous chromosomes during meiosis). The closer the loci are to each other, the less likely is recombination to occur between them. Thus, when the marker and the disease gene are linked, or co-inherited (as evidenced from a large enough lod score at a small recombination frequency), the marker signals the nearby presence of the disease gene and its approximate chromosomal location. At small recombination frequency, 1% recombination is equivalent to a distance of 1 centimorgan (one million nucleotides). The demonstration of linkage provides conclusive proof of single-gene inheritance since gene markers, by definition, have a mendelian mode of inheritance.

To locate particular genes, the markers are used to trace their pattern of inheritance in families. Linkage studies are most efficient in extended pedigrees with high density of illness. An alternative approach, known as the sib pair method, is based on pairs of affected siblings; it is easier to implement because it does not require multigeneration families, however, it is generally considered less efficient than the pedigree linkage strategy. Genetic markers can also be studied for association with the disorder of interest at the population level; for instance, studies of patients as compared with control groups. Such associations can be attributed to a causal relationship between the marker locus and the disease; alternatively, they can point to another gene nearby that may confer susceptibility to the illness.

These issues are discussed in greater detail elsewhere (4,32).

The "New Genetics"

Recent advances in molecular biology have opened new vistas for genetic marker studies. Prior to the introduction of recombinant DNA technology, inherited variations that could be used in these studies were confined to the classic or conventional markers, such as red blood cell antigens (i.e., blood groups), leukocyte antigens (HLA system), and serum proteins. These markers were of limited use owing to their paucity and small degree of polymorphism. Molecular genetic techniques have led to a dramatic expansion in the number of polymorphic genetic markers. These new DNA markers, also known as restriction fragment length polymorphisms (RFLPs), have generated a dense genomic map of genetic variations detectable by molecular genetic techniques (16). This new development virtually ensures the localization and, ultimately, identification of all major loci involved in genetic diseases. The powerful new techniques can eventually lead to (a) characterization of the faulty gene, (b) elucidation of its biological product, (c) refinement of diagnosis, and (d) improved genetic counseling.

Noteworthy advances using these methods are the localization of the genes for the neuropsychiatric disorders Huntington's disease and a familial form of Alzheimer's dementia, and the identification and characterization of the genes for Duchenne muscular dystrophy, neurofibromatosis, and cystic fibrosis. The genes for numerous other genetic conditions have been mapped in recent years using the new DNA technology.

Several categories of DNA markers can be considered: (a) Random or arbitrary polymorphic DNA sequences used in a systematic search throughout the human genome with no prior hypothesis concerning the disorder in question. (b) Candidate genes, namely, the genes encoding proteins of neurobiological significance (e.g., neuroreceptors, neurotransmitter enzymes, proteins that distinguish diseased from normal brains. (c) Markers selected from "candidate" chromosomal regions (e.g., cytogenetic abnormalities, such as deletions or translocation, found to segregate with the illness, may point to the location of the disease gene; epidemiological data on sex differences in prevalence and familial transmission would suggest the X-chromosome as a candidate region for the putative gene). These and related issues are reviewed in greater detail elsewhere (5,7,21,26,31,33).

Recent Findings

Genetic marker studies in bipolar affective illness have been in evidence for nearly two decades. However, most of these studies are of limited utility due to the paucity of polymorphic markers and potential methodological pitfalls concerning ascertainment of pedigrees, diagnostic issues, and statistical genetic techniques (see Methodological Issues section). As reviewed (8,30,38), these studies have led to inconsistent or equivocal results.

The recent convergence of modern diagnostic techniques, systematic methods for the collection of family data, molecular genetics, and advanced statistical methods for linkage analysis herald a new era in psychiatric genetics. Two recent studies may be perceived as the harbingers of the new era. These are the chromosome 11 linkage study in the Old Order Amish (17) and the X-linkage finding in a non-Ashkenazi Israeli population (10).

Aside from exploiting the new methdological advances, the two studies utilized populations particularly suitable for genetic linkage studies. Specifically, both the Amish and the non-Ashkenazi Israeli population are characterized by high geographic concentration, large extended pedigrees, stability and accessibility, and low rates of alcoholism and drug abuse, conditions known to confound the psychiatric diagnosis. The Amish, in addition, are a closed community descended from a small number of progenitors with little or no migration into or out of the community. Thus, they likely are genetically homogeneous. On the one hand, this should facilitate the search for the putative disease gene; on the other, the generalizability of genetic findings in this population can be questioned since the disease mutation may be unique to that particular gene pool.

Amish Study

The linkage study was based on one large composite family comprised of three interrelated families. The sample included 81 subjects including 19 affected and 62 mentally well members. Of the 19 affected subjects, 13 had some form of bipolar illness, one had atypical psychosis, and five had unipolar major depression. An additional five individuals were diagnosed with minor psychiatric conditions and were considered unaffected in the genetic analysis.

Using two DNA markers on the short arm of chromosome 11, insulin (INS), and the cellular oncogene Ha-ras-1 (HRAS1), the maximum lod score obtained in the Amish pedigree was 4.9. The investigators concluded that the affective disorder gene in their population is tightly linked to the HRAS1 locus (17). They further proposed that the structural gene encoding tyrosine hydroxylase (a major enzyme in the dopamine synthesis pathway) is a potential candidate gene for affective illness by virtue of its location in the same region as INS and HRAS1.

Unfortunately, the chromosome 11 finding has not fulfilled its initial promise. A subsequent extension and reanalysis of the linkage data have led to substantially reduced evidence of linkage (23). The outcome of the reanalysis has been attributed to changes in psychiatric status due to new illness onset, ambiguous or otherwise uninformative marker typing in the original analysis, and newly studied pedigree branches in which the purported gene does not segregate. In the light of this reanalysis, it may not be surprising that all efforts to replicate the chromosome 11 findings in other populations have failed (15,18,20,22,27).

X-Linkage Study

The X-linkage hypothesis of bipolar affective illness dates back nearly half a century. An excess of affected women and reduced rates of male-to-male transmission have been observed in some, but not all epidemiological and family studies. Both circumstances are compatible with X-linked dominant inheritance. Thus, the X-chromosome constitutes a plausible "candidate" genomic region for linkage analysis of bipolar illness.

Most linkage studies with X-chromosome classic markers have been either anecdotal or inconclusive. Additionally, methodological uncertainties concerning ascertainment, statistical analysis, and the X-chromosome map may have cast doubt on some of the early findings. The data and the methodological issues involved were discussed in detail elsewhere (8,38). Nevertheless, these early indications have generated sufficient impetus for pursuing this intriguing hypothesis.

To redress these methodological problems and to reexamine the X-linkage hypothesis, we have applied rigorous methodology to a new series of pedigrees (10). Five multigeneration families with high illness density were identified from a large sample of psychiatric patients in Israel. The families contained 161 adult individuals, 47 of whom were ill with bipolar illness or related affective disorder. Twenty-two of the affecteds had some form of bipolar illness; the remainder had unipolar depression or schizoaffective-depressed disorder. Four of the five pedigrees were non-Ashkenazi (of Mediterranean or Asian origin), and one pedigree was Ashkenazi (of European extraction). The pedigrees segregated color blindness or glucose-6-phosphate dehydrogenase (G6PD) deficiency, two classical genetic markers located in close proximity on the distal long arm of the X-chromosome (Xq28 region). The results of the linkage analysis showed close linkage of bipolar affective illness to the color blindness-G6PD region. The maximum lod score ranged from 7.52 (assuming homogeneity of the sample) to 9.17 (assuming heterogeneity). Only the non-Ashkenazi pedigrees displayed linkage thus leading to the speculation that X-linkage is more pronounced in the non-Ashkenazi and, possibly, other Mediterranean and Asian populations.

A subsequent study of a Belgian population (29) showed linkage between bipolar disorder and a Factor IX (F9) DNA marker in the Xq27 region. Although the F9 locus is in the same general region as the color blindness-G6PD loci, it is separated from that region by 30 to 40 centimorgans. To determine the compatibility of the Israeli and Belgian findings, it will be necessary to study additional DNA markers spanning the Xq27-28 region. It may also be that the F9 linkage represents a second, independent locus for bipolar illness on the X-chromosome.

Taken together, the various X-linked pedigrees reported to date strongly support X-linked transmission in a subset of bipolar affective illness. The evidence is reviewed in more detail elsewhere (5,6,8,38).

METHODOLOGICAL ISSUES

Bipolar affective illness, much like other complex disorders, poses challenges for the genetic researcher. Several methodological issues need to be taken into account. Foremost among these are diagnostic uncertainties, unclear mode of inheritance, etiological heterogeneity, cohort effect, and assortative mating.

The bipolar spectrum displays variable expressivity and its diagnostic boundaries are unclear. Bipolar-related conditions encompass bipolar I (depression and frank mania), bipolar II (depression and hypomania), schizoaffective, and unipolar depressive disorder. Minor affective conditions, such as cyclothymia, are also considered part of the spectrum. These disorders aggregate in the families of bipolar probands. However, with the possible exception of bipolar-I disorder, generally regarded as the "core phenotype," these clinical syndromes are likely heterogeneous and include diagnostic misclassifications also known as phenocopies or false positives (e.g., cases erroneously considered affected). False negatives (e.g., cases misclassified as unaffected) comprise the other type of phenotypic misclassifications. Both types of diagnostic misclassification can lead to spurious linkage findings and to biased estimates of genetic parameters. By and large, false positives have a greater impact on the outcome of linkage analysis in that they may reduce the lod score and generate false negative linkage results (i.e., missing a genuine linkage finding). False negatives can have an undue influence on the analysis especially at high penetrance and age values. The question of the phenotype is compounded by comorbidity (the coexistence of affective and other conditions, such as anxiety, panic, and eating disorders) and clinical variation within diagnostic categories (e.g., age of onset, symptom profile, response to treatment), which may contribute to phenotypic uncertainties.

As discussed earlier (see Genetic Markers section), linkage analysis requires specification of mode of inheritance (specifically, the assumption that the disease is caused by a single mendelian locus) and related genetic parameters, such as penetrance and allele frequency. Since the correct mode of inheritance parameters is not known for bipolar illness, these parameters will likely be misspecified in the lod score analysis. Another possible scenario is an interaction of alleles at more than one locus (i.e., the joint action of several genes). The primary effect of such misclassifications is to reduce the lod score, thereby diminishing the evidence of linkage (should linkage be present).

Etiologic heterogeneity, especially when the proportion of linked pedigrees is small, complicates linkage analysis. Specifically, genuine linkage may be missed entirely unless a large sample of families can be studied. Etiologic heterogeneity may thus lead to reduced evidence of linkage and failed attempts to replicate positive linkage findings. Since bipolar affective illness is considered etiologically heterogeneous, this methodological issue is of paramount significance.

Finally, some observations concerning bipolar disorder that confound genetic marker studies are cohort effect and assortative mating. Cohort effect refers to the increased rate of the illness over time or across generations. It has been ascribed, among other factors, to interaction between genetic vulnerability and environmental or cultural effects. Assortative mating refers to marriages in which both partners (or their relatives) are affected. The overall effect of these phenomena would be to mask the presence of linkage—cohort effect by leading to misspecified mode of inheritance parameters (specifically the penetrance), and assortative mating by increasing the extent of genetic heterogeneity within pedigrees through the genetic input from persons marrying in.

These methodological issues and their specific relevance to bipolar illness are reviewed in detail elsewhere (11,32,34).

IMPLICATIONS AND FUTURE COURSE

Recent advances in diagnostic nomenclature, statistical genetic techniques, and molecular biology portend well for psychiatric genetics. Some of the recent linkage findings attest to the potential embedded in these new approaches. The implications of these advances for future studies can by summarized as follows.

Some of the aforementioned methodological problems can be rectified (11). For example, diagnostic misclassifications involving phenocopies (false positives) can be minimized by focusing on a narrow definition of the phenotype (i.e., bipolar-I disorders). It may also be fruitful to incorporate estimates of phenotypic uncertainty based, for example, on clinical predictors of diagnostic stability (35) in the linkage analysis (12). The question of false negatives resulting from variable penetrance can be obviated by using a "penetrance-free" model whereby unaffected individuals are practically excluded from the analysis.

As for etiologic heterogeneity and uncertain mode of inheritance, new mathematical models are being developed to address these questions. These include simultaneous search (24), a method that utilizes a complete RFLP map of the human genome to determine if several loci can jointly account for the genetics of the disorder being studied; interval mapping (24), designed to determine if a complex disorder maps in a particular genomic interval; and an extension of the sib pair method (39), which includes features of the lod score method while retaining some robustness with respect to uncertain estimates of genetic parameters.

Statistical methods for incorporating cohort effect in linkage analysis (for instance, by introducing penetrances dependent on cohort) are available (11,42). Methods concerning assortative mating are also evolving. However, at the present time, a conservative approach would entail exclusion of pedigree branches with evidence of bilineal transmission.

The introduction of these methods will likely avert spurious linkage results and will facilitate replication of linkage findings. Once linkage has been found, the following course of action may be considered.

First, replication in other pedigrees would be most desirable. However, in the event of substantial heterogeneity, replication will likely entail a lengthy and laborious process requiring considerable genetic resources. To increase confidence in the reported linkage, other steps can be entertained, such as typing adjacent DNA markers in the genomic region thought to contain the putative gene, extending the pedigrees to determine if linkage exists in other family branches, and updating the clinical material as a safeguard against diagnostic misclassifications. Interestingly, similar measures have led to the demise of the linkage finding in the Old Order Amish (23).

Second, the genetic boundaries encompassing the disease gene can be delineated by saturating the region with RFLPs and defining the smallest possible genetic region in which the putative gene lies. As X-linkage is the only viable linkage remaining at the time of writing, current efforts in our laboratory aim at fine resolution genetic and physical mapping of the candidate genomic region on the distal long arm of the X-chromosome. This, in turn, will be followed by more focused attempts at isolating the gene, such as screening for subtle chromosomal aberrations (e.g., microdeletions that may involve the putative gene) by Southern blotting of standard and pulsed field DNA gels and looking for candidate transcripts. A variety of methods are currently available at several levels for homing in on disease genes, and rapid advances are almost routine. The X-chromosome is a host to numerous disease-related genes; the information gathered so far, coupled with evolving methodologies, will likely expedite our efforts (25). The isolation and cloning of the disease gene will have major implications for prevention and treatment. It should also provide a powerful tool for (a) genetic diagnosis, (b) genetic counseling, and (c) assessing the proportion of a particular genetic type in the ill population, thereby unraveling etiological heterogeneity.

Third, a linkage finding can be instrumental in refining the clinical diagnosis. For example, the diagnostic boundaries used to define the linked phenotype can be broadened to determine if other clinical or personality features are part of the genetic spectrum. Also, the genetically linked form of the illness may have unique clinical features that sets it apart from other genetic or nongenetic forms. Thus, genetic tools can be used for dissecting the phenotype and shedding light on etiologic heterogeneity. Preliminary evidence from our ongoing studies indicates that the X-linked form of bipolar affective illness may represent a more severe form of the disease as evidenced, for example, from early age of onset (12).

Fourth, aside from elucidating genetic etiology, gene markers can provide insights into gene-environment interaction through prospective studies of at-risk individuals identified by the linked marker. Such studies can be used to discern specific environmental factors that interact with the genetic predisposition to prevent or trigger the development of the illness.

Finally, the identification of a particular linkage should not supplant the search for other disease genes that may account for the (nonallelic) genetic heterogeneity of bipolar illness. Other susceptibility genes may act independently or interact with genes residing elsewhere in the genome; a complete genomic map could furnish a broad perspective on the mechanisms underlying the various genes that confer susceptibility for bipolar affective disorder.

SUMMARY

The bipolar affective spectrum is clinically heterogeneous and genetically complex. Current methods for assessment and analysis of familial traits with variable phenotypic expression and unclear mode of inheritance are reviewed. Recent evidence for a major gene localized on the X-chromosome is presented and other linkage findings are discussed. The limitations and prospects of psychiatric genetics are discussed in the light of recent advances in diagnostic nomenclature, statistical genetic techniques, and molecular biology. Methodological uncertainties notwithstanding, the powerful new techniques in genetic research portend well for unraveling the genetics of bipolar affective illness.

ACKNOWLEDGMENT

Supported by grants MH42535, MH44115, MH36963, MH43979, and a Research Scientist Development Award MH00176 from the NIMH, and grant No. 3350 from the U.S.-Israel Binational Science Foundation.

GLOSSARY

Genetic probe Sequence of DNA or RNA used to identify genetic markers.
LOD score A statistical measure of linkage.

REFERENCES

1. Andreasen, N. C., Rice, J., Endicott, J., Coryell, W., Grove, W. M., and Reich, T. (1987): Familial rates of affective disorder: a report from the National Institute of Mental Health Collaborative Study. *Arch. Gen. Psychiatry*, 44:461–469.
2. Baron, M. (1983): Polarity and sex effect in genetic transmission of affective disorders: the single major locus hypothesis. *Hum. Hered.*, 33:112–118.
3. Baron, M. (1986): Genetics of schizophrenia. I. Familial patterns and mode of inheritance. *Biol. Psychiatry*, 21:1051–1066.
4. Baron, M. (1986): Genetics of schizophrenia. II. Vulnerability traits and gene markers. *Biol. Psychiatry*, 21:1189–1211.
5. Baron, M. (1989): Molecular genetic studies of affective disorders. In: *Neuropsychopharmacology*, edited by W. E. Bunney, Jr., H. Hippius, G. Laakmann, and M. Schmauss, pp. 108–116. Springer-Verlag, New York.
6. Baron, M. (1989): X-linkage studies in affective disorders. In: *New Directions in Affective Disorders*, edited by B. Lerer and S. Gershon, pp. 188–191. Springer-Verlag, New York.
7. Baron, M., and Rainer, J. D. (1988): Molecular genetics and human disease: implications for modern psychiatric research and practice. *Br. J. Psychiatry*, 152:741–753.
8. Baron, M., Rainer, J. D., and Risch, N. (1981): X-linkage in bipolar affective illness: perspective on genetic heterogeneity, pedigree analysis and the X-chromosome map. *J. Affect. Dis.*, 3:141–157.
9. Baron, M., Risch, N., Levitt, M., and Gruen, R. (1985): Genetic analysis of platelet monoamine oxidase activity in families of schizophrenic patients. *J. Psychiatr. Res.*, 19:9–22.
10. Baron, M., Risch, N., Hamburger, R., et al. (1987): Genetic linkage between X-chromosome markers and bipolar affective illness. *Nature*, 326:289–292.
11. Baron, M., Endicott, J., and Ott, J. Genetic linkage in mental illness: limitations and prospects. *Br. J. Psychiatry (in press)*.
12. Baron, M., Hamburger, R., Sandkuyl, L. A., et al. X-linked manic depression: phenotypic variation and gene localization. *Acta Psychiatr. Scand. (in press)*.
13. Bertelsen, A. (1979): A Danish twin study of manic-depressive disorders. In: *Origin, Prevention and Treatment of Affective Disorders*, edited by M. Schou and E. Stromgren, pp. 227–245. Academic Press, London.
14. Bucher, K. D., and Elston, R. C. (1981): The transmission of manic-depressive illness. I. Theory, description of the model and summary of results. *J. Psychiatr. Res.*, 16:53–63.
15. Detera-Wadleigh, S., Benettini, W. H., Goldin, L., Boorman, D. G., Anderson, S., and Gershon, E. S. (1987): Close linkage of C-Harvey-ras-1 and the Insulin gene to affective disorder is ruled out in three North American pedigrees. *Nature*, 325:806–808.
16. Donis-Keller, H., Helms, C., Green, P., et al. (1989): A human genome linkage map with more than 500 RFLP loci and average marker spacing of 6 centimorgans. *Cytogenet. Cell Genet.*, 51:991 (A2039).
17. Egeland, J. A., Gerhard, D. S., Pauls, D. L., et al. (1987): Bipolar affective disorders linked to DNA markers on chromosome 11. *Nature*, 325:783–787.
18. Gerhard, D. S., Todd, R., Devor, E., and Reich, T. (1988): Linkage analysis of polymorphic markers on two chromosomes with affective disorder. *Am. J. Hum. Genet.*, 43:A144.
19. Gershon, E. S., Hamovit, J., Guroff, J. L., et al. (1982): A family study of schizoaffective, bipolar I, bipolar II, unipolar, and normal control probands. *Arch. Gen. Psychiatry*, 39:1157–1167.
20. Gill, M., McKeon, P., and Humphries, P. (1988): Linkage analysis of manic depression in an Irish family using H-ras-1 and INS DNA markers. *J. Med. Genet.*, 25:634–635.
21. Gurling, H. M. D. (1985): Application of molecular biology to mental illness. Analysis of genomic DNA and brain mRNA. *Psychiatr. Dev.*, 3:257–273.

22. Hodkinson, S., Sherrington, R., Gurling, H., et al. (1978): Molecular genetic evidence for the heterogeneity in manic depression. *Nature*, 325:805–806.
23. Kelsoe, J. R., Ginns, E. I., Egeland, J. A., et al. (1989): Reevaluation of the linkage relationship between chromosome 11p loci and the gene for bipolar affective disorder in the Old Order Amish. *Nature*, 342:238–243.
24. Lander, E., and Botstein, D. (1986): Strategies for studying heterogeneous genetic traits in humans by using a linkage map of restriction fragment length polymorphisms. *Proc. Natl. Acad. Sci. USA*, 83:7353–7357.
25. Mandel, J.-L., Willard, H. F., Nussbaum, R. L., Romeo, G., Puck, J. M., and Davies, K. E. (1989): Report of the committee on the genetic constitution of the X chromosome. *Cytogenet. Cell Genet.*, 51:384–437.
26. Martin, J. B. (1987): Molecular genetics: application to the clinical neurosciences. *Science*, 238: 765–772.
27. Mellon, C. D., Byerley, W. F., Holik, J. J., Leppert, M., and White, R. (1989): Linkage analysis of the 11 pter region in manic-depressive illness. 142nd Annual Meeting of the American Psychiatric Association, San Francisco.
28. Mendlewicz, J., and Rainer, J. D. (1977): Adoption study supporting genetic transmission in manic-depressive illness. *Nature*, 268:32–35.
29. Mendlewicz, J., Simon, P., Sevy, S., et al. (1987): Polymorphic DNA markers on X-chromosome and manic depression. *Lancet*, 2:1230–1232.
30. Nurnberger, J. I., Jr., and Gershon, E. S. (1983): Genetics of affective disorders. In: *Handbook of Affective Disorders*, edited by E. Paykel, pp. 126–145. Churchill Livingstone, London.
31. Orkin, S. H. (1986): Reverse genetics and human disease. *Cell*, 47:845–850.
32. Ott, J. (1985): *Analysis of Human Genetic Linkage*. The Johns Hopkins University Press, Baltimore.
33. Pearson, P. L., Kidd, K. K., and Willard, H. F. (1987): Report of the committee on human gene mapping by recombinant DNA techniques. *Cytogenet. Cell Genet.*, 46:390–566.
34. Rice, J., and Risch, N. (1989): Genetic analysis of the affective disorders: summary of Genetic Analysis Workshop (GAW) 5. *Genet. Epidemiol.*, 6:161–177.
35. Rice, J., Endicott, J., Knesvich, M. A., and Rochberg, N. J. (1987): The estimation of diagnostic sensitivity using stability data: an application to major affective disorder. *J. Psychiatr. Res.*, 21: 397–346.
36. Rice, J., Reich, T., Andreasen, N. C., et al. (1987): The familial transmission of bipolar illness. *Arch. Gen. Psychiatry*, 44:441–447.
37. Rieder, R. O., and Gershon, E. S. (1978): Genetic strategies in biological psychiatry. *Arch. Gen. Psychiatry*, 35:866–873.
38. Risch, N., and Baron, M. (1982): X-linkage and genetic heterogeneity in bipolar-related major affective illness: re-analysis of linkage data. *Ann. Hum. Genet.*, 46:153–166.
39. Sandkuyl, L. A. (1989): Extended sib-pair analysis of disease with a complex mode of inheritance. First World Congress on Psychiatric Genetics, Cambridge, England.
40. Thompson, E. A. (1986): *Pedigree Analysis in Human Genetics*. The Johns Hopkins University Press, Baltimore.
41. Tsuang, M. T., Winokur, G., and Grove, R. (1980): Morbidity risks of schizophrenia and affective disorders among first-degree relatives of patients with schizophrenia, mania, depression and surgical conditions. *Br. J. Psychiatry*, 137:497–504.
42. VanErdewegh, P. (1989): Linkage analysis with cohort effects: an application to X-linkage. *Genet. Epidemiol.*, 6:271–276.

Genes, Brain, and Behavior, edited by
P. R. McHugh and V. A. McKusick.
Raven Press, Ltd., New York © 1991.

Behavioral Genetics

Robert Plomin

Center for Developmental and Health Genetics, College of Health and Human Development, The Pennsylvania State University, University Park, Pennsylvania 16802

> A devil, a born devil, on whose nature
> Nurture can never stick; on whom my pains
> Humanely taken, all, all lost, quite lost.
>
> Shakespeare, *The Tempest*

Nearly 400 years ago, Shakespeare brought the words *nature* and *nurture* into juxtaposition in *The Tempest* with Prospero speaking of Caliban. This example of nurture in conflict with nature became the thrust of the alliterative phrase, "nature-nurture," which was coined by Francis Galton, Darwin's cousin, over a century ago. Joining the two words created a fission that exploded into the longest-lived controversy in the behavioral sciences. As with Shakespeare, the hyphen in nature-nurture connoted the implicit conjunction *versus*. The appropriate conjunction is *and*.

Behavioral genetics is the study of nature and nurture in relation to behavior. Behavior is a *phenotype*, that is, an observable characteristic we can measure. The basic principles of heredity are the same regardless of the phenotypes we choose to study. On the other hand, behavior is not just another phenotype. Because behavior involves the functioning of the whole organism rather than the action of a single molecule, a single cell, or a single organ, behavior is the most complex phenomenon that can be studied genetically. Unlike some physical characteristics, behavior is dynamic, changing in response to the environment—indeed, behavior is at the cutting edge of evolution for this very reason.

Behavior is especially difficult for genetic analysis for three additional reasons. Unlike the characteristics that Mendel studied in the edible pea such as smooth versus wrinkled seeds, most behaviors and behavioral problems are not distributed in either-or dichotomies—we are not either smooth or wrinkled psychologically. Second, unlike classic mendelian disorders such as Huntington disease that are caused by a single gene with little effect of genetic or environmental background, most behavioral traits appear to be influenced by many genes, each with small effects. The third reason is that behavior is substantially influenced by nongenetic factors.

The purpose of this chapter is to provide an introduction to the theory, methods, and results of behavioral genetics that focuses on these issues and to consider their implications for molecular biology approaches to the study of behavior. But, first, why study behavior if it is so complex? The answer lies in the importance of behavior rather than in its usefulness for revealing how genes work. Some of society's most pressing problems are behavioral problems such as drug abuse, mental illness, and mental retardation. Behavior is also key in health as well as illness, in abilities as well as disabilities, and in the personal pluses of life such as sense of well-being, love, and work.

THEORY AND METHODS

Although the effects of major genes and chromosomal abnormalities on behavior have been studied, most behavioral genetic research employs the theory and methods of quantitative genetics. Quantitative genetics emerged in the early 1900s from disagreements between the mendelians, who rediscovered Mendel's laws of inheritance, and the biometricians, who believed that Mendel's laws, derived from experiments with qualitative characteristics in lower organisms, were not applicable to complex characteristics of higher organisms, characteristics that are nearly always distributed continuously in a normal, bell-shaped curve. Both sides were right and wrong. The mendelians were correct in arguing that heredity works the way Mendel said it worked, but they were wrong in assuming that complex characteristics will show simple mendelian patterns of inheritance. The biometricians were right in arguing that complex characteristics are distributed quantitatively, not qualitatively, but they were wrong in arguing that Mendel's laws of inheritance did not apply to higher organisms. The resolution to the disagreement, and the essence of quantitative genetic theory developed by Fisher (21) over 70 years ago, is that Mendel's laws of discrete inheritance also apply to normally distributed complex characteristics if we assume that many genes, each with a small effect, combine to produce observable differences among individuals in a population.

The methods derived from this theory are referred to as quantitative genetic because they identify genetic influence even when many genes affect a behavior and when nongenetic factors are also important. In quantitative genetics, the phrase "genetic influence" refers to genetic variability among individuals that accounts for observed variability in behavior, that is, it does not address the genetic constants of nonvarying DNA that play the same role for everyone in our species. Quantitative genetic studies write the "bottom line" of heritable genetic influence on behavior, regardless of the complexity of genetic modes of action or the number of genes involved. They do not, however, tell us which genes are responsible for genetic influence. In the last section of this chapter, the use of molecular biology techniques to begin to identify specific genes responsible for genetic variance on behavior is discussed.

Quantitative genetic methods employed to study animal behavior include artificial selection and comparisons among inbred strains. Selection studies provide the clearest evidence for genetic influence: If a trait is heritable, it can be successfully bred, as animal breeders have known for centuries. The results of artificial selection can be seen most dramatically in differences in behavior as well as physique among dog breeds, differences that testify to the great range of genetic variability within a species. Selection studies in the laboratory still provide the most convincing demonstrations of genetic influence on behavior. For example, one of the largest and longest selection studies of mice selected high and low lines for activity in a brightly lit open field, which is an aversive situation for nocturnal rodents and thought to assess emotional reactivity (12). After 30 generations of selection, a 30-fold difference exists between the activity of the high and low lines and there is no overlap between them. Similar results have been found for most mouse behaviors subjected to selection in the laboratory; many behaviors of rats and *Drosophila* have also been bred successfully (47).

Inbred strains are created by mating brother to sister for at least 20 generations. This intensive inbreeding eliminates heterozygosity, which results in animals that are virtually identical genetically. Because inbred strains differ genetically from each other, genetically influenced traits will show average differences between inbred strains reared in the same laboratory environment. Comparisons among inbred strains also point to significant genetic influence for most behaviors that have been examined.

For human behavior, no methods as powerful as selection or strain studies exist because the human gene pool cannot be manipulated experimentally nor can humans be reared under controlled laboratory conditions. Human behavioral genetic research relies on family, adoption, and twin designs and combinations of these designs. Family studies assess the extent of resemblance for genetically related individuals, although they cannot disentangle possible environmental sources of resemblance. That is the point of adoption studies. Genetically related individuals adopted apart assess the extent to which familial resemblance is due to hereditary resemblance. For example, for height, first-degree relatives, whose coefficient of genetic relatedness is 0.50, correlate about 0.45, whether reared together or adopted apart.

Twin studies are like natural experiments in which the resemblance of genetically identical pairs of individuals, identical twins, is compared to the resemblance of first-degree relatives, fraternal twins. If heredity affects a behavior, identical twins must be more similar than fraternal twins. For example, identical twins correlate about 0.90 for height and the correlation for fraternal twins is 0.45.

As in studies of nonhuman animals, family, adoption, and twin data can be used to go beyond assessing the statistical significance of genetic influence to estimate the magnitude of genetic effects (the effect size). For example, adoption and twin data for height suggest that heritability, the proportion of phenotypic variance that can be accounted for by genetic factors, is 90%. For details of the methods of behavioral genetics and their problems, as well as important recent advances such as model-testing, multivariate, and longitudinal analyses, see (47).

EVIDENCE FOR GENETIC INFLUENCE ON HUMAN BEHAVIOR

What do these methods tell us about the role of inheritance in human behavior? This section provides a very brief overview of results of family, twin, and adoption studies emphasizing focal areas of research in cognitive abilities and disabilities, personality, and psychopathology. For details and documentation, see (47).

Cognitive Abilities and Disabilities

For general cognitive ability (IQ), first-degree relatives living together correlate about 0.40, adopted-apart first-degree relatives correlate about 0.20, and adoptive parents and their adopted children correlate about 0.20 (7). In over 30 twin studies involving more than 10,000 pairs of twins, identical and fraternal twin correlations average 0.85 and 0.60, respectively. These results, and model-fitting analyses that analyze all of the data simultaneously, are consistent with heritabilities of about 50% (10).

Specific cognitive abilities such as verbal ability and spatial ability show as much genetic influence as IQ; some types of memory ability appear to be less influenced by heredity than other specific cognitive abilities (44). Measures of academic achievement also show genetic influence, and recent multivariate research suggests that genetic effects on academic achievement tests overlap substantially with genetic effects on cognitive abilities (57). Surprisingly, there are no twin or adoption studies on the important problem of mental retardation.

Personality

Twin and adoption studies of personality questionnaires typically yield heritability estimates in the range of 20% to 50%. Traits such as activity level, emotional reactivity (neuroticism), and sociability/shyness (extraversion) have accumulated the best evidence for significant genetic influence (8,17). For example, four twin studies in four countries involving over 30,000 pairs of twins yield heritability estimates of about 50% for neuroticism and extraversion (33). Adoption studies of first-degree relatives suggest lower estimates of heritability for these traits than do twin studies—about 30% rather than 50% heritability. This may be due to nonadditive genetic variance (especially higher order interactions among loci called epistasis) that covaries completely for identical twins but contributes little to the resemblance of first-degree relatives (46).

Psychopathology

In the past, most research on psychopathology focused on schizophrenia; attention has now turned to the affective disorders, which include major depressive disorder and manic-depressive disorder.

In 14 studies involving nearly 20,000 first-degree relatives of schizophrenics, their risk for schizophrenia was 8%, eight times greater than the risk for individuals chosen randomly from the population (23). Twin studies suggest that familial resemblance for schizophrenia is due to heredity rather than to shared family environment. For example, the largest and most recent twin study involves all male twins who were veterans of World War II (29). Twin concordances were 30.9% for 164 pairs of identical twins and 6.5% for 268 pairs of fraternal twins. The same study indicates that genetic influence on schizophrenia exceeds that for common medical conditions such as diabetes mellitus (18.8% concordance for identical twins vs 7.9% for fraternal twins), ulcers (23.8% vs 14.8%), chronic obstructive pulmonary disease (11.8% vs 8.2%), hypertension (25.9% vs 10.8%), and ischemic heart disease (29.1% vs 18.3%). Adoption studies of schizophrenia support the twin findings of genetic influence (23,28).

The goal of much current research in psychopathology is to break down the apparent heterogeneity of psychoses in order to find etiologically distinct subtypes. For example, it is widely accepted that the classical subtypes of schizophrenia do not breed true (20), as seen most dramatically in a follow-up of the Genain quadruplets who were concordant for schizophrenia but showed variable symptoms (14).

Genetic effects on schizophrenia appear to be independent of genetic effects on the affective disorders, and unipolar depression appears to be distinct from manic-depressive disorder (60). The most recent family study of unipolar depression involved 235 probands with major depressive disorder and their 826 first-degree relatives (48). Major depression was diagnosed for 13% of the male relatives and for 30% of the female relatives. The familial risk for bipolar illness is lower, 5.8% in seven studies of 2,500 first-degree relatives of bipolar probands, with no gender difference in risk. A recent family study of 187 families of bipolar probands reported a 5.7% risk of bipolar illness in 557 first-degree relatives as compared with a risk of 1.1% in a control sample (49). Twin results for affective disorders suggest greater genetic influence than for schizophrenia, but adoption studies indicate less genetic influence (34). In the most recent adoption study, affective disorders were diagnosed in only 5.2% of biological relatives of affectively ill adoptees, although this risk is greater than the risk of 2.3% found in the biological relatives of control adoptees (62).

Much less behavioral genetic research has considered psychopathology other than schizophrenia and the affective psychoses. For example, we know that alcoholism runs in families—about 25% of the male relatives of alcoholics are themselves alcoholics, as compared with fewer than 5% of the males in the general population, but surprisingly little is known about the relative contributions made by nature and nurture to this familial resemblance. Although twin studies of normal drinkers show substantial genetic influence on the amount of alcohol consumed, no twin studies of diagnosed alcoholism have been reported. Adoption studies suggest that alcoholism may run in families for genetic reasons, at least for males (6). Other areas of current research in behavioral genetics include anorexia, antisocial personality disorder, anxiety disorder, attention deficit disorder, autism, somatization disorder, which involves multiple and chronic physical complaints of unknown origin, and Tourette's syndrome, which is characterized by chronic motor and phonic tics (34).

EVIDENCE FOR NONGENETIC INFLUENCE

The term *quantitative genetics* is misleading because the theory and its methods are as informative about environmental components of variance as they are about genetic factors. This feature of behavioral genetic research yields an important lesson for research on behavior: The same data reviewed above provide the best available evidence for the importance of nongenetic factors in the etiology of individual differences in behavior. Heritability estimates for selection and strain studies of animal behavior and for twin and adoption studies of human behavior rarely exceed 50% (47), meaning that nongenetic factors are at least as important as genetic factors in producing behavioral variability. It is difficult to assess the heritability of disorders such as schizophrenia because the data are cast as dichotomies and expressed in terms of concordance. Nonetheless, nongenetic factors are at least as important here. Consider schizophrenia. Although first-degree relatives are 50% similar genetically, over 90% of schizophrenics have no schizophrenic first-degree relative. Identical twins make this point even more dramatically. The risk of 30% for an identical cotwin of a schizophrenic far exceeds the population risk of 1%, but it is a long way from the 100% concordance expected if schizophrenia as currently diagnosed were entirely a transmissible genetic disorder. There is no way to explain such substantial discordance for identical twins for schizophrenia other than by nongenetic factors.

MULTIPLE GENES

Another implication of quantitative genetic analyses of behavior is that genetic influence appears to involve many genes rather than one or two major genes. The strongest evidence for multiple-gene influence on behavior comes from selection studies. Despite intense selection pressure, response to selection continues unabated during the course of most selection studies of behavior. If only one or two major genes were responsible for genetic effects on these behaviors, the relevant alleles would be sorted into the high and low lines in a few generations.

Family studies of mice have also provided test crosses used to explore transmission consistent with a single-gene model. Hundreds of single-locus, recessive mutations have been found that result in neurological defects such as the gene responsible for head shaking and rapid circling in "waltzer" mice. However, normal behavioral variability has not shown major-gene effects. These results broach an important issue: Although any one of many genes can disrupt behavioral development, the normal range of behavioral variation appears to be orchestrated by a system of many genes, each with small effect.

Crosses and backcrosses between inbred strains and their progeny have also been used to find patterns of inheritance consistent with single-gene transmission, but this approach in fact has little power to discriminate single-gene from multiple-gene transmission. A powerful strategy to uncover major-gene effects in animal behavior is the recombinant inbred (RI) strain method (1). The word "recombinant" here does not refer to recombinant DNA—RI lines were developed before recombinant DNA was known. RI lines are different inbred strains that were derived from separate brother-sister pairs from the same genetically segregating F_2 generation (crosses among hybrid offspring of two inbred strains). They are called recombinant inbred strains because the F_2 generation from which they are derived has recombined parts of chromosomes from the parental strains. If a single gene is responsible for a behavior that differs between the two parental strains, half of the RI strains should be like one parent and half like the other. In other words, there should be no intermediate phenotypes if just one locus is involved, because each RI strain will be homozygous for the allele of either one or the other parental strain. In line with results of selection studies, few behaviors studied in recombinant inbred strains have indicated major-gene effects.

The most direct evidence for multiple-gene influences on complex characteristics comes from research on plants. For example, the results of a study of associations between 20 electrophoretic genetic markers and 82 quantitative traits in maize (18) can be summarized as follows: (a) Significant associations were found for each of the 82 quantitative traits; (b) the maximum variance of any quantitative trait explained by a single marker was 16%; (c) over half of the significant associations accounted for less than 1% of the trait variance; (d) only 5% of the marker loci accounted for more than 5% of the variance; and (e) together, the genetic markers predicted between 8% and 37% of the variance of a subset of 25 relatively independent traits, which is most of the genetic variance for these traits. It seems unlikely that behavior is any less complex than these quantitative traits in plants.

Such powerful approaches to the identification of major-gene effects are not available for human behavior, but as in selection and RI strain analyses of the behavior of nonhuman animals, human behavioral variation in the normal range shows no evidence of major-gene effects. However, as in the mouse studies of behavior, many rare genes have been found that disrupt normal cognitive development in humans. For example, of the thousands of single-gene effects identified for human beings, more than 100 list lowered IQ scores as a clinical symptom (36). Although these recessive alleles have devastating effects for homozygous individuals, they are rare and thus can account for only a minuscule portion of IQ variance in the population. For example, the fragile-X marker, which accounts for the excess of mild mental retardation in males (39), cannot account for much IQ variance in the population because its incidence is less than 1 in 1,000 and many males with the fragile-X marker do not show lowered IQ (2). A better example is phenylketonuria (PKU). PKU occurs in the homozygous recessive condition only in about 1 in 10,000 births, and the severe retardation that would develop for these individuals is thwarted by dietary intervention. However, about 1 in 50 births are heterozygous carriers and there is evidence that heterozygotes have a slight lowering of IQ (3).

Thus, the PKU allele might account for a small portion of variation in IQ scores in the normal range.

The hundred or more rare recessive alleles that can in the homozygous condition dramatically lower IQ scores are probably just the most easily noticed tip of the iceberg of genetic variability. We can expect that many more alleles nudge cognitive development up or down and do not show such striking single-gene effects for certain individuals. That is, genetic variation on normal cognitive development is likely to involve more than just the sum of many single-gene disorders that seriously disrupt normal cognitive development of a few individuals. It is not the case that we are identical genetically with the exception of major mutational flaws: Many loci are polymorphic and many of these are likely to contribute to normal variability in behaviors as complex as cognitive abilities and disabilities. The statement made earlier in relation to mouse behavior bears reiteration: Although any one of many genes can disrupt behavioral development, the normal range of behavioral variation appears to be orchestrated by a system of many genes, each with small effect.

Continuing with IQ scores as an example, there is evidence that severe retardation (IQ lower than 50) differs etiologically from mild retardation (IQ between 50 and 70 [45]). For example, severely retarded children have siblings with IQs in the normal range, whereas mildly retarded children have siblings who are mildly retarded on average (38). The lack of familial resemblance for severe retardation suggests that unique genetic and environmental trauma is at work such as spontaneous mutations, chromosomal anomalies, and perinatal accidents. Mild retardation, on the other hand, appears to be just the low end of the IQ distribution, with the same familial resemblance and presumably the same mix of genetic and environmental influences as the rest of the IQ distribution. Here, it makes more sense to think about heritable influences that involve the joint action of many genes each with small effects, and perhaps different sets of genes for different individuals.

In addition to such conceptual arguments is the lack of evidence for major-gene effects on normal variability in behaviors such as cognitive ability. For example, earlier reports of sex linkage for spatial ability have been disconfirmed (13). Common cognitive problems such as reading disability have also shown no evidence of major-gene effects. For example, an early report of linkage for reading disability on chromosome 15 (53) is in doubt (31), with only 1 in 21 families showing near-significant LOD scores (54). The domain of personality has also yielded no evidence for major-gene effects from segregation, pedigree, or linkage studies.

Major-gene linkages have, however, been reported for psychopathology. The most well-known report of linkage for a behavioral disorder using RFLP markers is the first: In 1987, manic-depressive illness was reported to be linked to a dominant gene on the short arm of chromosome 11 in an Amish pedigree of 81 individuals, 19 of whom were affected (19). Two other reports published at the same time failed to find the linkage (15,25) and other failures to replicate have been reported subsequently. The Amish results have now essentially been withdrawn (27) because follow-up work on the original Amish pedigree yielded two new diagnoses of manic-depressive illness that reduced the evidence for linkage to nonsignificance, and an extension of the original pedigree has also failed to replicate the original result.

For schizophrenia, linkage to a dominant gene on chromosome 5 was reported in 1988 for five Icelandic and two English families with a high incidence of schizophrenia (52). Several failures to replicate the linkage have been reported (16,30,56; cf. 9), and as yet no positive replication has appeared.

It can be argued that such conflicting results are due to genetic heterogeneity— different major genes may be responsible for schizophrenia in different families. In other words, even if there are no major genes for schizophrenia in the population, certain families may have their own unique major gene, which recommends the current strategy of studying a few large pedigrees with many affected individuals. In this view, polygenic influence is seen at the population level because of the concatenation of different major genes in different families. The opposing view suggested by a quantitative genetic perspective is that for each individual many genes—perhaps different genes for different individuals—make small contributions toward schizophrenic vulnerability. It is possible that, by focusing on single large pedigrees with a high incidence of otherwise rare disorders, linkage might be found for a major mutation in a particular family that does not occur in the rest of the population. Genetic effects of this type might be useful in studies of gene-behavior pathways, although it is also possible that mechanisms uncovered in this way prove to be idiosyncratic and ungeneralizable. Other problems with linkage studies such as ascertainment biases, diagnoses, and significance levels are beginning to raise researchers' consciousness concerning the possibility of false positive results when pedigrees are selected because of a certain pattern of inheritance or because early linkage results begin to look positive. An April 1989 workshop on psychiatric genetics sponsored by the MacArthur Foundation concluded that replication must be a requirement for establishing linkage in psychiatric genetics—not just replication in a different pedigree but in a different laboratory as well (37). Using this criterion, no linkage for psychopathology has yet been established.

One might also argue that we have not yet tried hard enough to find major-gene linkages. This is a promissory note that can be cashed in during the coming decades because closely spaced genetic markers are available for nearly all human chromosomes and make it possible to exclude linkage for major genes. Although only a small portion of the genome in only a few families has been excluded for psychopathology, I predict that such exclusions will eventually provide the best evidence that human behavioral disorders are not due to major genes. My fear is that when this comes to pass it will be interpreted to mean that genes do not affect human behavior, whereas it will really only demonstrate that genetic influence on behavioral variability is not due to major-gene effects.

An approach to linkage that is more generalizable than studies of single large pedigrees is the affected-sib-pair method (43,61). This method attempts to identify linkages between genetic markers and disorders by assessing marker alleles for sibling pairs in which both siblings are affected. The essence of the method is that if a major gene is tightly linked to a marker, a pair of affected siblings will be concordant for the marker; if the marker and disorder are not linked, the siblings will inherit the same marker allele from the same parent only half of the time. Unlike the pedigree approach, the affected-sib-pair method does not require *a priori* specification of the mode of inheritance of the disorder and can detect linkage in the presence of heterogeneity. Similar to the pedigree approach, however, the affected-sib-pair method can only detect major-gene effects. The approach has not yet demonstrated linkage for behavior or behavioral disorders, although a recent report suggests linkage to chromosome 9 for broadly defined depressive spectrum (63).

MOLECULAR BIOLOGY AND BEHAVIOR

Quantitative genetic techniques, which have been the mainstay of behavioral genetic research, do not assess genetic variation directly. They use quasi-experimental designs such as inbred strain and selection studies for nonhuman animals and twin and adoption studies for humans to estimate the extent to which interindividual variability is due to genetic differences among individuals. This has been and will continue to be a source of great strength because quantitative methods address the "bottom line" of genetic influences on behavioral variability, the sum impact of genetic variability of any kind, regardless of its molecular source.

Behavioral genetic research is at the dawn of a new era in which specific DNA variation can be identified that accounts for variation in behavior (4). The preceding overview of behavioral genetic research draws two conclusions that have important implications for the application of molecular biology techniques to the study of behavior. First, nongenetic sources of variance are as important as genetic ones. Second, genetic influence on behavioral dimensions and disorders appears to involve many genes rather than one or two major genes.

Current pedigree approaches to linkage are only able to detect a gene that accounts for the majority of the variance of a behavioral trait. Large-pedigree linkage studies clearly represent a powerful strategy for identifying the chromosomal location of a disorder caused by a single gene that has its effect regardless of environmental or genetic background (41). For example, Huntington disease, which has long been known to be a single-gene characteristic, was the first disorder to be linked using this approach (24). However, reliance on large-pedigree linkage approaches for the analysis of behavior—as in the manic-depressive illness and schizophrenia examples described above—may be an example of the story of losing one's wallet in the dark alley but looking for it in the street because the light is better there. That is, applications of molecular biology techniques to the study of behavior are unlikely to succeed if they assume that a single major gene is largely responsible for genetic variation or that nongenetic influence is unimportant. The point is *not* that behavior is too complex for molecular biology, but rather that we need to bring the light of molecular biology into the dark alley of behavior. Strategies are needed to identify genes that account for a very small amount of variance in the presence of substantial nongenetic variance.

If behavioral variability is due to many genes and much nongenetic influence, the problem is not just finding a needle in the haystack but finding many needles in many haystacks. That is, for a particular behavior, several needles—perhaps scores of genes—need to be found among the stalks of polymorphic DNA. Furthermore, different needles may be lurking in different haystacks—genes that affect a behavior might differ across individuals. Widespread success in finding such needles in the haystacks of behavior will probably depend on the development of new techniques. For example, it may be possible to use subtractive hybridization (59) like a magnet to pull out most of the needles from the haystacks by identifying genes that differ between groups or even between individuals, yielding a set of quantitative trait loci (QTL) that could be used as probes in association and linkage studies. The human genome project is another example. One of the benefits of the project will be the identification of many more markers and genes that might play a role in genetic variation in behavior. Moreover, the human genome project is likely to yield technological spin-offs that will facilitate the mass production needed to find these needles in haystacks in studies with large sample sizes. One example of such an advance is the use of the polymerase chain reaction and automated sequencing equipment to work with sequence-tagged sites that will obviate the need to receive biological material for probes (40).

In the meantime, population association studies may be useful for finding these needles in haystacks because the sample size can be increased to provide adequate power to detect small effects. Association refers to covariation between allelic variation in a marker and phenotypic variation among individuals in a population. For example, in the first application of RFLPs to mammalian disease, a RFLP discovered about 5 kilobases from the [beta]-globin locus (26) showed a strong association with sickle cell anemia—the RFLP occurs 87% of the time when the sickle cell gene is present and only 3% of the time when the normal [beta]-globin gene is present. The goal of an association approach for traits that are not single-gene traits such as sickle cell anemia is to identify a battery of QTL markers (22), that in concert (including interactions among genes) accounts for genetic variability responsible for behavioral variation. The use of genetic markers to study associations with complex traits is not new (32)—the first association between genetic markers and quantitative traits was found over 60 years ago (50). Many associations were reported even before the widespread use of RFLP markers (58). However, the approach is enhanced by the great increase in available markers that permits QTL interval mapping—assessing associations with many closely spaced RFLPs simultaneously using the interval between markers rather than the markers themselves (42). This method was used to identify six QTLs that together accounted for 58% of the variance of fruit mass in a backcross between a domestic tomato and a wild green-fruited tomato.

Plant research uses F_2 populations because, as explained earlier, their chromosomes segregate as units broken up only by two exposures to recombination. As a result, in F_2 populations a marker indexes a region of millions of base pairs. In contrast, among individuals in outbred populations including humans, many generations of recombination have eliminated the linkage between alleles on the same chromosome so that the range of a marker is limited to a very small stretch of DNA not broken up by recombination, probably no more than a few hundred thousand base pairs. For this reason, trying to find associations between markers and human behavior is very much like trying to find tiny needles in huge haystacks. Nonetheless, a blood marker (HLA A9) has been found that appears to be associated with paranoid schizophrenia (35). Perhaps because the marker accounts for only a small portion of variance, linkage studies have not yet found evidence for linkage between the marker and schizophrenia.

Instead of using random RFLPs to look stalk by stalk through the human haystacks, a more efficient initial strategy is to screen candidate genes with known function, especially neurologically relevant genes, for their individual and joint contributions to behavior (5). For example, an association has recently been found between alcoholism and alleles of the aldehyde dehydrogenase locus (11). The likelihood of finding some needles in the haystacks could be increased by studying several behaviors for individuals screened for candidate genes that affect behavior. Another strategy is to look for haystacks most likely to contain needles by studying extreme individuals who presumably have more of the alleles associated with a trait.

Although new techniques are needed to isolate DNA polymorphisms responsible for small amounts of behavioral variability in the population, it is clear that the power of molecular biology techniques can be harnessed even for behavior. These techniques will become a standard part of the tool kit of behavioral geneticists of the future.

CONCLUSIONS

Just 15 years ago, the idea of genetic influence on complex human behavior was anathema to most behavioral scientists. In one of the most dramatic shifts in science, the role of inheritance in behavior has now become widely accepted, even for sensitive domains such as IQ (55). Indeed, acceptance of genetic influence has begun to outstrip the data in some cases such as alcoholism (51). For most domains of behavior, too few twin and adoption studies have been conducted to answer the basic question of whether genetic influence is significant. Only for a handful of behaviors is it possible to estimate effect size with reasonable certainty, estimates that one might expect to be prerequisite to exploring the relative importance of individual genes. More quantitative genetic research is needed, too, because such research can go well beyond the basic question of the relative importance of nature and nurture. For example, new developments include multivariate analyses of the genetic covariance among behaviors or between biology and behavior, consideration of age-to-age change as well as continuity of genetic effects as they unfold during development, and exploration of the interface with the environment (47).

The wave of acceptance of genetic influence on behavior is growing into a tidal wave that threatens to engulf an equally important conclusion from behavioral genetic research: Nongenetic sources of variance must be taken seriously because genetic variance rarely accounts for as much as half of the variance of behavioral traits. That is, evidence for significant genetic influence is often implicitly interpreted as if heritability were 100%, whereas heritabilities for behavior seldom exceed 50%. A second conclusion with far-reaching implications for molecular biology is the absence of evidence for the widely held assumption that genetic influence on behavior is primarily due to one or two major genes. It seems more reasonable to hypothesize that many genes, each with small effects are involved.

If it is the case that behavioral variation involves many genes and much environmental influence, linkage analyses that require the presence of a major gene with little nongenetic variance are unlikely to be successful. The search for the needles in haystacks will require strategies that can isolate DNA polymorphisms responsible for small amounts of variance in the population. Quantitative genetic research will be important in this endeavor to assess the extent to which individual genes account for genetic variance and the extent to which genetic variance accounts for phenotypic variance.

In conclusion, molecular biology techniques will revolutionize behavioral genetics, and the quantitative genetic perspective of behavioral genetics will transform our use of these techniques as we continue to explore the role of inheritance in the most complex of phenotypes, behavior.

ACKNOWLEDGMENTS

Preparation of this chapter was supported in part by grants from the National Science Foundation (BNS-8806589), the National Institute of Child Health and Human Development (HD-10333 and HD-18426), the National Institute of Mental Health (MH-43373 and MH-43899), and the John D. and Catherine T. MacArthur Foundation Program on Successful Aging.

GLOSSARY OF GENETIC TERMS

Adoption study Comparison between adopted-apart biological relatives to estimate the influence of heredity.
Association In contrast to linkage, association refers to a direct effect of a particular gene or genetic marker on a phenotype for individuals in a population.
Inbred strain Animals mated brother to sister (inbred) for many generations, which results in a strain in which all members are virtually identical genetically.
Linkage The occurrence of two genes close together on the same chromosome.

Model-fitting Statistical technique used in quantitative genetic analysis to test the fit between a genetic model and observed data.

Multivariate analysis Analyzing the covariance (association) among traits rather than the variance of each trait considered individually (i.e., univariate analysis).

Multifactorial inheritance Inheritance of traits that are affected by many genes (polygenic) as well as nongenetic factors.

Phenotype Measured characteristic (in contrast to genotype).

Polygenic "Many" ("poly")-gene influence—traits that are affected by many genes, each with small effects.

Quantitative genetics A theory and set of methods to decompose phenotypic (observed) variance into genetic and environmental components.

Quantitative trait loci Measured polygenic markers.

Restriction enzyme A class of enzymes that recognize a specific sequence of 4, 5, or 6 nucleotide bases and cuts DNA wherever that sequence is identified.

RFLP Restriction fragment length polymorphism—genetic marker of polymorphic (variable) DNA created by cutting DNA with restriction enzymes.

Selection study Breeding animals for a trait by intermating the "best" scorers to create a "high" line and intermating the "worst" scorers to create a "low" line.

Specific cognitive abilities In addition to general cognitive ability or IQ, mental tests yield separate abilities, most notably, verbal, spatial, memory, and perceptual speed.

Twin study Comparison between identical and fraternal twins to estimate the influence of heredity.

REFERENCES

1. Bailey, D. W. (1971): Recombinant inbred strains. *Transplantation*, 11:325–327.
2. Barnes, D. M. (1989): "Fragile X" syndrome and its puzzling genetics. *Science*, 243:171–172.
3. Bessman, S. P., Williamson, M. L., and Koch, R. (1978): Diet, genetics, and mental retardation interaction between phenylketonuric heterozygous mother and fetus to produce nonspecific diminution of IQ: evidence in support of the justification hypothesis. *Proc. Natl. Acad. Sci. USA*, 78:1562–1566.
4. Bodmer, W. F. (1986): Human genetics: the molecular challenge. *Cold Spring Harbor Symp. Quant. Biol.*, 51:1–14.
5. Boerwinkle, E., Chakraborty, R., and Sing, C. F. (1986). The use of measured genotype information in the analysis of quantitative phenotypes in man. *Ann. Hum. Genet.*, 50:181–194.
6. Bohman, M., Cloninger, R., Sigvardsson, S., and von Knorring, A.-L. (1987): The genetics of alcoholism and related disorders. *J. Psychiatr. Res.*, 21:447–452.
7. Bouchard, T. J., Jr., and McGue, M. (1981): Familial studies of intelligence. *Science*, 212:1055–1059.
8. Buss, A. H., and Plomin, R. (1984): *Temperament: Early Developing Personality Traits*. Lawrence Erlbaum, Hillsdale, NJ.
9. Byerley, W. F. (1989): Genetic linkage revisited. *Science*, 340:340–341.
10. Chipuer, H. M., Rovine, M., and Plomin, R. (1990): LISREL modeling: genetic and environmental influences on IQ revisited. *Intelligence*, 14:11–29.
11. Crabb, D. W., Edenberg, H. J., Bosron, W. F., and Li, T.-K. (1989): Genotypes for aldehyde dehydrogenase deficiency and alcohol sensitivity. *J. Clin. Invest.*, 83:314–316.
12. DeFries, J. C., Gervais, M. C., and Thomas, E. A. (1978): Response to 30 generations of selection for open-field activity in laboratory mice. *Behav. Genet.*, 8:3–13.
13. DeFries, J. C., Johnson, R. C., Kuse, A. R., et al. (1979): Familial resemblance for specific cognitive abilities. *Behav. Genet.*, 9:23–43.

14. DeLisi, L. E., Mirsky, A. F., Buchsbaum, M. S., van Kammen, D. P., and Berman, K. F. (1984): The Genain quadruplets 25 years later: a diagnostic and biochemical followup. *Psychiatr. Res.*, 13:59–76.
15. Detera-Wadleigh, S. D., Berrettini, W. H., Goldin, L. R., Boorman, D., Anderson, S., and Gershon, E. S. (1987): Close linkage of c-harvey-ras-1 and the insulin gene to affective disorder is ruled out in three North American pedigrees. *Nature*, 325:806–808.
16. Detera-Wadleigh, S. D., Goldin, L. R., Sherrington, R., et al. (1989): Exclusion of linkage to 5q11-13 in families with schizophrenia and other psychiatric disorders. *Science*, 340:391–393.
17. Eaves, L. J., Eysenck, H. J., and Martin, N. (1989): *Genes, Culture and Personality*. Academic Press, New York.
18. Edwards, M. D., Stuber, C. W., and Wendel, J. F. (1987): Molecular-marker-facilitated investigations of quantitative-trait loci in maize. I. Numbers, genomic distribution and types of gene action. *Geneticae*, 116:113–125.
19. Egeland, J. A., Gerhard, D. S., Pauls, D. L., Sussex, J. N., and Kidd, K. K., (1987): Bipolar affective disorders linked to DNA markers on chromosome 11. *Nature*, 325:783–787.
20. Farmer, A. E., McGuffin, P., and Gottesman, I. I. (1984): Searching for the split in schizophrenia: a twin study perspective. *Psychiatr. Res.*, 13:109–118.
21. Fisher, R. A. (1918): The correlation between relatives on the supposition of Mendelian inheritance. *Trans. R. Soc. Edinburgh*, 52:399–433.
22. Gelderman, H. (1975): Investigations on inheritance of quantitative characters in animals by gene markers. I. Methods. *Theoret. Appl. Genet.*, 46:319–330.
23. Gottesman, I. I., and Shields, J. (1982): *Schizophrenia: The Epigenetic Puzzle*. Cambridge: Cambridge University Press.
24. Gusella, J. F., Wexler, N. S., Conneally, P. M., et al. (1983): A polymorphic DNA marker genetically linked to Huntington's disease. *Nature*, 306:234–238.
25. Hodgkinson, S., Sherrington, R., Gurling, H., Marchbanks, R., and Reeders, S. (1987): Molecular genetic evidence for heterogeneity in manic depression. *Nature*, 325:805–806.
26. Kan, Y. W., and Dozy, A. M. (1978): Antenatal diagnosis of sickle-cell anemia by DNA analysis of amniotic-fluid cells. *Lancet*, 2:910–912.
27. Kelsoe, J., Ginns, E. I., Egeland, J. A., et al. (1989): Re-evaluation of the linkage relationship between chromosome 11p loci and the gene for bipolar affective disorder in the Old Order Amish. *Nature*, 342:238–243.
28. Kendler, K. S., and Gruenberg, A. M. (1984): An independent analysis of the Danish Adoption Study of Schizophrenia. *Arch. Gen. Psychiatry*, 41:555–564.
29. Kendler, K. S., and Robinette, C. D. (1983): Schizophrenia in the National Academy of Sciences-National Research Council twin registry: a 16-year update. *Am. J. Psychiatry*, 140:1551–1563.
30. Kennedy, J. L., Giuffra, L. A., Moises, H. W., et al. (1988): Evidence against linkage of schizophrenia to markers on chromosome 5 in a northern Swedish pedigree. *Nature*, 336:167–170.
31. Kimberling, W. J., Fain, P. R., Ing, P. S., Smith, S. D., and Pennington, B. F. (1985): Linkage analysis of reading disability with chromosome 15. *Behav. Genet.*, 15:597–598.
32. Kloepfer, H. W. (1946): An investigation of 171 possible linkage relationships in man. *Ann. Eugenics*, 13:35–47.
33. Loehlin, J. C. (1989): Environmental and genetic contributions to behavioral development. *Am. Psychol.*, 44:1285–1292.
34. Loehlin, J. C., Willerman, L., and Horn, J. M. (1988): Human behavior genetics. *Annu. Rev. Psych.*, 39:101–133.
35. McGuffin, P., and Sturt, E. (1986): Genetic markers in schizophrenia. *Hum. Hered.*, 36:65–88.
36. McKusick, V. A. (1988): *Mendelian Inheritance in Man*, 8th ed. Johns Hopkins University Press, Baltimore, MD.
37. Merikangas, K. R., Spence, M. A., Kupfer, D. J., and Kety, S. (1989): Linkage studies of bipolar disorder: summary of MacArthur Foundation workshop. Paper presented at the First World Congress on Psychiatric Genetics, Cambridge, August.
38. Nichols, P. L. (1984): Familial mental retardation. *Behav. Genet.*, 14:161–170.
39. Nussbaum, R. L., and Ledbetter, D. H. (1986): Fragile X syndrome: a unique mutation in man. *Ann. Rev. Genet.*, 20:109–145.
40. Olson, M., Hood, L., Cantor, C., and Botstein, D. (1989): A common language for physical mapping of the human genome. *Science*, 245:1434–1435.
41. Ott, J. (1985): *Analysis of Human Genetic Linkage*. Johns Hopkins University Press, Baltimore, MD.

42. Paterson, A. H., Lander, E. S., Hewitt, J. D., Peterson, S., Lincoln, S. E., and Tanksley, S. D. (1988): Resolution of quantitative traits into Mendelian factors by using a complete linkage map of restriction fragment length polymorphisms. *Nature*, 335:721–726.
43. Penrose, L. (1935): The detection of autosomal linkage in data which consists of pairs of brothers and sisters of unspecified parentage. *Ann. Eugenics*, 6:133–138.
44. Plomin, R. (1988): The nature and nurture of cognitive abilities. In: *Advances in the Psychology of Human Intelligence*, edited by R. J. Sternberg, pp. 1–33. Lawrence Erlbaum, Hillsdale, NJ.
45. Plomin, R. Genetic risk and psychosocial disorders: links between the normal and abnormal. In: *Biological Risk Factors for Psychosocial Disorders*, edited by M. Rutter and P. Caesar. Cambridge University Press, London (*in press*).
46. Plomin, R., Chipuer, H., and Loehlin, J. C. (1990): Behavioral genetics and personality. In: *Handbook of Personality Theory and Research*, edited by L. A. Pervin, pp. 225–243. Guilford Press, New York.
47. Plomin, R., DeFries, J. C., and McClearn, G. E. (1990): *Behavioral Genetics: A Primer*, 2nd ed. W. H. Freeman, New York.
48. Reich, T., Van Eerdewegh, P., Rice, J., Mullaney, J., Endicott, J., and Klerman, G. L. (1987): The familial transmission of primary major depressive disorder. *J. Psychiat. Res.*, 21:613–624.
49. Rice, J. P., Reich, T., Andreasen, N. C., et al. (1987): The familial transmission of bipolar illness. *Arch. Gen. Psychiatry*, 41:441–447.
50. Sax, K. (1923): The association of size differences with seed coat pattern and pigmentation in *Phaseolus vulgarus*. *Genetics*, 8:552–560.
51. Searles, J. S. (1988): The role of genetics in the pathogenesis of alcoholism. *J. Abnorm. Psychol.*, 97:153–167.
52. Sherrington, R., Brynjolfsson, J., Petursson, H., et al. (1988): Localization of a susceptibility locus for schizophrenia on chromosome 5. *Nature*, 336:164–167.
53. Smith, S. D., Kimberling, W. J., Pennington, B. F., and Lubs, H. A. (1983): Specific reading disability: identification of an inherited form through linkage analysis. *Science*, 219:1345–1347.
54. Smith, S. D., Pennington, B. F., Kimberling, W. J., and Ing, P. S. Familial dyslexia: use of genetic linkage data to define subtypes. *J. Am. Acad. Child Psychiatry (in press)*.
55. Snyderman, M., and Rothman, S. (1988): *The IQ Controversy, the Median and Public Policy*. Transaction Books, New Brunswick, NJ.
56. St. Clair, D., Blackwood, D., Muir, W., et al. (1989): No linkage of chromosome 5q11-q13 markers to schizophrenia in Scottish families. *Nature*, 339:305–308.
57. Thompson, L. A., Detterman, D. K., and Plomin, R. Associations between cognitive abilities and scholastic achievement: genetic overlap but environmental differences. *J. Educ. Psychology (in press)*.
58. Thompson, J. N., Jr., and Thoday, J. M. (Eds.) (1979): *Quantitative Genetic Variation*. Academic Press, New York.
59. Travis, G. H., and Sutcliffe, J. G. (1988): Phenol emulsion-enhanced DNA-drive subtractive cDNA cloning: isolation of low-abundance monkey cortex-specific mRNAs. *Proc. Natl. Acad. Sci. USA*, 85:1696–1700.
60. Vandenberg, S. G., Singer, S. M., and Pauls, D. L. (1986): *The Heredity of Behavior Disorders in Adults and Children*. Plenum Press, New York.
61. Weeks, D. E., and Lange, K. (1988): The affected-pedigree-member method of linkage analysis. *Am. J. Hum. Genet.* 42:315–326.
62. Wender, P. H., Kety, S. S., Rosenthal, D., Schulsinger, F., Ortmann, J., and Lunde, I. (1986): Psychiatric disorders in the biological and adoptive families of adopted individuals with affective disorders. *Arch. Gen. Psychiatry*, 43:923–939.
63. Wilson, A. F., Tanna, V. L., Winokur, G., Elston, R. C., and Hill, E.M. (1989): Linkage analysis of depression spectrum disease. *Biol. Psychiatry*, 26:163–175.

ated by
Genes, Brain, and Behavior, edited by
P. R. McHugh and V. A. McKusick.
Raven Press, Ltd., New York © 1991.

The Psychopathology of Huntington's Disease

Susan E. Folstein

Department of Psychiatry, Division of Psychiatric Genetics, The Johns Hopkins University School of Medicine, Baltimore, Maryland 21205

Huntington's disease (HD) has fascinated workers in genetics, psychiatry, neurology, and the neurosciences since the beginning of this century. The study of HD patients and their families has provided a model of true autosomal dominant inheritance (1), suggested clues to the functioning of the subcortical motor system (2), revealed a subcortical component of cognitive function (3), and suggested a neural mechanism for mood (4). Moreover, the at-risk family members of HD patients provide an opportunity for psychologists to observe the functioning of humans who know they have one chance in two to develop a fatal disease during early adult life.

This chapter reviews research by the Hopkins HD research group that illustrates what can be learned about mood and behavior from the study of the psychiatric features of HD patients and their at-risk offspring. Evidence will be presented that major affective disorder, when seen in HD families, often signifies the presence of the HD gene and its neuropathology. Conversely, antisocial conduct is related to the disruption in the family environment caused, in part, by the HD gene. Thus, we will conclude that the HD gene and the environment it can create are associated with different psychiatric disorders and that these associations in HD are relevant to the mechanisms underlying affective disorder and antisocial conduct in the general population.

CLINICAL FEATURES OF HD

HD is inherited as an autosomal dominant, which means that each offspring of an affected parent is at 50% risk for having the disease. While the gene is inherited at conception, clinical signs and symptoms are delayed usually until middle adult life, although symptoms may begin at any time between childhood and old age. The illness lasts an average of 18 years from onset until death, which usually results directly or indirectly from the inability to swallow food—aspiration pneumonia or suffocation (5). The most constant feature of neuropathology is atrophy and neuronal loss in the neostriatum, i.e., the caudate and putamen.

There are three cardinal clinical features of HD—abnormalities of movement, cognition, and mood. The motor disorder is characterized mainly by chorea early in the course of the disease. Chorea worsens over the first 10 years of illness and then gradually wanes. Problems with voluntary motor control gradually increase throughout the course, beginning with clumsiness and mild ataxia and progressing to an akinetic mute state with hypertonia, myoclonus, and other long tract signs (5).

Early in the course, cognition is affected by an inefficiency of thought and difficulty in accessing memories at will (6). Later in the course, there is a more global dementia. Comprehension of speech is usually preserved, although patients have increasing difficulty in initiating speech until, finally, they are no longer able to utter a word except when they are extremely excited (7).

The third cardinal feature of HD, emotional disorder, is the focus of this chapter and will be described more fully. Affective disorder has been part of the definition of HD since Huntington's original description (8). He said that patients had a "tendency to insanity . . . especially that form of insanity that leads to suicide." As part of a statewide survey of HD in Maryland (9,10), our group attempted to document each patient's psychiatric disorder using current diagnostic criteria, DSM III (11). When possible, patients and their informants were interviewed with a structured interview. In some additional cases, informants alone or medical records were judged to provide adequate psychiatric information. Diagnoses (shown in Table 1) could be made for 186 of the 217 HD patients affected in Maryland on April 1, 1980. These are lifetime diagnoses; not all patients were symptomatic at the time of interview. We did not follow the DSM III guidelines that require patients with a brain disease to be classified as "organic" psychiatric disorder. This approach limits both the number of diagnoses that may be made and the detail with which a disorder may be specified. Affective disorder was the most common disorder, followed by an irritable state, which was sometimes severe enough to meet DSM III criteria for intermittent explosive disorder.

TABLE 1. *Distribution of psychiatric disorder in black and white HD subjects*

DSM III diagnosis	No. (%) of subjects with diagnosis		
	Black (N = 50)	White (N = 136)	Total (N = 186)[a]
None	23 (46.0)	33 (24.3)	56 (30.1)[b]
Affective disorder	5 (10.0)	56 (41.2)	61 (32.8)[b]
Dysthymic disorder	5 (10.0)	4 (2.0)	9 (4.8)
Intermittent explosive disorder	10 (20.0)	47 (34.6)	57 (30.6)[b]
Alcoholism	9 (18.0)	20 (14.7)	29 (15.6)
Schizophrenia	1 (2.0)	7 (5.2)	8 (5.9)
Antisocial personality	5 (10.0)	6 (4.4)	11 (5.9)
Other	4 (8.0)	15 (11.0)	19 (10.2)

[a]Totals exceed the number of patients because a number of patients met criteria for more than one DSM III diagnosis.
[b]Racial difference in proportions significant at $P<0.05$.
From ref. 10.

FEATURES OF AFFECTIVE DISORDER SUGGESTING ITS RELATIONSHIP TO HD NEUROPATHOLOGY

We have studied affective disorder and its association with HD in some detail. Naturally, there has been some question about the cause of affective disorder in HD. Is it the result of HD neuropathology, or is it an understandable reaction to tragic adversity? There is no question that HD patients are distressed at their illness—having observed the disorder in family members, most are only too well aware of its eventual outcome. However, despite this, many patients maintain hope for the future and are surprised at the question, "Does life seem worth living?" Even those patients suffering from episodes of major affective disorder are generally able to enjoy life between the episodes. Several types of data suggest that major affective disorder, with its dysphoria and feelings of hopelessness, worthlessness, and guilt, is likely to be the result of HD neuropathology.

First, affective disorder usually precedes the cognitive and motor signs in HD, often by several years, and it never begins late in the course of illness. It does not appear to be precipitated by worry about HD and is often seen in persons who have either minimal awareness of their risk for HD or none at all. This sequence has been examined in two separate samples (Table 2), using a semistructured interview to document the year of onset of both affective disorder and motor signs. In both samples, affective disorder usually preceded the onset of motor signs.

Second, affective disorder in HD is phenomenologically similar to ordinary affective disorder in several ways. Early in our work, we reviewed the case notes of patients whose major affective disorder had gone untreated (Table 3). Although a few patients remained chronically depressed, most experienced episodes of depression, lasting about 6 months. For the most part, episodes appear to come and go without regard to patients' life events; many comment on their inability to appreciate why they are depressed. About 10% of HD patients are manic, certainly not an understandable reaction to HD (12). The manic symptoms are typical, with increased sexual interest, excessive energy and talk, unusual optimism, and overspending. Some patients are delusional, both during depression and mania. A recent

TABLE 2. Affective disorder usually precedes onset of motor symptoms

N = 56	
Age at onset of AD	35 years (± 10)
Age at onset of chorea	45 years (± 12)
T = 4.6, $p<0.006$	
N = 44	
AD preceded chorea	23
AD concurrent chorea	6
AD followed chorea	6
Mean = -5.5 years	

AD, affective disorder.

TABLE 3. *Population study of HD and major affective disorder duration of episodes of affective disorder*

Duration (months)	No. of patients
< 6	13
7–12	4
>12	4

patient believed that she was bleeding from her gastrointestinal tract; another that he was cheating the government by collecting disability because he did not deserve to receive it. One chronically manic patient proudly tells everyone she is pregnant with twins; another is convinced that her HD has been cured by gin and tonic. Although we have not carried out a formal clinical trial, clinicians who care for HD patients generally agree that tricyclic antidepressants are usually effective in treating affective disorder in HD. Mania is sometimes responsive to lithium but more often to carbamazepine.

A third aspect of affective disorder in HD suggesting that it may result from neuropathology is its familial aggregation. In one study, we selected five kindreds for having a HD proband with bipolar affective disorder. Most other affected members of these kindreds also had affective disorder (13). In five other kindreds selected by a proband with HD and no other psychiatric disorder, most of the other affected relatives in the kindred also were without affective disorder. The association was not attributable to affective disorder on the side of the family unaffected by HD; affective disorder was found in 2% of spouses and their siblings. Minor dysphoria, not meeting criteria for major affective disorder, was common in spouses and was associated in time with the burden of caring for family members with HD.

A fourth feature of HD suggesting the influence of neuropathology is its relationship to age at onset. The HD kindreds with affective disorder had a later onset of illness than those without. This was confirmed in the Maryland survey where we again showed that patients with affective disorder had a significantly later onset of movement disorder than other patients.

A final reason for suspecting an association with neuropathology is that affective disorder is quite uncommon in blacks with HD. This observation may be related to the fact that blacks have a significantly earlier age at onset than whites (10).

POSSIBLE NEUROPATHOLOGICAL CORRELATES OF AFFECTIVE DISORDER IN HD

If affective disorder in HD is understandable in light of neuropathology, is it related to striatal pathology or to cortical dysfunction or pathology? This question needs to be approached from an understanding of the major fiber connections of the striatum, and the answer is likely to be related to the direct connections between the striatum and specific areas of the cortex.

The striatum forms one segment of a cortical-subcortical circuit (Fig. 1), which begins in diverse cortical areas, provides excitatory stimulation to the striatum, the output of which goes to the pallidum, on to the thalamus, and back to the cortex, closing the circuit. However, the returning fibers do not distribute themselves widely in the cortex but return only to the prefrontal cortex (14). There is not just one circuit, but a series of at least five parallel cortical-subcortical circuits. Each circuit serves a specific function and is restricted to its own cortical and subcortical areas. The motor circuit involves the putamen; eye movement, and cognitive, and

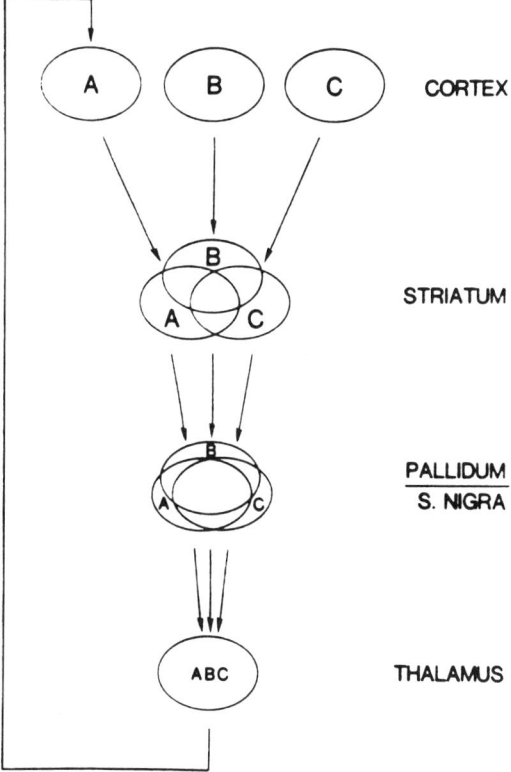

FIG. 1. Generalized basal ganglia-thalamocortical circuit. "Skeleton" diagram of the proposed basal ganglia-thalamocortical circuits. Each circuit receives output from several functionally related cortical areas (A, B, C) that send partially overlapping projections to the globus pallidus and substantia nigra, which in turn project to a specific region of the thalamus. Each thalamic region projects back to one of the cortical areas that feeds into the circuit, thereby completing the "closed loop" portion of the circuit. (From ref. 14.)

emotional functions involve various areas of the caudate. Fibers from the limbic cortex are particularly prominent in the medial caudate and in the ventral striatum (15).

Von Sattel et al. (16) have demonstrated that neuropathology in HD usually begins medially in the head of the caudate at the ventricular surface. It then proceeds laterally to involve the lateral caudate and the putamen (Table 4). The timing of affective disorder—always early in the illness and usually prior to cognitive or motor signs—suggests that the medial caudate and its cortical connections are the most likely candidates for the site of neuropathology related to affective disorder in HD.

The striatum is not a uniform structure, but is composed of a matrix surrounding a labyrinth, which appears cross-sectionally as patches (17). The incoming cortical fibers into the matrix areas are separate from those providing input to the labyrinth. The input from the cortex to the medial striatal *matrix* is mainly from the lateral prefrontal cortex. The more inferior parts of this lateral prefrontal area are selectively hypometabolic on deoxyglucose positron emission tomography (PET) scans in depressed parkinsonian patients, but normal in euthymic parkinsonian patients (18). We have now made identical observations in depressed HD patients (Mayberg et al., *in preparation*).

The labyrinthine system is also a likely candidate for involvement in depression in HD. The labyrinth is the site of entry to the caudate of a particular subset of dopamine fibers and fibers from the limbic cortex (20). The labyrinth is particularly prominent in the medial caudate and fades out toward the putamen and is high in enkephalin (17).

It is not clear why affective disorder is not found in all HD patients, but there are several possibilities. There are a number of age-related differences in the expression of HD, and it may be that older HD patients are more vulnerable because of age-related changes in neurochemical relationships (21). Also, despite the usual pattern of neuropathological progression described by Von Sattel (16), HD neuropathology

TABLE 4. *Atrophy and neuronal depletion in HD medial to lateral*

Atrophy grade	Medial caudate		Lateral caudate		Putamen		Lateral pallidum		Medial pallidum		Nucleus accumbens	
	A	ND	A	ND	A	ND	A	ND	A	ND	A	ND
0	0	0	0	0	0	0	0	0	0	0	0	0
I	0	1–2	0	0–1	0	0	0	0	0	0	0	0
II	1	2	1	1	1	1–2	0	0	0	0	0	0
III	2–3	3	2–3	2	2	2–3	1	1	0–1	0–1	0–1	0–1
IV	4	4	4	4	3	4	2	1–2	2	1–2	1	0–1

A systematic examination of a series of HD brains chosen for variability in the overall severity of neuropathologic findings (grades 0–IV) demonstrated that atrophy (A) and neuronal degeneration (ND) begin in the medial caudate and proceed laterally to the putamen and then to the pallidum. Ventral areas (e.g., the nucleus accumbens) are normal except in grade-III and -IV brains.
From refs. 7,16.

is surprisingly variable. For example, the putamen is sometimes first affected (22); we have examined the brains of several black patients who had only modest caudate involvement after many years of illness (10,23). This kind of variability is the rule rather than the exception in dominantly inherited disorders (see Pyeritz, *this volume*).

IS THERE A SUBCORTICAL TRIAD?

Huntington's disease is not the only subcortical disorder in which affective disorder is prominent. Affective disorder is quite common in Parkinson's disease (24). Not only do depressed parkinsonian patients show hypometabolic inferior lateral prefrontal cortex, but they also have hypometabolic caudate nuclei, as of course do HD patients. About half the patients with Fahr's syndrome or calcification of the basal ganglia of other etiologies suffer from disorders of mood, and mania is occasionally reported (25,26). Depression is also prominent in patients with left striatal strokes (27,28). Depression was most common in those with lesions in the head of the caudate. A recent report provides documentation of the association between affective disorder and Wilson's disease.

These disorders not only share depression as a clinical feature, but they also have overlapping types of motor and cognitive features. This triad of features—disorders of motor function, cognition, and mood—present in subcortical, and particularly striatal, disorders suggest that there is some necessary relationship among them related to the anatomical connections within the striatum (30). We have suggested these three features be designated the "subcortical triad" (31).

Perhaps "functional" affective disorder should be added to our list of subcortical conditions having this triad of features. There is a disorder of mood, a disorder of memory similar to that of HD with cognitive inefficiency, and the inability to access memories (32) as well as disordered motor function with bradykinesia or motor agitation. Evidence is beginning to accumulate from PET studies suggesting that the caudate may be dysfunctional in major affective disorder. Glucose metabolism, as measured by caudate-to-hemisphere ratio is decreased in patients with unipolar affective disorder (33,34). Drevets et al. (35) recently reported decreased cerebral blood flow, using PET, in the left caudate in patients with unipolar depression, both in the depressed and euthymic states. While the caudate is the first brain area affected in HD, and always predominates, the effect of striatal pathology on its cortical connections is important in understanding the emerging data on the relationship between mood and striatal disease. The striatum is part of a cortical-subcortical circuit, and when one segment of the circuit is affected, it has distant effects on the firing of neurons in other parts of the circuit. These issues are clearly reviewed by Albin et al. (2). Another principle of the circuits is that lesions in one segment (e.g., striatum) of a particular circuit may often produce signs and symptoms similar to those produced by lesions in another segment (e.g., cortical) of the same circuit (36). This may explain why glucose PET scans demonstrate hypometabolism in both caudate and inferior lateral prefrontal cortex in depressed HD and parkinsonian patients. The same is likely to be true for unipolar affective disorder although studies available at this time have not looked specifically at particular prefrontal areas.

EMOTIONAL DISORDER IN PERSONS AT RISK

Not all psychiatric disorder seen in HD patients is attributable to neuropathology. One example is antisocial behavior, which is quite common in at-risk adolescents and young adults. In adolescence, conduct disorder is characterized by truancy, lying, stealing, and chronic disregard for family and school-based rules of conduct (DSM III-R). Criteria for antisocial personality disorder are similar but require continuance into adult life and more serious offenses. Antisocial conduct disorder is to be clearly distinguished from the irritable (and occasionally aggressive) state seen in HD patients. The latter is associated in time with the onset of motor and cognitive signs in HD, usually in a person who has not had a lifelong history of aggressive behavior. This disease-related irritability is usually directed toward family members and caregivers and is not ordinarily associated with antisocial behavior such as stealing and other types of law breaking. There has been some confusion on this point in the literature.

We studied the psychiatric disorders in 112 offspring of 34 consecutively ascertained HD patients who were parents and had at least one child aged 15 or older (37). The two psychiatric conditions common in this sample of offspring were affective disorder (18%) and conduct disorder (25%). We investigated the relationship of these two disorders in the at-risk offspring to two possible causative factors: (a) as indicators of the onset of HD and (b) as indicators of having a disorganized family environment.

A disorganized family environment was defined as one in which the family structure had broken down so that there was no consistent discipline or expectations (e.g., children attending school, being home by dark, eating regular meals, etc.). In some instances there was more blatant neglect or abuse of the children and some children had been in foster care.

There were different associations for affective disorder and conduct disorder. Adolescents and young adults with affective disorder were more likely to have clear or suspicious signs of HD by the time of this study (Table 5). Their affected parent was also likely to have had major affective disorder. There was no association between affective disorder and family turmoil or disorganization.

Adolescent conduct disorder, on the other hand, did not predict the later onset of HD. While some at-risk persons with conduct disorder went on to have HD, many did not. As their lives stabilized in adulthood, their conduct improved, for the most part, although some have continued in their antisocial behavior.

Conduct disorder was strongly related to the presence of family disorganization. Families of children with conduct disorder tended to be large, and the parent was usually affected with HD while the children were still young. These features did not

TABLE 5. *Association of HD status with psychiatric diagnosis in offspring*

	At risk (N=86)		Certain or possible HD (N=26)		P
	No.	(%)	No.	(%)	
Antisocial personality or conduct disorder	18	(21)	10	(38)	N.S.
Major affective disorder	12	(14)	8	(31)	<0.05

N.S., not significant.
From ref. 13.

predict conduct disorder if the family remained well organized, however. Furthermore, abnormal parenting by the affected parent did not predict conduct disorder in their children. The failure of the *unaffected* parent to maintain the family environment and structure was the one feature uniting the families whose children had conduct disorder.

The correlation between conduct disorder and family turmoil is what one might expect from earlier research in conduct disorder. For example, Rutter et al. (38) have shown in two population-based studies that disordered conduct in children and adolescents is associated with large families, family turmoil, broken homes, and being in foster care. It has also been shown that conduct disorder is not common if *one* of the two parents is stable and nurturing. This was the case in the HD families whose children did well even though the affected parent was unpredictable and often punitive, the presence of a stable and nurturing unaffected parent predicted a good outcome for the children.

It is clear that conduct disorder in HD families is related to family turmoil and not to the presence of the HD gene in the offspring with the disorder. However, it should not be concluded that genetic factors are not involved. Clearly, there is a genetic predisposition to antisocial conduct (40), and antisocial behavior was present in several of the unaffected parents who were unable to maintain their families. The mechanism here may be one of gene-environment interaction like that described by Crowe (40) in an adoption study of the children of female offenders. Their adopted-away offspring did not have conduct disorder if their adoptive environments were stable and nurturing. However, if their adoptive environments were unstable, they were highly likely to develop antisocial behavior. This is in contrast to the adopted controls whose biological parents did not have antisocial behavior. Even when these adoptees were subjected to unfavorable adoptive environments, they did not develop antisocial behavior.

SUMMARY AND CONCLUSIONS

Our findings suggest that HD can cause psychiatric disorder in two ways. First, by the direct action of the gene on striatal neurons, and second, by the indirect effect of the disordered family environment on the children, regardless of whether they have inherited the HD gene. The gene and the environment created by the gene caused different psychiatric disorders.

The correlates of conduct disorder in HD correspond to those expected from principles already established by psychiatric research. The association of affective disorder and HD suggests two hypotheses: (a) affective disorder is part of a subcortical triad and will be present whenever there is subcortical (striatal) pathology and (b) functional affective disorder may be an example of a subcortical disorder with abnormalities of mood, memory, and movement and emerging indications of striatal pathology.

ACKNOWLEDGMENTS

Support for this grant was provided, in part, by the Research Center Without Walls for Huntington's Disease #5 PO1 MS16735.

REFERENCES

1. Wexler, N., et al. (1987): Homozygotes for Huntington's disease. *Nature*, 326:194–197.
2. Albin, R. L., Young, A. B., and Penny, J. B. (1989): The functional anatomy of basal ganglia disorders. *TINS*, 12:366–375.
3. Brandt, J., and Butters, N. (1986): The neuropsychology of Huntington's disease. *TINS*, 9:118–120.
4. Folstein, S. E., et al. The subcortical triad of Huntington's disease: a model for a neuropathology of depression, dementia, and dyskinesia. *Am. Psychopathol. Assoc. (in press)*.
5. Folstein, S. E. (1989): The motor disorder. In: *Huntington's Disease: A Disorder of Families*. The Johns Hopkins University Press, Baltimore, pp. 13–31.
6. Brandt, J. (1985): Access to knowledge in the dementia of Huntington's disease. *Dev. Neuropsychol.* 1:335–348.
7. Folstein, S. E. (1989): The cognitive disorder. In: *Huntington's Disease: A Disorder of Families*. The Johns Hopkins University Press, Baltimore, pp. 32–48.
8. Huntington, G. (1872): On chorea. Reprinted in *Adv. Neurol.*, 1:33–35.
9. Folstein, S. E., et al. (1986): The diagnosis of Huntington's disease. *Neurology*, 36:1279–1283.
10. Folstein, S.E., et al. (1987): Huntington's disease in Maryland: clinical aspects of racial variation. *Am. J. Hum. Genet.*, 41:168–179.
11. DSM III. (1987): American Psychiatric Association, Washington, D.C.
12. Peyser, C. E., and Folstein, S. E. Huntington's disease as a model for mood disorder: clues from neuropathology and neurochemistry. *J. Neurochem. Pathol. (submitted)*.
13. Folstein, S. E., et al. (1983): The association of affective disorder with Huntington's disease in a case series and in families. *Psychol. Med.*, 13:537–542.
14. Alexander, G. E., DeLong, M. R., and Strick, P. L. (1986): Parallel organization of functionally segregated circuits linking basal ganglia and cortex. *Annu. Rev. Neurosci.*, 9:357–381.
15. Gerfen, C. R., Baimbridge, K. G., and Thibault, J. (1987): The neostriatal mosaic: III. Biochemical and developmental dissociation of patch-matrix mesostriatal systems. *J. Neurosci.* 7:3935–3944.
16. Von Sattel, J. P., et al. (1985): Neuropathological classification of Huntington's disease. *J. Neuropathol. Exp. Neurol.*, 44:559–577.
17. Graybiel, A. M. (1984): Neurochemically specified subsystems in the basal ganglia. In: *Functions of the Basal Ganglia*, edited by D. Evered, pp. 114–149. Ciba Foundations Symposium 107. Pitman, London.
18. Mayberg, H. S., et al. Selective inferior frontal lobe hypometabolism in depressed patients with Parkinson's disease. *Ann. Neurology (in press)*.

19. Deleted at proofs.
20. Gerfen, C. R., et al. (1987): The neostriatal mosaic: II. Patch- and matrix-directed mesostriatal dopaminergic and non-dopaminergic systems. *J. Neurosci.*, 7:3915–34.
21. Wong, D. F., et al. (1984): Effects of age on dopamine and serotonin receptors measured by positron tomography in the living human brain. *Science*, 226:1393–1396.
22. Carrasco, L. H., and Mukherji, C. S. (1986): Atrophy of corpus striatum in normal male at risk of Huntington's chorea. *Lancet*, 2:1388–1389.
23. Zweig, R. M., et al. (1989): Linkage to the Huntington's disease locus in a family with unusual clinical and pathological features. *Ann. Neurology*, 26:78–84.
24. Taylor, A. E., et al. (1986): Parkinson's disease and depression: a critical re-evaluation. *Brain*, 109:279–292.
25. Konig, P., et al. (1986): Bilateral symmetrical calcifications and the basal ganglia—a morphological change responsible for a high incidence of affective organic psychosis (Abstract). Proceedings of Society of Biological Psychiatry.
26. Trautner, R. J., et al. (1988): Idiopathic basal ganglia calcification and organic affective disorder. *Am. J. Psychiatry* 145:350–353.
27. Starkstein, S. E., Robinson, R. G., and Price, T. R. (1987): Comparison of cortical and subcortical lesions in the production of poststroke mood disorders. *Brain*, 110:1045–1059.
28. Starkstein, S. E., et al. (1988): Differential mood changes following basal ganglia vs thalamic lesions. *Arch. Neurology*, 45:725–730.
29. Dening, T. R., and Berrios, G. E. (1989): Wilson's disease: psychiatric symptoms in 195 patients. *Arch. Gen. Psychiatry*, 46:1126–1134.
30. McHugh, P. R. The neuropsychiatry of basal ganglia disorders: a triadic syndrome and its explanations. *J. Neuropsychiatr. Neuropsychol. Behav. Neurol. (in press)*.
31. Folstein, S. E., et al. The subcortical of Huntington's disease: a model for a neuropathology of depression, dementia, and dyskinesia. American Psychopathological Association. Raven Press: New York *(in press)*.
32. Wolfe, J., et al. (1987): Verbal memory deficits associated with major affective disorders: a comparison of unipolar and bipolar patients. *J. Affective Disord.*, 13:83–92.
33. Baxter, Jr., L. R., et al. (1985): Cerebral metabolic rates for glucose in mood disorders: studies with positron emission tomography and fluorodeoxyglucose F 18. *Arch. Gen. Psychiatry*, 42:441–447.
34. Buchsbaum, M. S., et al. (1986): Frontal cortex and basal ganglia metabolic rates assessed by positron emission tomography with ^{18}F-2-deoxyglucose in affective illness. *J. Affective Disord.*, 10:137–152.
35. Drevets, W. C., et al. (1989): Trait and state cerebral blood flow abnormalities in depression. *Soc. Neurosci. Abstr.*, 15:18.10.
36. Alexander, G. E., Witt, E. D., and Goldman-Rakic, P. S. (1980): Neuronal activity in the prefrontal cortex, caudate nucleus and mediodorsal thalamic nucleus during delayed response performance of immature and adult rhesus monkeys. *Soc. Neurosci. Abstr.*, 10:515.
37. Folstein, S. E., et al. (1983): Conduct disorder and affective disorder among the offspring of patients with Huntington's disease. *Psychol. Med.*, 13:45–52.
38. Rutter, M., et al. (1976): Isle of Wight Studies, 1964–1974. *Psychol. Med.*, 6:313–332.
39. Masten, A. S., Garmezy, N., Tellegen, A., Pellegrin, D. S., Larkin, K., and Larsen, A. (1988): Competence and stress in school children: the moderating effects of individuals and family qualities. *J. Child Psychol. Psychiatry*, 29:745–764.
40. Crowe, R. R. (1974): An adoption study of antisocial personality. *Arch. Gen. Psychiatry*, 31:785–791.

Genes, Brain, and Behavior, edited by
P. R. McHugh and V. A. McKusick.
Raven Press, Ltd., New York © 1991.

Molecular Genetic Analysis of Phenylketonuria and Mental Retardation

Savio L. C. Woo

Howard Hughes Medical Institute, Department of Cell Biology and Institute for Molecular Genetics, Baylor College of Medicine, Houston, Texas 77030

CLINICAL AND BIOCHEMICAL BASIS OF PHENYLKETONURIA

Classical phenylketonuria (PKU) is caused by a deficiency of the hepatic enzyme phenylalanine hydroxylase (PAH) and is a typical example of inborn errors in amino acid metabolism. The disorder causes severe mental retardation in affected children who excrete large quantities of phenylpyruvate in the urine (7). A year after the discovery of the disease, Penrose (21) observed that it is a genetic disorder transmitted as an autosomal recessive trait. A dozen years afterward, it was shown that the administration of phenylalanine to normal humans led to prompt elevation in serum tyrosine and the response is absent in patients with PKU (8). Subsequently, he was able to demonstrate that postmortem liver samples from normal individuals were able to convert phenylalanine to tyrosine *in vitro*, while those from PKU patients could not, thereby defining the biochemical basis of phenylketonuria (9).

MOLECULAR CLONING OF RAT AND HUMAN PAH cDNAs AND THEIR PRIMARY STRUCTURES

PAH mRNA was purified from rat liver by polysome immunoprecipitation and used for the cloning of its cDNA. The authenticity of the cDNA clone was established by hybrid-selected translation (22) and confirmed by matching the nucleotide sequence with the partial amino acid sequence of the purified enzyme (23). Using the cloned rat PAH cDNA as a specified hybridization probe, a human liver cDNA library comprising of 10^7 independent recombinants was screened. A full-length human PAH cDNA clone was obtained (designated phPAH247) and sequenced in its entirety. The clone contains an inserted DNA fragment of 2,448 base pairs, including 19 bases of poly A at the 3' end (10). The first methionine codon occurs at nucleotide position 223, followed by an open reading frame of 1,353 base pairs encoding 451 amino acids. The predicted amino acid sequence of the human enzyme was deduced from the nucleotide sequence of phPAH247 and shown to be

90% homologous with the amino acid sequences of the corresponding rat enzyme reported by Robson et al. (23).

THE PKU LOCUS IN HUMANS IS ON CHROMOSOME 12

Chromosomal assignments for human genetic loci can be made using cloned genes as probes in molecular hybridization studies to genomic DNA isolated from human/rodent cell hybrids that contain different assortments of human chromosomes. A panel of mouse/human hybrid cell lines bearing an assortment of human chromosomes was analyzed by Southern blot using the human PHA cDNA clone as the hybridization probe. Results indicated that the PAH-hybridizing human DNA bands were consistent with only human chromosome 12, providing strong evidence that the human PAH locus is on chromosome 12 (15). Subsequently the regional map position of PAH on human chromosome 12 was defined by deletion chromosome mapping as well as *in situ* hybridization. It was observed that the hybridized grains were highly concentrated in the 12q22–q24.1 region (16). Since the cDNA contains all the genetic information necessary for expression of phenylalanine hydroxylase, which is the enzyme deficient in PKU (11), the PKU locus in humans has also been mapped to 12q22–q24.1.

CLASSICAL PKU IS NOT CAUSED BY DELETION OF THE ENTIRE PAH GENE

Genomic DNAs were isolated from two PKU cell lines obtained from the Human Mutant Cell Repository (GM934 and GM2406) and from two normal individuals. The DNA preparations were digested with restriction enzymes followed by Southern hybridization using the human PAH cDNA clone as the specific probe. Identical hybridization signals were obtained from all four DNA preparations after digestion with a number of restriction enzymes (27). These results indicated that the PAH gene was not only present in the genome of cells derived from the PKU patients, but the overall organization of the gene also remained unchanged. Comparison of densitometer tracings of the gel lanes containing normal and PKU DNAs has shown that the hybridization signals generated by the PKU DNA samples were not the result of compound heterozygotes with deletions in nonoverlapping regions of the two PAH alleles present in each cell line. Consequently, it could be concluded that classical PKU, at least in these two cases, is not caused by deletion of the entire PAH gene. Subsequently this observation has been extended to include several hundred PKU chromosomes. Deletion mutations were found to represent only a very minor fraction of total PKU alleles.

THE MOLECULAR STRUCTURE OF THE HUMAN PAH GENE

In order to effectively study the molecular genetics of PKU, the structural organization of the PAH gene needs to be established. A human genomic DNA library was constructed using a cosmid vector (pCV107). The library was screened with the PAH cDNA probe and the corresponding genomic sequences were isolated. Four overlapping PAH cosmid clones, spanning more than 125 Kb of the genetic locus, were used for structural analysis of the gene. The structural gene is about 90 Kb in length and contains 13 exons, with intron sizes ranging from 1 to 23 Kb (3). The human PAH gene codes for a mature RNA of approximately 2.4 Kb and has one of the highest ratio's of noncoding to coding DNA found among eukaryotic genes, possibly attributing to its extensive polymorphic nature.

EXTENSIVE RESTRICTION FRAGMENT LENGTH POLYMORPHISMS IN THE HUMAN PAH LOCUS

Genomic DNAs isolated from 20 random Caucasians were analyzed by Southern hybridization using the full-length human PAH cDNA clone and a battery of restriction enzymes. Enzymes that yielded polymorphic patterns in the PAH locus identified in this manner include BglII, PvuII, EcoRI, XmnI, MspI, HindIII, and EcoRV (17,27). The frequencies of these restriction fragment length polymorphisms (RFLPs) among Caucasians are such that the observed heterozygosity in the population is about 90%. Using these enzymes to perform RFLP analysis in PKU families, it was demonstrated that the segregation of the PKU alleles and the disease state are concordant. Thus, the RFLP analysis of the human PAH locus can be applied to prenatal diagnosis of the hereditary disorder in most PKU families (26,28,29).

The RFLPs identified in the PAH locus were assayed in 33 nuclear PKU families from Denmark. RFLP haplotype analysis of 66 normal chromosomes and 77 chromosomes bearing PKU mutation demonstrated two clusters of RFLPs: (a) BglII, PvuIIa, and PvuIIb at the 5' end of the PAH gene, and (b) EcoRI, MspIa, MspIb, XmnI, HindIII, and EcoRV at the 3' end. Having determined the exact map positions of the RFLPs by structural analysis of the PAH gene (3), a relationship between the physical distance and RFLP linkage map was established. The RFLP sites within each cluster have a significant tendency to segregate as a group ($p < 0.001$), a process referred to as "linkage disequilibrium." The RFLP sites in the 5' and 3' clusters, however, are randomly associated.

PRENATAL DIAGNOSIS OF PKU

The polymorphism detected with HindIII is inherited in a mendelian fashion and was used for prenatal diagnosis of PKU for the first time since the discovery of PKU by Folling in 1934 (18). Both parents in a family at risk were heterozygous for the HindIII polymorphism containing the 4.2-Kb and 4.0-Kb alleles. DNA analysis revealed that the affected child in this family inherited the PAH gene containing the 4.0-Kb HindIII fragment from both parents. The mutant genes are therefore associated with the 4.0-Kb allele in this family. Analysis of DNA isolated from amniocytes revealed that the fetus was homozygous for the 4.0-Kb fragment. The fetus has the same genotype as the affected child and was consequently diagnosed as having PKU. After delivery, this diagnosis was confirmed by the phenotype of the infant.

The extensive polymorphic nature of the human PAH locus permits the use of eight restriction enzymes for prenatal diagnosis of PKU. However, the polymorphisms generated by various enzymes tend to segregate as groups in PKU families. Consequently, it was determined that PvuII, XmnI, and EcoRV (detecting RFLPs in the 5', middle, and 3' regions of the gene) will establish disease status in about 85% of PKU families at risk and these are the useful enzymes for future prenatal diagnosis of PKU (2,14).

MOLECULAR AND GENETIC ANALYSIS OF PREVALENT PKU ALLELES

Prenatal diagnosis of PKU by RFLP analysis is applicable only to families with a previously affected child whose RFLP pattern serves as the reference for fetal DNA analyses. Its ability to predict the incidence of PKU in a given population is thus limited, since the majority of PKU infants are born to couples without prior family PKU history. However, if PKU is caused by a limited number of mutations in the PAH gene, diagnosis and carrier detection could be achieved by direct analysis of the mutation sites in the gene within the population. We have observed the existence of multiple RFLP haplotypes in the human PAH gene from various European populations (1), and a strong association of PKU alleles among distinct RFLP haplotypes in that population (Fig. 1). Close associations between RFLP haplotypes of the β-globin locus and specific β-thalassemia mutations in different ethnic populations have previously been reported by other laboratories (for review, see [20]). The association of RFLP haplotypes and specific PKU mutations, if any, can be verified by isolation and sequencing of PKU genes. Having established the molecular structure and RFLP linkage map of the PAH gene, this important issue can be addressed by cloning the mutant alleles of the predominant RFLP haplotypes.

The PAH gene of a prevalent PKU haplotype (i.e., haplotype 3) was isolated by molecular cloning. Sequence analysis demonstrated a single-base substitution in this gene (G to A) involving the 5' donor splice site of intron 12 (4). Expression analysis after site-directed mutagenesis had verified that this nucleotide substitution is indeed a PKU mutation and constitutes the first mutant PAH gene ever characterized (19). An oligonucleotide specific for the splicing mutation was synthesized and hybridized to cloned PAH DNA in order to test the feasibility of using this probe as a tool for direct analysis of the mutation. The mutant oligonucleotide probe specifically hybridized to the mutant donor splice site, while a corresponding normal oligonucleotide probe hybridized with only the normal sequence. Genomic DNAs isolated from Danish PKU individuals with previously defined haplotypes were analyzed by hybridization using the mutant and normal oligonucleotide probes. These analyses have demonstrated that all haplotype 3 mutant alleles in the Danish population bear the same splicing mutation and none of the nonhaplotype 3

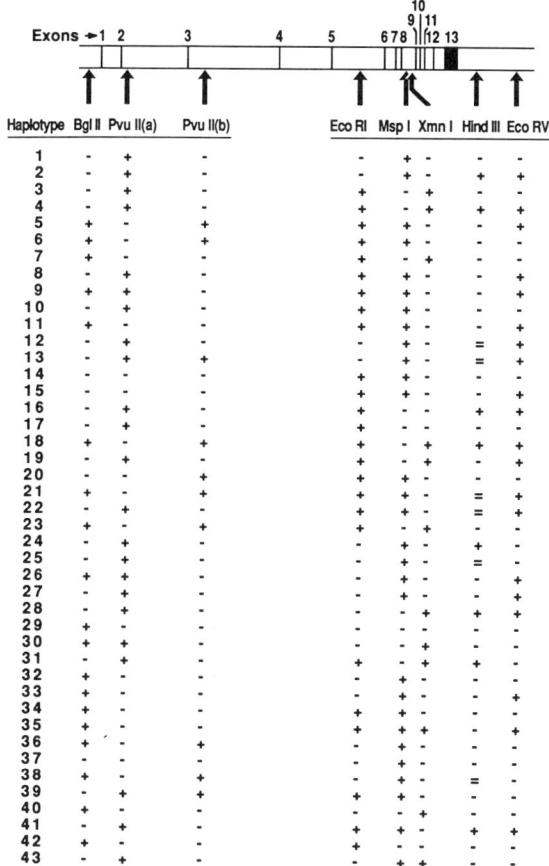

FIG. 1. Structure of the human PAH gene and RFLP haplotypes at the human PAH locus. The molecular structure of the human PAH gene is shown schematically with its 13 axons encompassing about 90 kb of DNA. The *heavy arrows* correspond to the polymorphic restriction sites in and immediately flanking the gene. + and − symbols are used to designate the presence and absence of a polymorphic restriction site, respectively. = is used to designate a 4.4-Kb HindIII allele. Contributing PKU centers in Europe include those in Denmark, Scotland, Switzerland, Germany, France, Italy, Hungary, and Czechoslovakia. (From ref. 15.)

mutant alleles bear that particular mutation (4). The absolute association between haplotype 3 mutant alleles and the splicing mutation must be the result of a recent mutational event on a haplotype 3 chromosome background that was spread in the population before there had been sufficient time for transfer of the mutant fragment into chromosomes of other haplotypes by cross-overs during meiosis. This is the first demonstration of linkage disequilibrium between a specific mutation and a particular haplotype in PKU.

Subsequently, a mutant haplotype 2 allele was cloned from a PKU individual. Sequence characterization of the gene showed that there is a C to T transition in exon 12, resulting in the substitution of Arg^{408} to Trp^{408} in the enzyme. Site-directed mutagenesis using specific oligonucleotides was performed in order to create the specific mutant allele in an expression vector. When the normal and mutant constructs were introduced into cultured mammalian cells, only the former produced immunoreactive protein and active enzyme in the cytoplasm, while both produced similar levels of PAH mRNA. Thus, the Arg to Trp substitution is a PKU mutation, which also creates a CRM⁻ phenotype (5). A specific oligonucleotide corresponding to the mutation sequence in the haplotype 2 allele was synthesized and used to determine if there is any association between mutation and haplotype. Results demonstrated there is a strong linkage disequilibrium, suggesting again that there was a recent mutation event on a normal haplotype 2 chromosome, which was then spread in the population (5).

DETECTION OF MUTANT HAPLOTYPE 2 AND 3 ALLELES USING THE POLYMERASE CHAIN REACTION AND ALLELE-SPECIFIC OLIGONUCLEOTIDES

The polymerase chain reaction (PCR) technique (24,25) was used to amplify exon 12 plus flanking introns of the human PAH gene for subsequent dot-blot hybridization analysis (6). Oligonucleotides specific for the haplotype 2 and 3 mutations were used as molecular probes to detect patients and carriers in the population. As shown in Fig. 1, the mutant haplotype 2 probe hybridized only with amplified genomic DNA from the haplotype 2 carriers and the compound heterozygotes bearing both mutant alleles (Fig. 2A). Similarly, the mutant haplotype 3 probe hybridized only with amplified genomic DNA from the haplotype 3 carriers and the compound heterozygotes (Fig. 2B). The sensitivity of the analysis was greatly increased through the use of PCR-mediated amplification, since no hybridization signal was detectable with unamplified DNA samples (Fig. 2 A,B), while the specificity of the analysis is demonstrated by the failure of either mutant oligonucleotide probe to hybridize with amplified normal genomic DNA samples.

IDENTIFICATION OF MUTATIONS ASSOCIATED WITH HAPLOTYPES 1 AND 4 OF THE PAH GENE

More recently, PCR-mediated amplification techniques have been applied to the characterization of the molecular lesions associated with haplotype 1 and 4 mutant alleles in the Swiss population. Exon-containing regions of the PAH gene from genomic DNA of a PKU patient bearing a haplotype 1 and a haplotype 4 mutant allele were amplified by PCR. The amplified DNA fragments were subcloned into M13 for sequence analysis. Missense mutations were observed in exons 5 and 7, resulting in the substitution of glutamine for arginine at residues 158 and 261 of the enzyme, respectively. Direct hybridization analysis of the point mutations using allele-specific oligonucleotide probes demonstrated that the exon 7 mutation is

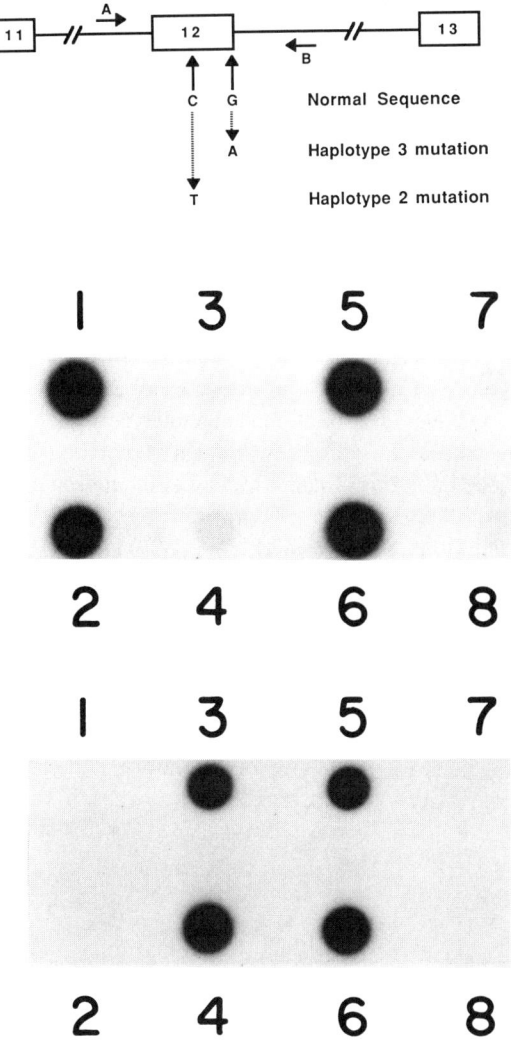

FIG. 2. Molecular analysis of PKU by PCR. **Upper panel:** Schematic representation of 245-bp DNA fragment containing exon 12 and flanking intronic sequences of the PAH gene. This segment contains both mutation sites for the mutant PAH alleles associated with haplotypes 2 and 3 that are prevalent among Caucasians of northern European ancestry. *Arrows A* and *B* represent primer oligonucleotides used for the PCR amplification reaction. **Lower panel:** Dot-blot analysis of PCR-amplified genomic DNA. **Panels A** and **B** are autoradiographs of the membranes after hybridization with the mutant haplotype 2 and 3 oligonucleotide probes, respectively. Dots 1 and 2, two mutant haplotype 2 carriers; dots 3 and 4, two mutant haplotype 3 carriers; dot 5 and 6, two haplotypes 2 and 3 compound heterozygotes; dots 7 and 8, two normal individuals. (From ref. 6.)

present in 13 of 18 haplotype 1 mutant alleles and the exon 5 mutation is present in two of six haplotype 4 mutant alleles in the Swiss population. These mutations were not detected among normal alleles or mutant alleles of other haplotypes. The results provide strong evidence for linkage disequilibrium between the mutant haplotypes and specific mutations in the PAH gene. Furthermore, they constitute conclusive evidence that haplotype 1 and 4 chromosomes bear multiple mutant PAH alleles in Caucasians.

POTENTIAL CARRIER SCREENING FOR PKU IN CAUCASIANS

Oligonucleotides specific for the four mutations were used to screen for these mutant PAH alleles among Caucasians in various European populations. The Arg^{261} to Gln^{261} mutation comprises 26% of all mutant haplotype 1 alleles, while the Arg^{158} to Gln^{158} mutation accounts for 48% of all mutant haplotype 4 alleles in the European population. Since haplotype 1 and 4 mutant PAH alleles account for 28% and 13%, respectively, of all PKU alleles in Europe, current carrier detection rates for haplotype 1 and 4 mutations are 26% × 28% = 7.3% and 48% × 13% = 6.2%, respectively. Combined with the haplotype 2 and 3 mutations, the overall potential for carrier screening of PKU at the present time is 48.3% of the European population using specific oligonucleotide probes to all four mutant alleles (see Table 1).

Characterization of the remaining prevalent mutant alleles in the Caucasian population will significantly increase the reliability of carrier screening programs. When 90% of all mutant PKU alleles are identified, reliable carrier screening programs may be implemented for the detection of PKU in the Caucasian population without prior family history.

ACKNOWLEDGMENTS

I wish to express my sincere gratitude to all my collaborators in Europe, for without their cooperation the population genetic analysis of PKU would not have been possible. I am also indebted to, and proud of, my previous and present associates, whose combined efforts have been the key to the molecular genetic analysis of PKU. I would also like to thank Mrs. Brenda Grossie for the typing of this manu-

TABLE 1. *Cumulative frequency of prevalent mutant PAH alleles in Europe*

Haplotypes	Mutations	Frequencies (%)
1	Arg^{261} tp Gln^{261}	26 × 28 = 7.3
2	Arg^{408} to Gln^{408}	100 × 21 = 21.0
3	$GT^{(12)}$ to $AT^{(12)}$	92 × 15 = 13.8
4	Arg^{158} to Gln^{158}	48 × 13 = 6.2
Cumulative frequency		48.3

script. This work was supported in part by NIH grant HD-17711 and the author is also an investigator of the Howard Hughes Medical Institute.

GLOSSARY

Autosomal recessive A genetic trait inherited on an autosome (not a sex chromosome) that has to be present on both chromosomes to be phenotypically expressed (not dominant).

Polysome immunoprecipitation Polysomes, short for polyribosomes, are engaged in protein synthesis; since the nascent polypeptide chain is still attached to them they can be precipitated with a specific antiserum.

cDNA Short for complementary DNA; a DNA copy obtained from mRNA by a process known as reverse transcription.

Hybrid-selected translation A pure mRNA species can be obtained by hybridization to a cloned probe (hybrid selection), the resulting mRNA can then be translated *in vitro* into protein and the product analyzed.

Hybridization probe Piece of DNA that is labeled (generally radio-labeled) allowing the specific detection of homologous DNA in a mixture.

Recombinant (clones) DNAs consisting of two parts: a "vector" for propagation (generally in *E. coli*) and an insert (often mammalian DNA).

Restriction enzyme Short for restriction endonuclease: an enzyme (generally of bacterial origin) that recognizes a specific DNA sequence (usually 4 or 6 bp long) and cleaves within that recognition sequence.

Southern (blotting) A tool for the analysis of DNA named after E. Southern: (a) DNA digested with a restriction enzyme is fractionated on an agarose gel and then (b) transferred to a solid support membrane that (c) can be annealed to a hybridization probe; the band(s) of interest are (d) finally revealed by autoradiography.

Alleles Different forms of a gene (polymorphisms are allelic forms of a gene).

RFLP Short for restriction fragment length polymorphism, pronounced riflip; a polymorphism involving the presence or absence of a restriction recognition site.

Linkage disequilibrium Cosegregation of independent genetic markers, i.e., coinheritance of genetic traits at a higher frequency than expected from independent segregation.

Haplotype Set of genetic markers on *one* chromosome.

Oligonucleotide A short (generally less than 30 nucleotides) piece of DNA.

PCR Short for polymerase chain reaction: a technique for the specific amplification of DNA segments of interest *in vitro* using a thermostable DNA polymerase in conjunction with oligonucleotide primers by repeating usually dozens of times a cycle consisting of (a) denaturation of the double stranded DNA by heat, (b) annealing of the specific primers and (c) extension of the primers by the DNA polymerase.

Dot-blot hybridization Variation of Southern blotting in which total DNA is spotted directly on a solid support without prior gel fractionation.

REFERENCES

1. Chakraborty, R., Lidsky, A. S., Daiger, S. P., et al. (1987): Polymorphic DNA haplotypes at the human phenylalanine hydroxylase locus and their relationship with phenylketonuria. *Hum. Genet.*, 76:40–46.
2. Daiger, S. P., Lidsky, A. S., Chakraborty, R., Koch, R., Güttler, F., and Woo, S. L. C. (1986): Effective use of polymorphic DNA haplotypes at the phenylalanine hydroxylase locus in prenatal diagnosis of phenylketonuria. *Lancet*, 1:229–232.
3. DiLella, A. G., Kwok, S. C. M., Ledley, F. D., Marvit, J., and Woo, S. L. C. (1986): Molecular structure and polymorphic map of the human phenylalanine hydroxylase gene. *Biochemistry*, 25:743–749.
4. DiLella, A. G., Marvit, J., Lidsky, A. S., Güttler, F., and Woo, S. L. C. (1986): Tight linkage between a splicing mutation and a DNA haplotype in phenylketonuria. *Nature*, 322:799–803.
5. DiLella, A. G., Marvit, J., Brayton, K., and Woo, S. L. C. (1987): An amino acid substitution in phenylketonuria is in linkage disequilibrium with DNA haplotype-2. *Nature*, 327:333–336.
6. DiLella, A. G., Huang, W. M., and Woo, S. L. C. (1988): Screening for phenylketonuria mutations by DNA amplification with polymerase chain reaction. *Lancet*, 1:497–499.
7. Fölling, A. (1934): Uber Ausscheidung von Phenylbrenztraubensaure in den Harn als Stoffwechselanomalie in Verbinding mit Imbezillitat. *Z. Physiol. Chem.*, 227:169–176.
8. Jervis, G. A. (1947): Studies on phenylpyruvic oligophrenia; position of metabolic error. *J. Biol. Chem.*, 169:651–656.
9. Jervis, G. A. (1953): Phenylpyruvic oligophrenia. Deficiency of phenylalanine oxidizing system. *Proc. Soc. Exp. Biol. Med.*, 82:514–515.
10. Kwok, S. C. M., Ledley, F. D., DeLella, A. G., Robson, K. J. H., and Woo, S. L. C. (1985): Nucleotide sequence of a full-length cDNA clone and amino acid sequence of human phenylalanine hydroxylase. *Biochemistry*, 24:556–561.
11. Ledley, F. D., Grenett, H. E., DiLella, A. G., Kwok, S. C. M., and Woo, S. L. C. (1985): Gene transfer and expression of human phenylalanine hydroxylase. *Science*, 228:77–79.
12. Ledley, F. D., Levy, H. L., and Woo, S. L. C. (1986): Molecular analysis of the inheritance of phenylketonuria and mild hyperphenylalaninemia in families with both diseases. *N. Engl. J. Med.*, 314:1276–1280.
13. Ledley, F. D., Grenett, H. E., and Woo, S. L. C. (1987): Biochemical characterization of recombinant human phenylalanine hydroxylase produced in E. coli. *J. Biol. Chem.*, 262:2228–2233.
14. Ledley, F. D., Koch, R., Jew, K., et al. (1988): Phenylalanine hydroxylase expression in liver of a fetus with phenylketonuria. *J. Pediatr.*, 113:463–468.
15. Lidsky, A. S., Robson, K., Chandra, T., Barker, P., Ruddle, F., and Woo, S. L. C. (1984): The PKU locus in man on chromosome 12. *Am. J. Hum. Genet.*, 36:527–533.
16. Lidsky, A. S., Law, M. L., Morse, H. G., et al. (1985): Regional mapping of the human phenylalanine hydroxylase gene and the PKU locus on chromosome 12. *Proc. Natl. Acad. Sci. USA*, 82:6221–6225.
17. Lidsky, A. S., Ledley, F. D., DiLella, A. G., et al. (1985): Molecular genetics of phenylketonuria: extensive restriction site polymorphisms in the human phenylalanine hydroxylase locus. *Am. J. Hum. Genet.*, 37:619–634.
18. Lidsky, A. S., Güttler, F., and Woo, S. L. C. (1985): Prenatal diagnosis of classical phenylketonuria by DNA analysis. *Lancet*, 1:549–551.
19. Marvit, J., DiLella, A. G., Brayton, K., Ledley, F. D., Robson, K. J. M., and Woo, S. L. C. (1987): GT to AT transition at a splice donor site causes skipping of the preceding exon in phenylketonuria. *Nucleic Acids Res.*, 15:5613–5628.
20. Orkin, S. H., and Kazazian, H. H. (1984): The mutation and polymorphism of the human beta-globin gene and its surrounding DNA. *Annu. Rev. Genet.*, 18:131–171.
21. Penrose, L. S. (1935): Inheritance of phenylpyruvic amentia (phenylketonuria). *Lancet*, 2:192–194.
22. Robson, K. J. H., Chandra, T., MacGillivray, R. T. A., and Woo, S. L. C. (1982): Polysome immunoprecipitation of phenylalanine hydroxylase mRNA from rat liver and cloning of its cDNA. *Proc. Natl. Acad. Sci. USA*, 79:4701–4705.
23. Robson, K. J. H., Beattie, W., James, R. J., Cotton, R. C. H., Morgan, F. J., and Woo, S. L. C. (1984): Sequence comparison of rat liver phenylalanine hydroxylase and its cDNA clones. *Biochemistry*, 23:5671–5673.

24. Saiki, R. K., Scharf, S., Faloona, F., et al. (1985): Enzymatic amplification of beta-globin genomic sequences and restriction site analysis for diagnosis of sickle cell anemia. *Science*, 230:1350–1354.
25. Saiki, R. K., Bugawan, T. L., Horn, G. T., Mullis, K. B., and Erlich, H. A. (1986): Analysis of enzymatically amplified beta-globin and HLA-DQ alpha DNA with allele-specific oligonucleotides. *Nature*, 324:163–166.
26. Speer, A., Dahl, H. H., Reiss, O., et al. (1986): Typing of families with classical phenylketonuria using three alleles of the Hindiii linked restriction fragment polymorphism, detectable with a phenylalanine hydroxylase cDNA probe. Family typing for PKU by linked Hing III RFLP. *Clin. Genet.*, 29:491–495.
27. Woo, S. L. C., Lidsky, A. S., Chandra, T., Güttler, F., and Robson, K. J. H. (1983): Cloned human phenylalanine hydroxylase gene allows prenatal diagnosis and carrier detection of classical phenylketonuria. *Nature*, 306:151–155.
28. Woo, S. L. C. (1984): Prenatal diagnosis and carrier detection of classic phenylketonuria by gene analysis. *Pediatrics*, 74:412–423.
29. Woo, S. L. C., Lidsky, A., Chandra, T., Güttler, F., and Robson, K. (1984): Prenatal diagnosis of classical phenylketonuria by gene mapping. *JAMA*, 251:1998–2002.

Genetic Contributions to Human Obesity

Albert J. Stunkard

*Department of Psychiatry, University of Pennsylvania,
Philadelphia, Pennsylvania 19104- 3246*

Recent discoveries in the field of genetics have transformed our understanding of human obesity. For many years obesity had been viewed as a disorder with strong behavioral determinants, primarily psychopathology manifested as overeating. This view has changed 180° in direction and the psychopathology of obese persons is now seen as consequence, rather than cause—a consequence of the prejudice and discrimination directed against obese people, particularly adolescent girls and young women.

But if psychopathology is not causing obesity, what is? Heredity is increasingly viewed as the major determinant of human obesity. This view will not come as a surprise to most Americans. Textbooks of medicine and endocrinology have long assured us of the power of genetic effects in human obesity. What is a surprise is how limited the evidence for this assurance has been. Most of our beliefs about human obesity have been extrapolated from animal studies. It is true that the *ob/ob* mouse and the Zucker fatty rat get very fat and primarily on a genetic basis (1,4). But the relevance of these unusual rodents to human obesity is not at all clear.

Most of the evidence for the importance of genetic factors in human obesity has been obtained in the past 4 years. It is based on the three traditional types of genetic studies: twin, adoption, and family.

TWIN STUDIES

The largest of the twin studies used the Twin Register of the National Academy of Sciences/National Research Council (6). This register contains information on 1,974 identical twin pairs and 2,097 fraternal twin pairs of men inducted into the Armed Forces of the United States between 1940 and 1955. The heights and weights of these twins were determined when they were 20 years of age and again when they were 45 years of age. From these heights and weights we calculated the body mass index (weight in kilograms/height in meters squared) and then arrayed the distribution from thinnest to fattest (16). At age 20 the distribution of body mass index of both identical and fraternal twins was essentially normal, with a peak at 21, corresponding to a normal body weight. At that age only 1.4% of twins were more than 30% overweight; 25 years later, at age 45, the distribution was shifted to the right, and 8.3% were more than 30% overweight.

The extent of the genetic influence on the body mass index was estimated by calculating its "heritability"—the percentage of the variance of a trait that can be attributed to genetic factors (5). It is calculated as $h^2 = 2(r_{MZ} - r_{DZ})$, where h^2 is the convention for heritability, r_{MZ} is the intrapair correlation coefficient of monozygotic (MZ or identical) twins and r_{DZ} is the intrapair correlation coefficient of the dizygotic (DZ or fraternal) twins.

Heritability of the body mass index calculated by the classic twin method at age 20 was 0.77 and at age 45 was 0.84, indicating that genetic factors accounted for 77% and 84% of the variance, respectively (16). These values are very high, and there is concern that heritability estimates exaggerate the influence of genetic factors. Nevertheless, these estimates make possible a more conservative measure—a comparison of the heritability of obesity with that of other disorders that have been studied by the twin method. The heritabilities of several of these disorders are listed in Table 1. Their rank ordering makes clear the importance of genetic factors in obesity as compared with genetic influences on other common disorders (16).

The concern that twin studies overestimate the influence of genetic factors derives in part from the possibility that the environment affects MZ twins differently from DZ twins. If the environment in which MZ twins were raised made them more alike than they otherwise would be, this similarity might incorrectly be attributed to heredity, and thereby inflate the estimate of heritability.

This kind of bias does not affect MZ twins reared apart and a separated twin study is a geneticist's dream. Such a study of genetic influences on the body mass index was made possible by the data of the Swedish Adoption/Twin Study of Aging and the generosity of its staff (8). It showed strong genetic effects on the body mass index and indicated that earlier studies that had used the classical twin design had overestimated the effect of genetic factors only slightly if at all (18).

The study enrolled 93 MZ twin pairs reared apart, 154 MZ twin pairs reared together, 214 DZ twin pairs reared apart, and 208 DZ twin pairs reared together. The sample was identified by use of the Swedish Twin Registry, which includes

TABLE 1. Heritability estimates from twin studies

Obesity (children)	0.77
Obesity (children)	0.88
Obesity (age 20)	0.80
Obesity (age 20)	0.77
Obesity (age 45)	0.84
Schizophrenia	0.68
Hypertension	0.57
Alcoholism	0.57
Cirrhosis	0.53
Epilepsy	0.50
Coronary	0.49

TABLE 2. *Heritability by gender estimated by three methods*

Calculation	Men	Women
$2(r_{MZT} - r_{DZT})$	0.82	0.78
$2(r_{MZA} - r_{DZA})$	1.10	0.82
r_{MZA}	0.70	0.66

MZ, monozygotic; DZ, dizygotic; A, twins reared apart; T, twins reared together.
From ref. 18.

25,000 pairs of same-sex twins born in Sweden between 1886 and 1958 (2). It comprised largely older persons, with a mean age and ($\pm$ S.D.) of 58.6 $\pm$ 13.6 years. Heritability was estimated for both the twins reared apart and those reared together by use of the classic twin method described above. Heritability of the male twins reared together was the same as that of the American male twins described above—0.82, with a similar value for women—0.78. Surprisingly, the heritability of the twins reared apart was no lower, although the value for men, 1.10, is clearly too high, an artifact of an unusually low intrapair correlation coefficient of DZ twins reared apart.

The most direct and probably the best estimate of heritability is that made possible for the first time by the Swedish sample—the intrapair correlation coefficient of MZ twins reared apart. This value, 0.70 for men and 0.66 for women, is only slightly lower than estimates yielded by the classic twin method in this and other studies (Table 2).

In addition to the estimates of heritability derived from correlations, the data were analyzed also by maximum likelihood model-fitting using LISREL-VI. This powerful approach is based on a simultaneous treatment of all of the information, which makes it possible not only to estimate heritability but also to partition it into additive and nonadditive components. Additive genetic effects are those in which genes that influence a trait sum according to gene doses and nonadditive effects are those that, because of dominance, do not sum according to gene doses.

In addition to estimating and partitioning genetic variance, the effects of three different kinds of environments were estimated: the shared rearing environment, other "correlated" environments, and "nonshared" environments that are unique to the individual. The study of twins reared apart makes it possible to estimate the effects of the shared rearing environment: one simply compares the resemblances between pairs reared together with those of twins reared apart. The difference between the two is ascribed to the shared rearing environment. Even twins reared apart could resemble each other on environmental grounds if their environments were similar in character, that is, if their environments were "correlated." Twin resemblances attributable to neither heredity nor the shared rearing environment may be attributed to correlated environments. For example, a correlated environment may be the result of "selective placement"—placing adopted children in homes that resemble those of their biological parents—or by contact between the twins in adulthood. The third form of environmental effects, "nonshared" environment unique to

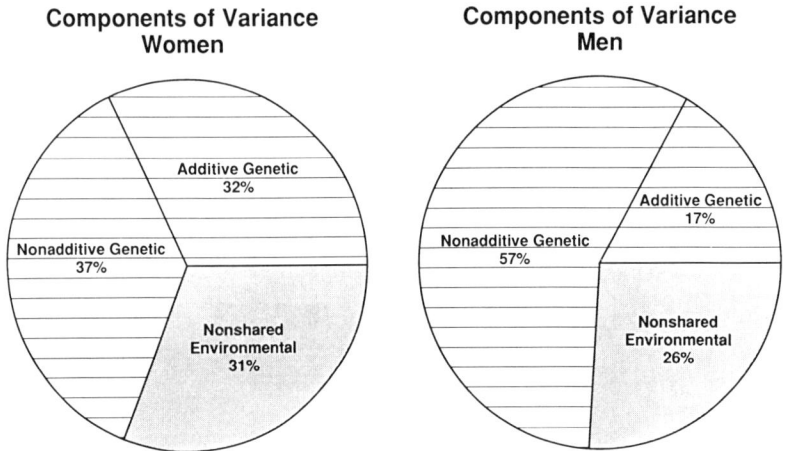

FIG. 1. Variance explained by genetic and environmental sources. Shared and correlated environmental contributions each account for less than 1% of the variances. (From ref. 18.)

the individual, consists of residual variance that cannot be explained by heredity, the shared rearing environment, or correlated environments. These latter environmental effects are those experienced by adults who are no longer associated with their twins or siblings.

The results of the model-fitting analyses are depicted in Fig. 1 and Table 3. The estimates of overall heritability were very similar to those derived from the MZ twins reared apart: 74% for men and 69% for women. Partitioning the variance revealed important nonadditive contributions: 57% for men and 37% for women. Additive genetic variance was 17% for men and 32% for women. The remaining variance (26% for men and 31% for women) can be attributed to nonshared environmental influences unique to the individual. Significantly, the parameters for shared rearing environment and correlated environments were trivial, accounting for less than 1% of the variance.

The finding of significant nonadditive genetic variance in this sample of older

TABLE 3. *Maximum likelihood model-fitting: parameter estimates, standard errors, and chi-square values*

	Parameter estimates ± S.E.					
	G_a	G_d	E_n	χ^2	d	p
Men						
Body mass index	0.34 ± 0.30	0.62 ± 0.16	0.42 ± 0.03	6.64	5	0.249
Variance (%)	17	57	26			
Women						
Body mass index	0.61 ± 0.22	0.65 ± 0.21	0.60 ± 0.04	11.35	5	0.045
Variance (%)	32	37	31			

G_a, additive genetic variance; G_d, nonadditive genetic variance; E_n, nonshared environment; S.E., standard error. Parameter estimates were squared before calculation of percentage of the total variance. (From ref. 18.)

Swedish twins raises the question as to whether such variance is due to age or to ethnicity. The cross-sectional nature of the Swedish study makes it impossible to assess the effects of age. The American twins, however, were measured twice, once at age 20 and again at age 45. At age 20 there was no evidence of nonadditive variance; at age 45 there was (16). These results make it appear that nonadditive variance exerts its effects on the body mass index only later in life.

The results of this study should be interpreted in the light of the concept of heritability (5). Heritability does not imply an invariant, immutable genetic influence such as occurs in the case of hair color or eye color. Instead it describes the genetic influences found among persons living in a particular range of environmental conditions. Under different environmental conditions, different estimates of heritability might be obtained. Adoption studies are a way of extending the understanding provided by twin studies, and adoption studies of human obesity have complemented the twin studies.

ADOPTION STUDIES

The rationale of adoption studies is straightforward. Adoptees are compared with both their biologic and their adoptive parents for the trait under consideration: schizophrenia, alcoholism, or obesity. The relationship between biologic parents and adoptees assesses genetic influences; the relationship between adoptive parents and adoptees assesses environmental influences.

The first full adoption study of human obesity made use of the Danish Adoption Register, which had been employed successfully in previous assessments of genetic influences on schizophrenia and alcoholism. We obtained information on the height and weight of 3,580 adoptees who were living in Copenhagen and whose average age was 42 years at the time of the study (17). Body mass index was calculated and a sample of 540 male and female adoptees was selected, representing four critical weight classes; the thinnest 4%, the fattest 4%, the next-to-fattest 4%, and the 4% at the median.

The heights and weights of both biologic and adoptive parents were then ascertained and compared with those of the adoptees. The relationship between biologic parents and adoptees indicated a genetic influence. The weight class of the adoptees was strongly related to the body mass index of their biologic parents ($p < 0.001$ for mothers; $p < 0.02$ for fathers) (Fig. 2).

A second finding provided firm support for a key finding of the separated twin study: there was no apparent effect of the early family environment. Figure 2 shows that the weight class of the adoptees was not related to the body mass index of their adoptive parents. Whatever the influence their adoptive parents may have had when the adoptees were children, no traces of it remained when the adoptees reached middle age. It appears that the dire consequences of faulty childhood eating habits, so often blamed for the development of obesity, have been, to say the least, exaggerated.

This study of the relationship between the Danish adoptees and their parents has

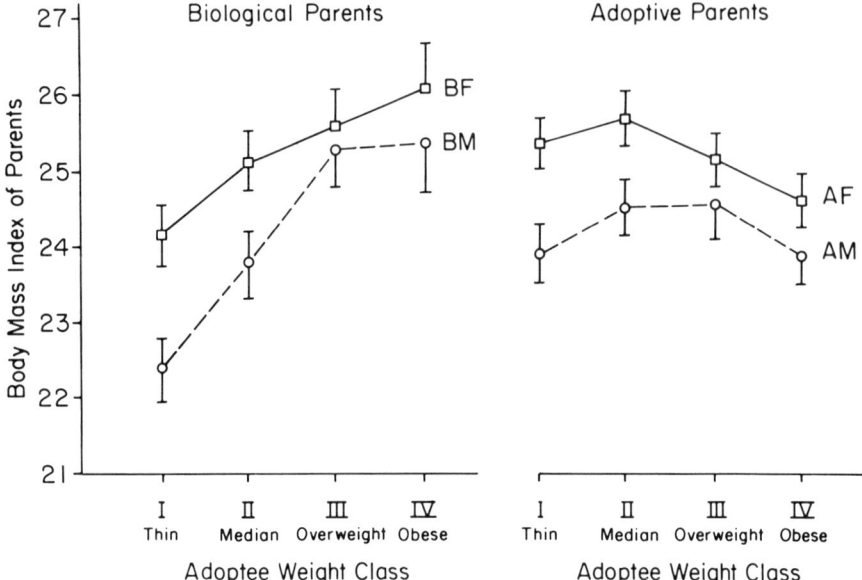

FIG. 2. Body mass index of the parents of the adoptees. On the horizontal axis is the weight class of the adoptees: thin, medium, overweight, and obese. On the vertical axis is the body mass index of the parents. As the adoptees proceed from thin to fat, both the biologic mothers and the biologic fathers become fatter, although the relationship with the mothers is stronger. The weight class of the adoptees is not related to the body mass index of the adoptive parents. (From ref. 17.)

recently been supplemented by one that examined the relationship between the adoptees and their siblings. The results of the two studies are similar.

The study of siblings compared the body mass index of 115 siblings and 850 half siblings with that of the adoptees in the same way as the body mass index of their parents had been compared with that of the adoptees (13). The body mass index of the siblings increased with increase in the weight class of the adoptees as had the body mass index of the parents (Fig. 3). There was, however, one important difference. As the weight class of the adoptees increased from overweight to obese, there was little or no increase in the body mass index of the parents. By contrast, the increase among the siblings was pronounced.

This striking difference between the relationship of the adoptees to their parents and their relationship to their siblings suggests an intriguing possibility—the presence of a major gene for obesity. If this gene were transmitted in a recessive manner, it would exert its effect only when present in two copies. Siblings would obtain the requisite two copies when they received one copy each from a heterozygous parent. The body mass index of these heterozygous parents, however, would not be related to that of their homozygous obese offspring with whom they share only one gene. The possibility of recessive transmission of obesity is heightened by recent evidence that the skewed distribution of body mass index is constituted by three component distributions that include an obese distribution (9).

The body mass index of the half siblings also increased with an increase in the

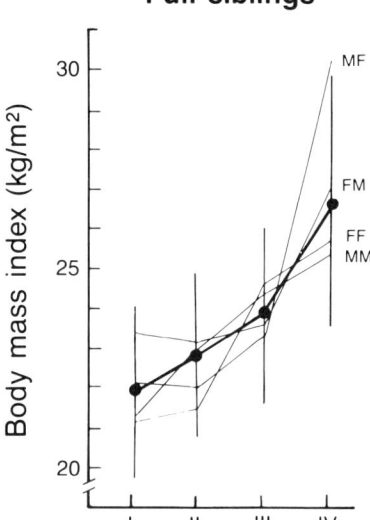

FIG. 3. Body mass index of the siblings of the adoptees. On the horizontal axis is the weight class of the adoptees: thin (I), medium (II), overweight (III), and obese (IV). On the vertical axis is the body mass index of the siblings. As the adoptee weight class proceeds from thin to fat, there is a monotonic increase in body mass index of the siblings, with a more pronounced increase between the overweight and obese classes. The thin lines show the contribution of different sex combinations to the overall relationship: MF, male adoptees/female siblings; FM, female adoptees/male siblings; FF, female siblings/female adoptee; MM, male siblings/male adoptees. Ns, the number of siblings; Na, the number of adoptees. (From ref. 14.)

weight class of the adoptees. Reflecting the lesser genetic relationship between the half siblings and the adoptees, however, this increase was less than that of the full siblings.

The results of the analyses of siblings and half siblings are compatible with two separate modes of inheritance. One is a major gene that determines frank obesity; the other is a polygenic influence exerted across the entire spectrum from thin to fat.

Both twin and adoption studies show that heredity influences human obesity. The classical twin studies, however, may have overestimated the importance of heredity while the adoption studies did not indicate precisely how important it was. A recent adoption study carried out in Iowa does estimate the extent of genetic influence.

Because the results of the Iowa study replicated those in Copenhagen to a remarkable degree, they can be generalized. The strong relationship between biologic parents and adoptees is shown in Table 4. The correlation coefficient between mothers and daughters of 0.40 indicates that a substantial portion of the variance in the body mass index may be genetic. Note, as in the Danish Adoption study, a stronger effect of biologic mothers than of biologic fathers and no relationship between adoptive parents and adoptees.

THE SIGNIFICANCE OF GENETIC INFLUENCES ON HUMAN OBESITY

Clearly genetic influences are major determinants of human obesity. But how are these influences exerted? Is human obesity determined at conception, like hair color

TABLE 4. *Correlation of residual body mass index adoptees and their biologic and adoptive parents*

Adoptee relatives	N	r^a
Daughters		
Biologic mother	123	0.40^b
Biologic father	62	0.18
Adoptive mother	161	0.06
Adoptive father	153	0.09
Sons		
Biologic mother	114	0.15
Biologic father	69	0.08
Adoptive mother	173	0.04
Adoptive father	164	−0.09

^{a}Pearson correlation, with age regressed out.
$^b p<0.001$.
From ref. 10.

and eye color? Can people do nothing to alter their fate? As far as obesity is concerned, are genes destiny?

The answer to all four questions is "No!" Obesity is not determined at conception. What is inherited is a liability that requires a suitable environment in order to be manifested. Our current understanding of this genetic liability provides no basis for personal despair or therapeutic nihilism. Countless formerly obese persons have shown how courage and determination can overcome even the most unpromising heritage. Increased understanding of genetic influences on human obesity will enable us to do even more. The first step is to identify people at increased risk and help them to cope in a more informed manner. Understanding their liability to obesity can be a prelude to better control. Prevention may well be the first activity to benefit from increased understanding of the genetics of human obesity.

A model proposed by Harry Harris (*personal communication*, May 1987) can help in understanding the nature of genetic vulnerability and environmental challenge. Figure 4 depicts this model, in which the small circle inside the larger one represents those with a genetic liability to a disorder. This area can be very small, as in the case of phenylketonuria, or very large, as in the case of scurvy to which all humans are vulnerable because of their inability to synthesize vitamin C. Our currents efforts are designed to determine the size of this circle for obesity. That 25% of Americans are obese suggests that this area may be quite large.

The wedge represents environmental circumstances that favor development of the disorder. Again, this area can be very small or very large. The environmental circumstances that contribute to obesity in the United States today are extensive and this area is a large one. Thus Americans consume a diet high in calories and expend few calories in physical activity. Our diet, in fact, has such a high fat content that it can produce obesity in genetically susceptible rats (4,11), and our labor-saving lifestyle is so efficient that we become obese on a diet that has 1,000 fewer calories per day than it did at the turn of the century.

Harris's model shows that the issue in human obesity is not one of heredity or environment, or heredity versus environment, but of heredity and environment, or

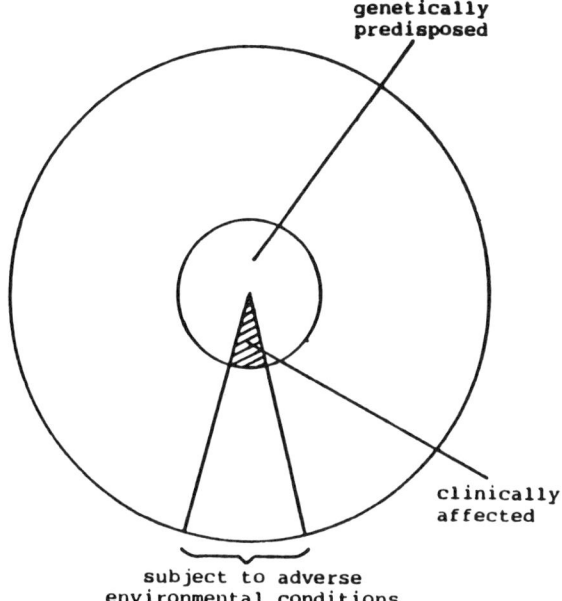

FIG. 4. Model showing the subset of the population that is affected by gene-environment interaction. See description in text.

genetic vulnerability and environmental challenge. This issue affects all of psychiatry, indeed all of medicine. It may well set the agenda for medical research for the foreseeable future. As so often in the past, research on obesity can serve as a model for understanding matters far beyond the field of obesity.

When we look more closely at the ways in which heredity and environment may influence the development of a trait such as obesity we see at least three different kinds of relationship: simple addition, interaction, and genetic control of exposure to the environment (7).

Additive Relationships

The Iowa adoption study (10) provides an example of a simple additive relationship, an environmental influence coexisting with a genetic influence. Even when the genetic effect was taken into account, there was also an environmental effect: adoptees who had been raised in a rural environment were more overweight than those who had been raised in an urban environment. The two types of influence did not interact statistically and presumably not genetically; they appeared to be simply additive. The effect was small and it could easily have been overlooked. That it was not is due to two factors. First is its theoretical importance and second the fact that it has just been replicated in a new study of Danish adoptees (14).

Interactive Relationships

A second type of relationship between heredity and environment is an interaction between them. Studies of experimental animals provide examples of such interaction in the case of obesity. Thus different strains of rats respond differently to the amount of fat in the diet. When receiving a high fat diet, some genetically vulnerable rats become very fat, whereas others with little genetic vulnerability show only a slight adiposity (4,11).

Sonne-Holm and Sørensen's (12) large-scale study of Danish draftees describes a phenomenon that is best explained by an interactive model. During a 30-year period there was no change in the average weight of these men, and for 17 years, from 1943 to 1960, the percentage who were severely obese remained constant at about 0.01%. Then, as shown in Fig. 5, in a 12-year period, during which the average body weight remained constant, there was a dramatic increase in the prevalence of severe obesity. In Copenhagen the rise was sevenfold, to 0.07%, and it was even greater in the less urban area adjacent to Copenhagen.

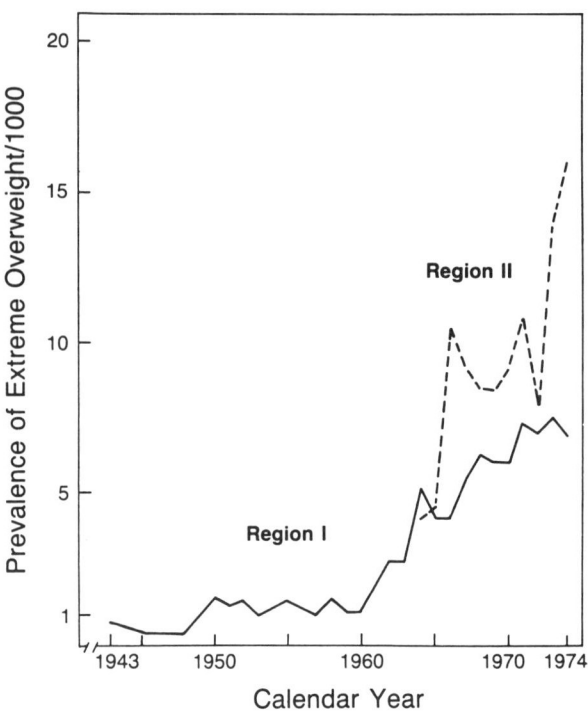

FIG. 5. Prevalence of severe overweight (body mass index of 31 or greater) in Danish young men in Region I (Copenhagen) and Region II (adjacent area of the island of Zealand). Note the rapid increase in prevalence beginning in the early 1960s. (Redrawn from data in ref. 12.)

It seems inconceivable that the Danish gene pool could have changed so much in such a short time. Far more likely is some change in the environment with a specific effect on a few genetically predisposed persons.

A recent analysis of the MZ twins of the American veterans sample described earlier provides support for an interactive relationship (9). A bivariate analysis of the body mass index of the MZ twins revealed an unexpected finding. The correlation in body mass index of normal weight twins was considerably higher than that for the overweight twins. This finding is illustrated in Fig. 6, with the distributions of MZ twins at age 20 on the left and at age 45 on the right. Each distribution is oriented with the upper tail facing the reader so that the overweight portion is clearly visible. The high correlation in body mass index of the twins is shown by the clustering of scores along the main diagonal. The finding of decreasing correlation is shown by the decreasing steepness of this ridge with increasing body weight. Quantitative estimates revealed that the intrapair correlation of twins in the first (thin and normal weight) distribution was 0.84 at age 20 and 0.77 at age 45. By contrast, the intrapair corrrelation of twins in the overweight distribution did not exceed 0.35. A decreasing concordance rate of MZ twins with increase in percentage overweight found in the American veterans sample also reflects the conclusion of the bivariate analysis; while the concordance for the prevalence of overweight in twins is high, the correlation in extent of overweight is low.

These findings suggest a model for the role of genes and environment in determining human obesity. Genetic influences may largely determine whether an individual becomes obese. Given this genetic vulnerability, it is environmental influences that determine how obese the person becomes.

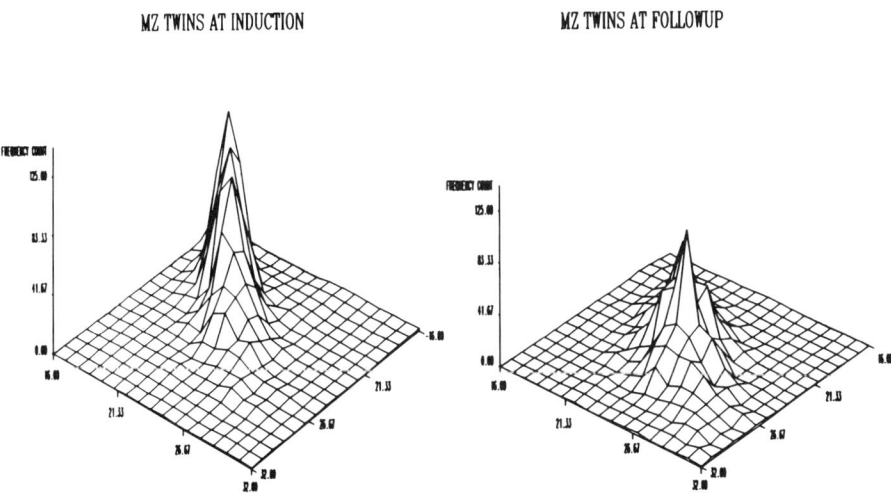

FIG. 6. Joint distribution of body mass index of MZ co-twins at age 20 and again at 45. (From ref. 9.)

Genetic Control of Exposure to the Environment

A third type of relationship between heredity and environment is one of genetic control of exposure to the environment. For example, bronchial carcinoma may show a strong familial aggregation and yet the bronchial mucosa of affected persons may be no more vulnerable to the carcinogens in cigarette smoke than is that of unaffected persons. Their differing liability to lung cancer may result from differing genetic vulnerabilities to addiction to nicotine. The bronchial mucosa may be nothing more than a hapless bystander.

An example of genetic control of exposure to the environment in human obesity is seen in the predisposition toward physical activity. Low physical activity may not cause obesity, but high physical activity could protect against it. Obese people may lack this protection because obese adults, and particularly obese women, are less active than are people of normal weight (3).

Another example of genetic control of exposure to the environment is the tendency for some persons to enter environments that foster overeating, particularly of foods with high fat content. We have noted the vulnerability of some genetically predisposed rats to diets high in fat (4,11). Some people are probably just as vulnerable, and some of them seem particularly likely to frequent environments rich in fatty foods. Such environments are provided by restaurants with "smorgasbord nights," during which customers can eat as much as they wish for a fixed price. Customers eat far more food on these nights than on nights when they must pay for each item of food separately, on an *à la carte* basis. Significantly, on smorgasbord nights there are two to three times more obese customers than there are on *à la carte* nights (15) (Fig. 7).

It is important to note that obese people did not eat more than nonobese people,

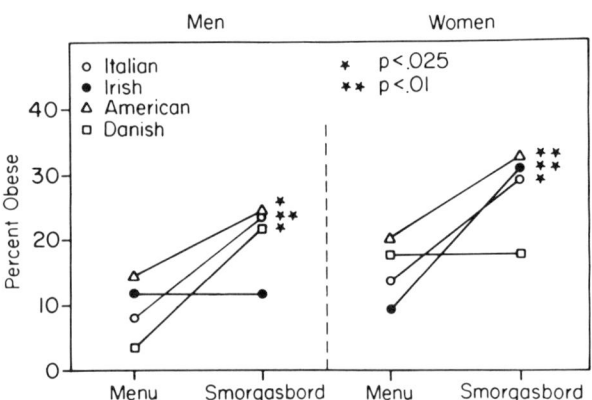

FIG. 7. Percentage of obese people at four restaurants under two conditions of food service. Significantly more obese men and women were present under smorgasbord conditions than under traditional menu service conditions. (From ref. 15.)

either on smorgasbord nights when everyone overate or on *à la carte* nights when very few people overate. Obese people were simply more likely to be found in environments that facilitated overeating.

SUMMARY AND CONCLUSIONS

Surprisingly, until the very recent past almost nothing had been known about genetic influences on human obesity. The powerful genetic effects described with such assurance in the textbooks were based almost entirely on extrapolation from animal studies. The first strong evidence of genetic influence on *human* obesity was obtained from an adoption study in Denmark that showed a high correlation of the body mass index of adoptees with that of their biological parents and no correlation with that of their adoptive parents. The body mass index of the adoptees was also highly correlated with that of their siblings and showed evidence of recessive transmission. These findings have been extended by a twin study that revealed very high heritabilities at both age 20 and age 45. A bivariate analysis of the identical twins of this population revealed high intrapair correlations among the normal weight twins and low correlations among the obese twins distributions, suggesting a strong environmental influence on the genetically vulnerable obese twins. The best estimate of heritability, the correlation coefficient of 93 identical twin pairs reared apart, from the Swedish Adoption Study of Aging, revealed high levels of heritability, indicating that traditional twin studies have overestimated the heritability of body mass index only slightly, if at all.

GLOSSARY

Nonadditive genetic variance Involves dominance (interactions between alleles at a locus) and epistasis (interactions among alleles at different loci).
Additive genetic variance The extent to which genes that influence a trait sum according to gene dosage.
Commingling analysis A type of segregation analysis that looks for differences in distributions in a population.
Heritability A measure of the extent to which a phenotype is influenced by the genotype.

REFERENCES

1. Bray, G. A., and York, D. A. (1979): Hypothalamic and genetic obesity in experimental animals: an autonomic and endocrine hypothesis. *Physiol. Rev.*, 59:719–809.
2. Cederlof, R., and Lorich, U. (1978): The Swedish Twin Registry. In: *Twin Research: Part C. Biology and Epidemiology*, edited by W. E. Nance, W. Allen, and P. Parisi, pp. 188–195. Allan R. Liss, New York.
3. Chirico, A. M., and Stunkard, A. J. (1960): Physical activity and human obesity. *N. Engl. J. Med.*, 263:935–940.

4. Cruce, J. A. F., Greenwood, M. R. C., Johnson, P. R., et al. (1974): Genetic versus hypothalamic obesity: studies of intake and dietary manipulation in rats. *J. Comp. Physiol. Psychol.*, 87:295–301.
5. Falconer, D. S. (1981): *Introduction to Quantitative Genetics*, 2nd ed., p. 113. Longman, New York.
6. Hrubec, Z., and Neel, J. V. (1978): The National Academy of Sciences—National Research Council Twin Registry: ten years of operation. *Prog. Clin. Biol. Res.*, 24:153–172.
7. Kendler, K. S., and Eaves, L. J. (1986): Models for the joint effect of genotype and environment on liability to psychiatric illness. *Am. J. Psychiatry*, 143:279–289.
8. Pedersen, N. L., Friberg, L., Floderus-Myrhed, B., McClearn, G. E., and Plomin, R. (1984): Swedish early separated twins: identification and characterization. *Acta Genet. Med. Gemollol. (Romo.)*, 33:243–250.
9. Price, R. A., and Stunkard, A. J. (1989): Commingling analysis of obesity in twins. *Hum. Hered.*, 39:121–135.
10. Price, R. A., Cadoret, R. J., Stunkard, A. J., and Troughton, E. (1987): Genetic contributions to human fatness: an adoption study. *Am. J. Psychiatry*, 144:1003–1008.
11. Sclafani, A. (1980): Dietary obesity. In: *Obesity*, edited by A. J. Stunkard, pp. 166–181. W. B. Saunders, Philadelphia.
12. Sonne-Holm, S., and Sorensen, T. I. A. (1977): Post-war course of the prevalence of extreme overweight among Danish young men. *J. Chronic Dis.*, 30:351–358.
13. Sorensen, T. I. A., Price, R. A., Stunkard, A. J., and Schulsinger, F. (1989): Genetics of obesity in adult adoptees and their biological siblings. *Br. Med. J.*, 298:87–90.
14. Sorensen, T. I. A., Teasdale, T. W., and Stunkard, A. J. (1990): Genetic and early environmental components in sociodemographic influences on adult body fatness. *Br. Med. J.*, 300:1615–1618.
15. Stunkard, A. J., and Mazer, A. (1978): Smorgasbord and obesity. *Psychosom. Med.*, 40:173–175.
16. Stunkard, A. J., Foch T. T., and Hrubec, Z. (1986): A twin study of human obesity. *JAMA*, 256:51–54.
17. Stunkard, A. J., Sorensen, T. I. A., Hanis, C., et al. (1986): An adoption study of human obesity. *N. Engl. J. Med.*, 314:193–198.
18. Stunkard, A. J., Harris, J., Pedersen, N., and McClearn, R. E. (1990): The body-mass index of twins who have been reared apart. *N. Engl. J. Med.*, 322:1483–1487.

Genes, Brain, and Behavior, edited by
P. R. McHugh and V. A. McKusick.
Raven Press, Ltd., New York © 1991.

The Genetics of Alcoholism

Donald W. Goodwin

Department of Psychiatry, Kansas University Medical Center, Kansas City, Kansas 66103

DEFINITION

There are numerous definitions of alcoholism. According to Charles Jackson, author of *The Lost Weekend*, "The alcoholic is a person who can take it or leave it, so he takes it." This may sound frivolous but actually captures two important features of alcoholism: denial and rationalization. It also conveys the gallows humor that alcoholics often engage in when talking about their illness.

For research purposes the *Diagnostic and Statistical Manual of the American Psychiatric Association* (DSM-III-R) (9) provides operational criteria for *alcohol dependence* (a term widely favored in official circles to alcoholism). As summarized in Table 1, these criteria are essential for research purposes but less useful clinically where clinical judgment rather than symptom-counting provides the best guidelines for treatment. By and large, the APA criteria can be condensed to a single sentence: *Alcoholism involves a compulsion to drink, causing injury to one's self and others*. The critical word is "compulsion," which suggests that addictive drinking is not entirely volitional—a view met with skepticism by many, including many physicians. In any case, this is what is meant by alcoholism when the term is used in this chapter. Some of the studies reviewed used operational criteria and some did not, but a clinical judgment that the person was alcoholic was made in each case. (There probably is a good deal of overlap between operational criteria and clinical judgment, although this has been little studied.)

RISK FACTORS

The etiology of alcoholism is not known. In Western European countries about 1 in 10 drinkers, at some point in their life, consume alcohol in amounts that usually causes damage to self or others and involves an element of compulsion (13). The selection process whereby 10% of drinkers, more or less, become alcoholic is not known. However, there is general agreement about the existence of risk factors. These include:

Sex. Men alcoholics outnumber women alcoholics by a factor of five to one (Some say three to one, but the facts favor the former figure.)

TABLE 1. *Diagnostic criteria for alcohol dependence*

Three or more manifestations required for diagnosis:
1. Alcohol often taken in larger amounts or over a longer period than intended
2. persistent desire or one or more unsuccessful efforts to control alcohol use
3. much time spent in activities necessary to get alcohol, taking the substance, or recovering from its effects
4. frequent intoxication or withdrawal symptoms when expected to fulfill role obligations at work, school, or home, (e.g., does not go to work because hung over, goes to school or work intoxicated, or intoxicated while taking care of his or her children), or when alcohol use is physically hazardous (e.g., drives when intoxicated)
5. important social, occupational, or recreational activities given up or reduced because of alcohol
6. continued alcohol use despite a recurrent social, psychological, or physical problem that is caused or exacerbated by the use of the substance
7. marked tolerance: need for increased amounts of the substance to achieve desired effect, or diminished effect with continued use of the same amount
8. characteristic withdrawal symptoms
9. alcohol often taken to relieve withdrawal symptoms

Adapted from ref. 9.

This gender differential apparently has existed throughout history and in all cultures. The explanation is unknown. Cultural factors are usually given credit for the difference, but, based on informal surveys by the author, more women than men are physiologically intolerant of alcohol. This intolerance, like the later described Oriental flush, may protect many women from becoming alcoholic.

Family history. Alcoholism runs in families, as will be discussed in the next section.

Ethnic background. Jewish people have a relatively low rate of alcoholism, and the Irish a high rate. Alcoholism appears to be more prevalent in northern parts of Western Europe than in southern climates. The French have a high cirrhosis rate compared to other Western European countries, but it is not clear whether the alcoholism rate is equally high. In short, cultural and ethnic differences are associated with different rates of alcoholism and medical consequences of drinking. These are difficult to attribute to genetic factors.

Vocation. Alcoholism is unevenly distributed among occupational groups. Bartenders and fiction writers have high rates, while ministers have a low rate. Judging from cirrhosis data, physicians have a relatively low rate of alcoholism.

Americans who have won the Nobel Prize for literature have a phenomenally high rate. Seven Americans have won the award, five of whom were alcoholic, for a rate of alcoholism of 71% (12). (The alcoholic writers were O'Neill, Faulkner, Hemingway, Lewis, and Steinbeck. The nonalcoholics were Pearl Buck and Saul Bellow.)

HEREDITY AND ALCOHOLISM

Three types of evidence support the possibility that heredity may contribute to alcoholism: family studies, adoption studies, and twin studies.

Family Studies

Alcoholism runs in families. An estimated 20% to 25% of sons of alcoholics become alcoholic and about 5% of the daughters (7). Estimates of the rate of alcoholism in the general population vary widely, but the rates for first-degree relatives of alcoholics are severalfold higher than most population estimates. Along with gender, a family history of alcoholism represents the strongest known risk factor for alcoholism.

Similarly, about 20% to 25% of male siblings of alcoholics become alcoholic and about 5% of female siblings. The observation that alcoholism runs in families dates to classical times and is one of the most documented facts in the field of substance abuse.

Not everything that runs in families is inherited. Languages, for example, run in families. For many years it was believed that alcoholism was "learned" in the same way that languages were learned. Twin and adoption studies tend to challenge this belief.

Adoption Studies

Studying adoptees is one way to separate nature from nurture. If there is alcoholism in the biological parents and the disorder has a partial genetic basis, one would predict that children of alcoholics adopted in infancy by nonalcoholics would still have a relatively high rate of alcoholism. Four such studies have been conducted.

The first by Roe (26) found no difference between children of alcoholics and children of nonalcoholics when both groups had been raised by adoptive parents who presumably were not alcoholic. There were no alcoholics in either group. The sample size was small and it was not clear that the biological parents would be classified as alcoholic today. Many had a history suggestive of antisocial personality. Also, the adoptees were young at the time they were studied and many had not entered the age of risk for alcoholism.

The 1970s saw a renewed interest in biological factors in alcoholism. Three adoption studies were conducted in three countries: Denmark, Sweden, and the United States (Iowa) (1,4,10). Although methodologically dissimilar, the three studies came to similar conclusions:

1. Grown-up children of alcoholics raised by nonalcoholic adoptive parents continued to have a high rate of alcoholism—about as high as that found in children of alcoholics raised by alcoholic parents.
2. Having an alcoholic biological parent apparently did not increase the risk of the adoptees having other psychiatric disorders.

In the Danish study, four groups of individuals were interviewed: sons and daughters of alcoholic parents who were adopted-out and raised by nonalcoholic, unrelated, adoptive parents, and their brothers and sisters raised by the alcoholic parent (13). No difference in alcoholism rates in same-sex siblings were found.

Nor did the adopted-out children of alcoholics have elevated rates of other psychiatric pathology compared to controls (adopted-out children of nonalcoholics). Daughters of alcoholics, when raised at home by their alcoholic biological parent, had an elevated risk of depression (11). Alcoholism ran true to type. Having an alcoholic parent did not even increase the chance of the adopted-out offspring being classified as heavy drinkers.

The Swedish (1) and Iowa studies (4) initially reported similar findings. In the Swedish study, criminality in the biological parents did not predict criminality in the offspring, nor did alcoholism predict criminality. The data were reanalyzed by Cloninger et al. (6) who identified environmental factors (e.g., income) as important in one group of adoptees but not in the other. In the first group (called Type-I alcoholism) both sexes were susceptible to what seemed a rather mild form of alcoholism and heredity seemed relatively unimportant. In Type-II alcoholism, men were mainly susceptible and there was a strong history of alcoholism in the biological parents. Also, Cloninger et al. reported that Type-II alcoholism was associated with antisocial personality.

Originally, the Iowa study also found that alcoholism ran true to type, that is, a family history of alcoholism in the biological parents did not increase the likelihood of other psychiatric illnesses occurring in the adopted-out offspring. Further study found a tendency for the adopted-out children to misuse drugs and also found that alcoholism in the adoptive parents somewhat raised the chance of alcoholism occurring in their adopted children (5). At present, the issue remains unclear about whether alcoholism in parents increases the chance of other psychiatric disorders occurring in their adopted-out offspring. Later in this chapter the concept of two alcoholisms will be examined further.

Twin Studies

Single-egg monozygotic twins share the same DNA and presumably have identical susceptibility to genetic illnesses. Twin-egg dizygotic twins share a familial susceptibility to genetic illnesses to the extent to which they share the same genes.

Four twin studies have examined drinking patterns and alcohol dependence. A Swedish study (17) found that identical twins were more concordant for alcoholism than fraternal twins. A large Finnish study (24) found similarities of drinking patterns, but no difference between identical and fraternal twins regarding "loss of control" (believed by some to be the *sine qua non* of alcoholism). However, there was a discrepancy in concordance rates for younger twins, with young identical twins more likely to be concordant for alcoholism than young fraternal twins. A review of Veterans Administration records in the United States lent support to a genetic factor (16), finding that identical twins were more often concordant for alcoholism than fraternal twins. Finally, an ongoing study in England has failed so far to find differences between identical and fraternal twins with respect to alcoholism (21).

Like the adoption studies, most of the twin data are consistent with the presence of genetic factors in alcoholism, but there are exceptions, and the relative importance of environmental and genetic factors remains to be ascertained.

TWO ALCOHOLISMS

Jack London, describing his own alcoholism, said there were two forms of alcoholism, a congenital and acquired form (19). He believed he had the acquired form. Thus the notion that alcoholism comes in two types—a familial and nonfamilial type—dates back many years. The idea was resurrected in the 1980s and has resulted in studies in which alcoholics with a family history of alcoholism are compared to alcoholics without such a history.

One consistent finding emerges. Familial alcoholism has an earlier onset than nonfamilial alcoholism (13). Most studies also find that familial alcoholism is particularly severe and difficult to treat. Here the agreement ends. One set of studies (10) suggest that familial alcoholism is "primary," meaning it is not usually accompanied by other psychiatric disorders. Other studies suggest that familial alcoholism is associated with adult antisocial personality and conduct disorder in adolescence (25,27). The conflict between these findings remains unresolved.

In work by Cloninger and associates (6), mentioned earlier, a reanalysis of Swedish adoption data suggested that alcoholism could be divided into two types. According to Cloninger's classification, Type-II alcoholism affects mainly men, involves a strong family history of alcoholism (particularly among males), has an early onset, and is associated with antisocial personality. Except for the latter feature, his Type-II alcoholism closely resembles what is described as familial alcoholism. His Type-I alcoholism involves a weaker family history of alcoholism, affects both sexes, and seems influenced by such environmental factors as poverty and low educational level. It is not clear whether this type corresponds to nonfamilial alcoholism or represents a heterogeneous group of alcohol abusers, many of whom perhaps would not be called alcohol dependent using current research criteria.

WHAT IS INHERITED?

The evidence presented above suggests that genetics may influence so-called familial or Type-II alcoholism. The mode of transmission remains speculative.

One aspect of alcoholism is definitely inherited: millions of people are physiologically intolerant of alcohol and thus largely "protected" from becoming excessive drinkers. After small amounts of alcohol, these people become ill. Adverse reactions to alcohol are most commonly seen in Orientals (28). Two-thirds or more of Orientals develop a cutaneous flush somewhat resembling measles or the hives after ingesting one drink or less. The so-called "Oriental flush" is accompanied by nausea and tachycardia, plus a marked disinclination to drink more alcohol. Oriental infants, given minute amounts of alcohol, also develop a cutaneous flush. Unquestionably the reaction is genetically determined (14). Among Caucasian men, only a few (perhaps 1% or 2%) develop a similar reaction. Thus most Caucasian men are relatively unprotected from becoming alcoholic. To this extent, alcoholism can definitely be said to be influenced by heredity. A larger proportion of Caucasian women appear to be physiologically intolerant—perhaps as many as 50%. Some develop a cutaneous flush; others feel dizzy or have a headache. Whatever the adverse reaction is, it may contribute to the lower rate of alcoholism among women than men.

SEROTONIN THEORY

A genetic tendency of alcoholism probably involves more than the protection provided by genetically determined adverse reactions. In general, two biochemical models have been proposed explaining why some individuals become alcoholic and most do not. One postulates a biochemical deficiency, the other an overproduction of "addictive substances."

Persons with a genetic propensity for alcoholism may be deficient in certain forms of biochemical activity required for optimal well-being. These persons, given available alcohol, a suitable culture, and an absence of countervailing traits, might discover that alcohol temporarily corrects this hypothetical deficiency, producing an intensity of mood change foreign to those without the deficiency. The model then requires that alcohol would have a biphasic effect, causing subsequent underactivity of the reward system.

There is some evidence that alcohol has a biphasic effect on serotonin metabolism that might correspond to the deficiency model (18). Alcohol appears to increase serotonergic activity during acute intoxication followed by a reduction of serotonin activity to subnormal levels during the postintoxication period. The "deficient" person then would have two reasons for drinking. He would first drink to correct the deficiency and then continue to drink to correct for an even greater deficiency resulting from the biphasic effect of alcohol on serotonin. Biochemically, this might explain the "addictive cycle" in which a person initially drinks to feel good and then later drinks to stop feeling bad from the substance that originally made him feel good. Evidence for the theory includes the following:

1. Animals bred to have a high preference for alcohol have lower levels of serotonin in the limbic system and centers regulating emotion than do animals bred to have a low preference for alcohol (20).

2. Alcoholics who first begin having symptoms before age 20 and have a family history of alcoholism have lower serotonin activity, as measured by a tryptophan-amino-acid ratio, than do people who become alcoholic after the age of 20 without a family history of alcoholism (3). This supports the proposal that there are two forms of alcoholism—one with an early onset and a family history of alcoholism and a second, perhaps more heterogeneous group of alcoholics, without a family history in whom genetic factors are relatively unimportant.

3. Pharmacologic agents have been developed for the treatment of depression that have a highly selective effect on serotonin activity. By blocking the reuptake of serotonin released into the synaptic cleft, more serotonin becomes available for postsynaptic receptors. Serotonin reuptake blockers cause reduced drinking in experimental animals (29) and, in three double-blind, placebo-controlled studies (23), reduce drinking in nondepressed heavy drinkers.

Thus, increasing evidence points to serotonin as having a critical role in consumption of alcohol and perhaps alcoholism.

THE ALKALOID THEORY

There is also the overproduction model. This theory holds that a genetic propensity to alcoholism involves the overproduction of substances that in some way facilitate addiction. For example, alcohol produces minute amounts of morphine-like compounds in the brain (8). One study found these compounds in the spinal fluid of alcoholics in greater quantities after alcohol ingestion than in nonalcoholics (2). Rats and monkeys drink increased amounts of alcohol when these substances are injected into the brain (22). Thus, the possibility exists that the genetic defect in alcoholism involves a reduced capacity of the brain to oxidize aldehydes, resulting in the overproduction of morphine-like alkaloid compounds (aldehyde condensation products), which may facilitate alcohol addiction.

OTHER THEORIES

Space does not permit elaboration on other theories explaining a possible role of genetic factors in alcoholism. These involve a variety of neurotransmitters, including norepinephrine and dopamine, prostaglandins; endorphins; and calcium channels associated with the benzodiazepine-GABA complex. At the present time none of these theories has as much supporting evidence as the serotonin theory, but this may change with further study.

REFERENCES

1. Bohman, M. (1978): Some genetic aspects of alcoholism and criminality: a population of adoptees. *Arch. Gen. Psychiatry*, 35:269–276.
2. Borg, S., Kvande, H., Magnusson, E., and Sjoquist, B. (1980): Salsolinol and salsoline in cerebrospinal lumbar fluid of alcoholic patients. *Acta Psychiatr. Scand. [Suppl.]*, 286:171–177.
3. Buydens-Branchey, L., Branchey, M. H., Noumair, D., and Lieber, C. S. (1989): Age of alcoholism onset: II. Relationship to susceptibility to serotonin precursor availability. *Arch. Gen. Psychiatry*, 46:231–236.
4. Cadoret, R. J., Cain, C. A., and Grove, W. M. (1979): Development of alcoholism in adoptees raised apart from alcoholic biologic relatives. *Arch. Gen. Psychiatry*, 37:561–563.
5. Cadoret, R. J., O'Gorman, T. W., Troughton, E., and Heywood, E. (1984): Alcoholism and antisocial personality: interrelationships, genetic and environmental factors. *Arch. Gen. Psychiatry*, 42:161–167.

6. Cloninger, C. R., Bohman, M., and Sigvardsson, S. (1981): Inheritance of alcohol abuse: cross-fostering analysis of adopted men. *Arch. Gen. Psychiatry*, 36:861–868.
7. Cotton, N. S. (1979): The familial incidence of alcoholism: a review. *J. Stud. Alcohol*, 40:89–116.
8. Davis, V. E., and Walsh, M. J. (1970): Alcohol, amines and alkaloids: a possible biochemical basis for alcohol addiction. *Science*, 167:1005–1007.
9. *Diagnostic and Statistical Manual of Mental Disorders* (Third Edition—Revised) (1987): The American Psychiatric Association, Washington, D.C.
10. Goodwin, D. W., Schulsinger, F., Hermansen, L., Guze, S. B. and Winokur, G. (1973): Alcohol problems in adoptees raised apart from alcoholic biological parents. *Arch. Gen. Psychiatry*, 28:238–242.
11. Goodwin, D. W., Schulsinger, F., Knop, J., Mednick, S., and Guze, S. B. (1977): Alcoholism and depression in adopted-out daughters of alcoholics. *Arch. Gen. Psychiatry*, 34:751–755.
12. Goodwin, D. W. (1988): *Alcohol and the Writer*. Andrews and McMeel, New York.
13. Goodwin, D. W. (1988): *Is Alcoholism Hereditary?* Ballantine, New York.
14. Harada, S., Agarwah, D. P., and Goedde, H. W. (1981): Aldehyde dehydrogenase deficiency as cause of facial flushing reaction to alcohol in Japanese. *Lancet*, 1:982.
15. Hesselbrock, V. M., Stabenau, J. R., Hesselbrock, M. N., Mayer, R. E., and Babor, T. F. (1982): The nature of alcoholism in patients with different family histories for alcoholism. *Neuro-Psychopharmacol. Biol. Psychiatry*, 6:607–614.
16. Hrubec, A., and Omenn, G. S. (1981): Evidence of genetic predisposition to alcoholic cirrhosis and psychosis: twin concordances for alcoholism and its biological end points by zygosity among male veterans. *Alcoholism Clin. Exp. Res.*, 5:207–215.
17. Kaij, L. (1960): *Studies on the Etiology and Sequels of Abuse of Alcohol*. University of Lund, Lund, Sweden.
18. Kent, T. A., Campbell, J. R., and Goodwin, D. W. (1985): Blood platelet uptake of serotonin in men alcoholics. *J. Stud. Alcohol.*, 46:357–359.
19. London, J. (1982): John Barleycorn. In: *Novels and Social Writings*. Macmillan, New York.
20. McBride, W. J., Murphy, J. M., Lumeng, L., and Li, T. K. (1989): Serotonin and ethanol preference. In: *Recent Developments in Alcoholism*, edited by M. Galanter, Vol. 7. Plenum Press, New York.
21. Murray, R. M., and Gurlin, C. C. (1983): Twin and alcoholism studies. In: *Recent Developments in Alcoholism*, edited by M. Galanter, Vol. 1. Gardner Press, New York.
22. Myers, R. D., McCaleb, M. L., and Ruwe, W. D. (1982): Alcohol drinking induced in the monkey by tetrahydropapaveroline (THP) infused into the cerebral ventricle. *Pharmacol. Biochem. Behav.*, 16:995–1000.
23. Naranjo, C. A., Sellers, E. M., Sullivan, J. T., Woodley, D. V., Kadlec, K., and Sykora, K. (1987): The serotonin uptake inhibitor citalopram attenuates ethanol intake. *Clin. Pharmacol. Ther.*, 41:266–274.
24. Partanen, J., Bruun, K., and Markkanen, T. (1977): Inheritance of drinking behavior: a study on intelligence, personality, and use of alcohol of adult twins. In: *Emerging Concepts of Alcohol Dependence*, edited by E. M. Pattison, M. B. Sobell, L. C. Sobell. Springer, New York.
25. Penick, E., Read, M., Crowley, P., and Powell, B. (1978): Differentiation of alcoholics by family history. *J. Stud. Alcohol*, 39:1944–1948.
26. Roe, A. (1944): The adult adjustment of children of alcoholic parents raised in foster homes. *Q. J. Stud. Alcohol*, 5:378–393.
27. Tarter, R. (1981): Minimal brain dysfunction as an etiological predisposition in alcoholism. In: *Evaluation of the Alcoholic: Implications for Research, Theory and Practice*, edited by R. Meyer, J. O'B. Glueck, T. Babor, J. Jaffe, and J. Stabenau. Research Monograph 5, U.S. Dept. of Health and Human Services, Washington, D.C.
28. Wolff, P. H. (1972): Ethnic differences in alcohol sensitivity. *Science*, 175:449–450.
29. Zabik, J. E., Binkerd, K., and Roache, J. D. (1985): Serotonin and ethanol aversion in the rat. In: *Research Advances in New Psychopharmacological Treatments for Alcoholism*, edited by C. A. Naranjo and E. M. Sellers. Elsevier Science, New York.

Subject Index

A

Abortion, spontaneous
  chromosome abnormality-related, 26,27, 29,30
  45, X-related, 27
  X-linked inheritance-related, 59
Acetylcholine, 87
Acetylcholinesterase, 87,91
N-Acetylglucosamine-6-sulfatase gene, 6
Achondroplasia, 53
a-Actinin, 124
Adenosine triphosphate (ATP), synthesis, 101
Adoption study
  alcoholism, 169,221–222
  antisocial behavior, 189
  behavioral genetics, 167
  bipolar affective disorder, 153,154
  obesity, 209–211,212
  personality, 168
  schizophrenia, 138,169
Affective disorder
  bipolar, 153–164
    adoption studies, 153,154
    assortative mating, 160,161
    biological markers, 155
    chromosome 5 marker, 141,142–143
    cohort effect, 160
    diagnostic misclassification, 159–161
    family studies, 153,157–159
    genetic markers, 155–159
    Huntington's disease-related, 182,183, 184–189,190
    incidence, 153
    linkage analysis, 157,158–160,161–162
    multifactorial-polygenic transmission, 154
    Parkinson's disease-related, 187
    single major focus transmission, 154
    twin studies, 153–154,169
    X-linkage, 156,158–159,161–162
  functional, 187
  unipolar, 187,188
Agnosia, Alzheimer's disease-related, 131
Albumin gene, 13
Alcohol intolerance, 223–224
Alcoholism
  aldehyde dehydrogenase marker, 176

definition, 219
genetics, 220–225
  adoption studies, 169,221–222
  alkaloid theory, 225
  familial alcoholism, 223–224
  family studies, 221
  serotonin theory, 224–225
  twin studies, 169,206,222–223
incidence, 219
nonfamilial, 223
occupational factors, 220
risk factors, 219–220
Aldehyde dehydrogenase, 176
Allele
  definition, 39
  of genetic markers, 137–138
  HbS, 49
  Mendel's law regarding, 47–48
  mutant, 8,10,48
    lethal, 51,53,56,57,58–59
  recessive, IQ and, 171–172
  recombination frequency, 156
  segregation, 48. *See also* Segregation analysis
  wild-type, 48
Alpha-6-iduronidase deficiency, 6
Alzheimer's disease
  autosomal dominant inheritance, 130–135
  dementia of, 79,129,131–132
  Down's syndrome relationship, 79, 86–88,133
    amyloid precursor protein, 93–94
    nerve growth factor, 92–93
    neuropeptide expression, 94–95
    trisomy 16 mouse model, 90–95,96
  familial, 79–81
    chromosome 21 loci, 79–81
    DNA marker, 79
    linkage analysis, 79–81
  familial risk, 130,131–132,133–135
  gene, 130,133,135,156–157
  genetic heterogeneity, 133
  genetic subtypes, 133
  incidence, 129,130
  linkage analysis, 79–81
  neuropathology, 79–80,87,93–94,130–131

Alzheimer's disease (contd.)
  parental age factor, 132–133,134–135
  phenotype, 130–131,133
  trisomy 21 and, 129,133
  twin studies, 129
Amish
  autosomal recessive inheritance, 55,56
  inbred populations, 3
  linkage study, 157–158,161,172–173
Amnesia, Alzheimer's disease-related, 130,131
Amylase, gene loci, 14
Amyloid plaque, 79,87,131
Amyloid precursor protein, 93–94
  gene, 79–80
Amyloid protein, 87–88
Anaphase, 44
Anemia
  hemolytic, 6–7
  sickle cell, 8,10,49,175
Aneuploidy
  causes, 26
  mental retardation and, 85
  of sex chromosomes, 27
  as somatic mosaic, 59–60
Angelman syndrome, 31,32
Anorexia, 169
Anticipation, 54
Antisocial behavior
  behavioral genetics research, 169
  Huntington's disease-related, 181,188,189
Anxiety disorder, 169
Aphasia, Alzheimer's disease-related, 131
Apolipoprotein, gene loci, 15
Apraxia, Alzheimer's disease-related, 131
Artificial selection, 166–167
Ashkenazi Jews, 10,11
Association study, 175
Assortative mating, 160,161
Ataxia
  Friedreich, 54
  ocular myopathy-related, 107
Attention deficit disorder, 169
Autism, 169
Autosomal dominance. See Dominance, autosomal
Autosomal recessive. See Recessiveness, autosomal
Autosome, 26

B

Beckwith-Wiedemann syndrome, 31
Behavior, as phenotype, 165
Behavioral genetics, 165–179
  cognitive ability, 168
  definition, 165
  methods, 166–167,176–177
  molecular biology and, 174–176
  multiple genes, 170–174
  nongenetic factors, 170
  personality, 168
  psychopathology, 168–170
  theory, 166
Bellow, Saul, 220
Beta-galactosidase deficiency, 6
Biochemical genetics, 1
Birth cohort effect, 54,160
Blood-brain barrier, 125
Blood group, as genetic marker, 156
  AB, 53
  Duffy, 11,12,14
  Xg, 16
Body mass index, heritability, 206–211,212,214–215,217
Brain
  in Alzheimer's disease
    amyloid plaque, 131
    amyloid precursor protein, 79–80,93–94
    neurofibrillary tangle, 79,131
  in Down's syndrome, 85–88
    amyloid precursor protein, 93–94
    nerve growth factor, 92–93
    neuropeptide expression, 94–95
    trisomy 16 mouse model, 90–95,96
  dystrophin localization, 123
  dystrophin-related protein, 125
B3 protein, 124–125
Buck, Pearl, 220

C

Cancer
  acquired chromosomal changes, 29–30
  chromosome theory, 18
Candidate gene analysis, 157
  behavioral genetics applications, 176
  schizophrenia, 143–147
Carbamazepine, as mania treatment, 184
Catechol-o-methyltransferase, 155
Centromere, 20,21
Cerebellum, in Down's syndrome, 86
Cerebrum, in Down's syndrome, 86
Character, 8,47
Charcot-Marie-Tooth disease, 53,56,58
Chiasma, 43,44
Choline acetyltransferase
  in Alzheimer's disease, 87
  in trisomy 16 mouse, 91–92,93
Cholinergic neuron
  in Alzheimer's disease, 87
  in Down's syndrome, 87,88
    nerve growth factor, 92–93
    in trisomy 16 mouse, 90–93
Chorea, Huntington's disease-related, 76,182
Chromatin, 19,20–21

SUBJECT INDEX

Chromosome(s)
  classification, 21
  crossing-over, 42–43,44
  mitochondrial, 63–64. *See also*
      Deoxyribonucleic acid (DNA),
      mitochondrial
  number, 19,20,26
    abnormal, 26–27
    homologue pairs, 39
    random distribution, 40
    recombination, 40–41,48
  structure, 19,20–21
    abnormal, 27–29
Chromosome abnormalities, 19,26–30
  cancer-related, 29–30
  deletion, 28,29
    dystrophin gene, 122
    length mutations, 11
  duplication, 28,29
    length mutations, 11
  frequency, 30
  inversion, 28
  isochromosome, 28
  numerical, 26–27
  ring, 28
  structural, 27–29
    frequency, 30
  translocation, 28–29
    Robertsonian, 29
Chromosome banding, 19,21–25
  C-banding, 22,23,25
  G-banding, 23,24,25
  Q-banding, 22,23
  R-banding, 23
Chromosome 1
  gene map, 14
  heterochromatin, 20
Chromosome 2, Burkitt's lymphoma-related
      translocation, 30
Chromosome 4
  Huntington's disease loci, 13,76–78
  short-arm deletion, 28
Chromosome 5
  bipolar affective disorder locus, 141,
      142–143
  major depression locus, 141
  psychosis locus, 141
  schizoaffective disorder locus, 141
  schizophrenia locus, 137,139–143,173
  short-arm deletion, 28
Chromosome 6, B3 protein, 124
Chromosome 7, isodisomy, 61
Chromosome 8, Burkitt's lymphoma-related
      translocation, 30
Chromosome 9
  heterochromatin, 20
  pericentric inversion, 28
  Philadelphia chromosome and, 29

Chromosome 11
  gene map, 15
  linkage analysis, 157–158
  major-depressive illness locus, 172
Chromosome 11q23, 145–146
Chromosome 12, phenylalanine hydroxylase
      locus, 194
Chromosome 14, Burkitt's lymphoma-related
      translocation, 30
Chromosome 15
  distamycin staining, 23
  gene map, 16
  reading ability linkage, 172
Chromosome 16
  Duffy blood group locus, 12
  haptoglobin locus, 12
  heterochromatin, 20
Chromosome 17, von Recklinghausen NF-I
      locus, 65
Chromosome 21. *See also* Trisomy 21
  Alzheimer's disease locus, 79–81,129,133
  Burkitt's lymphoma-related translocation, 30
  Philadelphia chromosome and, 29
Chromosome X. *See also* X-linkage
  heterochromatin, 21
Chromosome XX, 26
Chromosome XXX, 27
Chromosome XXY, 27
Chromosome XY, 26
  crossing-over, 42
Chromosome XYY, 27
Chromosome Y. *See also* Y-linkage
  distamycin staining, 23
  heterochromatin, 20
  testis-determining factor, 1
Chronic obstructive pulmonary disease, twin
      study, 169
Clinical genetics
  definition, 2
  principles, 65–69
c-myc oncogene, 30
Codominance, 53
Coffin-Lowry syndrome, 58
Cognitive function
  genetic basis, 168
  in Huntington's disease, 181,182,183,
      185–186
  in Parkinson's disease, 187
  recessive alleles, 171–172
  twin study, 168
Cohort effect, 54,160
Collagen, type-1, 7
Color blindness
  as bipolar affective disorder marker, 159
  gene locus, 16
Commingling analysis, 217
Conduct disorder, Huntington's disease-
      related, 188–189

Consanguinity, 55
Contiguous gene syndromes, 31
Cortex
  in Down's syndrome, 86,87
  in Huntington's disease, 184–186,188
  in Parkinson's disease, 186,188
Cri du chat syndrome, 28
Crossing-over, chromosomal, 42–43,44
Cystathionine beta-synthase deficiency, 68
Cystic fibrosis
  gene, 157
    locus, 13
    mutations, 69
    size, 13
  isodisomy and, 61
Cytogenetics, historical background, 1–2
Cytoskeleton
  dystrophin association, 123–124
  proteins, 123–125

D

D_2 dopamine receptor gene, as schizophrenia candidate gene, 144–147
Deletion, 28,29
  dystrophin gene, 122
  muscular dystrophy-associated, 11
Delusions, Huntington's disease-related, 183–184
Dementia
  Alzheimer's disease-related, 79,129, 131–132
  retinitis pigmentosa-related, 104
Deoxyribonuclease (DNase) I, hypersensitive sites, 20
Deoxyribonucleic acid (DNA)
  genomic, 20
  hybridization
    in situ, 11–12,24–25
    subtractive, 175
  iatrogenic lesions, 9–10
  markers, 11
  methylation, 63
  mitochondrial, 101–119
    ATP production, 101–102
    chromosome, 63–64
    oxidative phosphorylation diseases, 102–109, 112–116
    oxidative phosphorylation genes, 109–112
  mutation detection, 53
  polymorphism, 176,177
    detection, 75
  recombination
    chromosomal crossing-over and, 42–43,44
    genetic marker alleles, 137–138
    genetic variance and, 41,42–43,44

replication, 42
structure, 8
of tumors, 18
Depression
  Huntington's disease-related, 183,186
  major. *See* Major depressive illness
  Parkinson's disease-related, 187
  unipolar, 153,169,187. *See also* Affective disorder, bipolar
Diabetes mellitus, twin study, 169
Diagnostic and Statistical Manual-III
  alcohol dependence diagnostic criteria, 219,220
  psychiatric disorder diagnostic criteria, 182
Diakinesis, 43
Dietary factors, in obesity, 212,214,216–217
DiGeorge syndrome, 31
Diploidy, 40,42,45
Diplotene, 43
Disease
  classification, 4–6,49
  multifactorial, 59
Disomy, 48
  biparental, 62
  uniparental, 60–61,62–63
Dispermy, 26
Dominance, 7–8
  autosomal, 49–54
    Alzheimer's disease, 130–135
    anticipation, 53
    characteristics, 49–50
    codominance, 52
    germinal mosaicism, 51–52
    homozygosity, 52
    Huntington's disease, 181
    incomplete dominance, 52
    parental age effects, 50–51
    penetrance, 51–52
Dopamine hypothesis, of schizophrenia, 144–147
Dopaminergic neurons, of trisomy 16 mouse, 91
Down's syndrome. *See also* Trisomy 21
  Alzheimer's disease relationship, 79, 86–88,133
    amyloid precursor protein, 93–94
    nerve growth factor, 92–93
    neuropeptide expression, 94–95
    trisomy 16 mouse model, 90–95,96
  brain weight, 86
  chromosomal abnormalities, 85,88
  HSA 21, murine chromosome 16 homology, 88–90,94,96
  IQ, 85
  mental retardation and, 85
  neurogenesis abnormalities, 86

Robertsonian translocation, 29
  trisomy 16 mouse model, 90–95,96
DRD2 gene. *See* D$_2$ dopamine receptor gene
Drosophila, behavioral genetics, 167
Duplication, 28,29
  length mutations, 11
Dysgenesis, gonadal, 27,28
Dystrophin
  brain localization, 123
  as fusion protein, 123,124
  gene, 157
    deletions, 11,122
    locus, 13
    locus size, 122
    muscular dystrophy diagnostic application, 121
  neuromuscular disease and, 123–124
  related proteins, 124–125
  structure, 122–123
Dystrophin-binding proteins, 124,125
Dystrophy, myotonic, 63

E

Ectrodactyly, 52
Ehlers-Danlos syndrome, 7
Emotional disorders, Huntington's disease-related, 182,188–189
Enzymopathy, 8–11,48,49
  red cell, 6–7
Epilepsy, myoclonic, 64,104
Erythremia, 7
Ethnic factors, in alcoholism, 220,223–224
Euchromatin, 20–21
  staining, 22,23
Extraversion, 168

F

F$_2$ generation, 171,175–176
Factor VIII gene, 13
Fahr's syndrome, 187
Family study
  alcoholism, 221
  behavioral genetics, 167
  bipolar affective disorder, 153,157–159,169
  depression, 169
  DNA markers, 11
  schizophrenia, 138
Faulkner, William, 220
Finger protein, 59
5p syndrome, 24
45,X, 27
47,XXX, 27
47,XXY, 27
47,XYY, 27
49,XXXXX, 27

49,XXXY, 27
Fragile X syndrome, 30,171
Fusion proteins, 123,124

G

Galton, Francis, 165
Gamete, 40–41
Gametogenesis, 42
  disomy during, 61,62
  sex differences, 45
Gamma-aminobutyric acid (GABA)
  as bipolar affective disorder marker, 155
  neuron, 87,91,95
Gangliosidosis GM1, 6
Gene(s). *See also* specific genes
  first description of, 47
  identification methods, 3–4
  linked, 48. *See also* Linkage analysis
  mendelizing phenotypes, 3–4,8
  numbers, 13
    mapped, 12–13
  size, 13
  syntenic loci, 48
  unlinked, 48
Gene mapping, 1
  clinical applications, 17–18
  development, 11–18
  Huntington's disease, 76–78
  in situ hybridization and, 25
  schizophrenia, 137
    candidate genes, 145–146
Genetic compound, 56
Genetic influence, 166
Genetic marker. *See also* Linkage analysis
  alleles, 137–138
  in association studies, 175
  definition, 137
  polymorphism, 156
Genetics. *See also* Clinical genetics; Medical genetics; Mendelian genetics; Quantitative genetics
  definition, 2
  "reverse," 17
Genocopy, 66
Genomic imprinting. *See* Imprinting
Genomics, 17–18
Genotype, 40
Geriatric disease, segregation analysis, 129–130
Globin gene, 13
Globin gene α, 10,13
Globin gene β
  sickle cell locus, 69
  β-thalassemia mutation locus, 196
Glucocorticoid receptor gene, 139,140

Glucose-6-phosphate dehydrogenase deficiency, 159
Glucose metabolism, 187–188
Glutamate decarboxylate, 91,95
Goltz syndrome, 58
Gonads, dysgenesis, 27,28
Growth retardation, isodisomy and, 61
Gs-alpha protein, 10

H

Haploidy, 40,42,45
Happy puppet syndrome. *See* Angelman syndrome
Haptoglobin, locus map, 12
Height, heritability, 167
Hemingway, Ernest, 220
Hemoglobin
  Constant Spring, 10
  Grady, 11
  variant, 9
Hemoglobinopathy, 7
Hemophilia A, 11,52
Hemophilia B, 11
Heparan sulfate, 6
Heritability
  of body mass index, 206–211,212, 214–215,217
  definition, 206,217
Heterochromatin, 20–21,22
  in chromosomal inversion, 28
  chromosome banding, 22,23
  heteromorphism, 25–26
Heterogeneity, 48,66–69
  Alzheimer's disease, 133
  definition, 39
  detection methods, 67–69
  identification methods, 4–5
  neurologic diseases, 68
  nonpenetrance and, 53
  sexual reproduction basis, 45–46
Heteromorphism, 25–26
Heterozygosity, 48
  lethal alleles and, 57
Histone, 19,20
Histone proteins, 19,20
HLA, 156,176
Homeostasis, metabolic, 48–49
Homocystinuria, 67–69,133
Homozygosity, 48
  dominant phenotype and, 53
  incomplete dominance and, 53
Human genetics, definition, 2
Human Genome Project, 13,175
Huntington's disease
  animal models, 79
  autosomal dominant inheritance, 181
  chromosome 4 loci, 13

definition, 76
genes, 156–157
  candidate genes, 78–79
  chromosomal location, 76–78
  DNA markers, 76–79
  DNA polymorphisms, 77–78
  gene mapping, 76–78
  linkage analysis, 76,79–81,174
homozygosity, 53
imprinting and, 63
onset age, 76,181,183,184
parental factors, 132
pedigree, 50
psychopathology, 181–191
  affective disorder, 182,183,184–189,190
  antisocial conduct, 181,188,189
  clinical features, 181–182
  emotional disorders, 182,188–189
  mood disorders, 181,182,187
  as subcortical disorder, 181,182, 184–189,190
  racial factors, 182,184,187
  sporadic mutation and, 51
Hurler syndrome, 4,6
Hybridization
  in situ, 11–12,24–25
  somatic cell, 11,12
  subtractive, 175
Hypercholesterolemia, familial, 11,53
Hyperlipidemia, type-I, 11
Hypertension, twin study, 169
Hypoplasia, focal dermal, 58
Hypothalamus, in Down's syndrome, 87

I

Imprinting, 19,31–32,48,61,63
Inbred strains, 166–167
  single-gene transmission, 170–171
Insertion, length mutations, 11
Insulin gene, 15,158
Intelligence quotient (IQ)
  in Down's syndrome, 85
  in phenylketonuria, 171–172
  recessive alleles and, 171–172
  twin study, 168
Inversion, 28
Ischemic heart disease, twin study, 169
Isochromosome, 28
Isodisomy, 61,63
Israel, X-linkage study, 157,158–159

K

Karyotype, 21–26
Kearns-Sayre syndrome, 107,109
Kinetochore, 42
Klinefelter syndrome, 1,27

L

Langer-Giedion syndrome, 31
Learning disability, von Recklinghausen NF-I-related, 66
Leptotene, 43–44
Leukemia, chromosomal changes, 29,30
Lewis, Sinclair, 220
Linkage, 48
Linkage analysis
　Alzheimer's disease, 79–81
　Amish studies, 157–158,161,172–173
　bipolar affective disorder, 157, 158–160,161–162
　definition, 12,155
　genetic basis, 75
　Huntington's disease, 76,79–81,174
　large-pedigree studies, 174
　LOD score, 139,140,141,155–156
　principles, 155–156
　requirements, 142–143
　schizophrenia, 137–152
　　applications, 138
　　candidate marker gene studies, 143–147
　　chromosome 5 marker, 137,139–143
　　gene mapping, 137
　　genetic heterogeneity, 138,141,142,143
Lipoprotein lipase, gene insertion, 11
Lisch nodule, 65,66
Lithium, as mania treatment, 184
Lithium transport, as bipolar affective disorder marker, 155
LOD score, 155–156
　in schizophrenia, 139,140,141
Low density lipoprotein, receptor gene, 13
Lung cancer, 18
Lymphoma, Burkitt's, 30

M

Major depressive illness
　familial risk, 169
　penetrance, 141
　restriction fragment length polymorphism, 172
Major histocompatibility antigens. *See also* HLA
　codominance, 53
Mania
　Huntington's disease-related, 183,184
　Parkinson's disease-related, 187
Manic depressive illness. *See* Affective disorder, bipolar
Marfan's syndrome, 67–68,133
Maroteaux-Lamy syndrome, 4
Medical genetics
　advances in, 1–18

gene mapping, 11–18
molecular defects, 8–11
definitions, 2–3
Meiosis, 39–46
　genetic variance and, 39–46
　chromosomal random distribution, 40
　chromosomal recombination, 40–41
　mitosis comparison, 42
　nondisjunction, 42
　prophase, 43–45
　sex differences, 45
　stages, 41
　mutation during, 51
Memory, 168
Mendel, Gregor, 7–8
Mendelian disorders
　mapped genes, 13,17
　molecular defects, 8–11
　iatrogenic lesions, 9–11
Mendelian genetics, 1,47–59
　dominance, 7–8,48–54
　　autosomal, 49–54
　recessiveness, 48–49
　　autosomal, 54–57
　X-linkage, 57–59
　Y-linkage, 59
Mendelian Inheritance in Man, 3–8
Mendel's law, 1,3,47–48,166
Menopause, 45
Mental retardation
　aneuploidy-related, 85
　contiguous gene syndromes-related, 31
　Down's syndrome-related, 85
　multiple-gene transmission, 172
　phenylketonuria-related, 172,193
　von Recklinghausen NF-I-related, 66
Metabolism, inborn errors, 48. *See also* Mendelian disorders
Metaphase, 22,44
　chromosome banding, 22,23–24
Methemoglobinemia, 7
3-Methoxy-4-hydroxy phenylglycol, 87
Methylation, DNA, 63
Miller-Dieker syndrome, 31
Mitochondrial genes, neuromuscular disease and, 109–119
　chronic external ophthalmoplegia plus, 107–109,115
　Kearns-Sayre syndrome, 107,109
　Leber's hereditary optic neuropathy, 102–104,113
　ragged-red fiber disease, 64, 104–106,107,113,114
　retinitis pigmentosa, 104,107
Mitochondrial inheritance, 63–64
Mitosis, 42
　disomy during, 61,62

Molecular biology, behavioral genetics and, 174–176
Monoamine oxidase
  as bipolar affective disorder marker, 155
  gene loci, 16
Monosomy 21, 26
Monosomy X, 30
Mood disorders, Huntington's disease-related, 181,182,187
Morquio syndrome, 4,6
Mosaicism, 27,29
  Down's syndrome-related, 85
  germinal, 51–52,59,60
  somatic, 51,59–60
Motor disorders, Huntington's disease-related, 181–182,183,186
Mucopolysaccharidoses, 4,6
Multifactorial-polygenic transmission model, 154
Muscular dystrophy
  Becker
    dystrophin gene deletion, 11,122
    muscle biopsy, 121,123
    mutations, 69
    X-linked recessive inheritance, 121
  Duchenne
    diagnosis, 121
    dystrophin gene, 13,122–123,157
    dystrophin gene deletion, 11,122
    germinal mosaicism and, 52
    muscle biopsy, 121,123
    mutations, 69
    X-linked inheritance, 57,58,121
Mutation
  allele, 8,10,48
  lethal, 51,53,56,57,58–59
  detection, 53
  disease-producing, 13
  frequency, 51
  length, 11
  "loss of function," 75
  point, 10
  somatic, 51
  somatic mosaicism and, 60
  sporadic, 50–51
Myopathy
  distal, 53
  ocular, 106–109

N

Nature-nurture, 165
Neoplasia, somatic mutation and, 60
Nerve cell
  cholinergic, 87,88,90–93
  dopaminergic, 91
  dystrophin association, 123–124
  GABAergic, 87,91,95
  serotonergic, 87

Nerve growth factor, 92–93
Neurofibrillary tangle, 79,131
Neurofibroma, 65,66
Neurofibromatosis, 63,157
Neurologic disease. *See also* specific neurologic diseases
  adult-onset, 53
  genetic heterogeneity, 68
Neuromuscular disease. *See also* specific neuromuscular diseases
  dystrophin and, 123–124
  mitochondrial genes, 101–119
    ATP production, 101–102
Neuropathy, Leber's hereditary optic, 64, 102–104,113
Neuropeptide Y, 94–95
Neuroticism, 168
Neurotransmitters. *See also* specific neurotransmitters
  in alcoholism, 225
  in Down's syndrome, 87–88
  in trisomy 16 mouse, 90–95,96
Nobel Prize winners, alcoholics as, 220
Nondisjunction, 42
Nonmendelian inheritance, 59–64
  imprinting, 61,63
  mitochondrial inheritance, 63–64
  somatic mosaicism, 59–60
  uniparental disomy, 60–61,62–63
Nonpenetrance, 52–53,56
Norepinephrine, 87
Nosography (Faber), 4–5
Nosology, genetic, 4–8
Nucleosome, 20
Nucleus organizing region, 21
  staining, 22,23

O

Obesity
  adoption studies, 209–211,212
  dietary factors, 212,214,216–217
  gene, 210
  genetic-environmental factor interaction, 206,207–209,212–217
  parental factors, 211,212
  twin studies, 205–209,211,215,217
Occupational factors, in alcoholism, 220
O'Neill, Eugene, 220
Oncogene
  chromosome rearrangement and, 29–30
  c-myc, 30
  definition, 3
  Ha-ras-one, 158
Oocyte, 45,46
  germ-line mosaicism, 52
  mutation, 51
Ophthalmoplegia, chronic external plus, 107–109,115

"Oriental flush," 223–224
Osteogenesis imperfecta, 7,11
Ova, 40,45,46
Ovulation, 45
Oxidative phosphorylation, mitochondrial
  DNA and, 64,101–119
  ATP production, 101–102
  genes, 109–112
  oxidative phosphorylation diseases,
    102–109,112–116

P

Pachytene, 43,44
Pallidum, in Huntington's disease, 185,186
Parental factors
  Alzheimer's disease, 132–133,134–135
  Huntington's disease, 132
  obesity, 211,212
Parkinson's disease
  affective disorder and, 187
  depression and, 187
  mania and, 187
  prefrontal cortex in, 186
Penetrance, 52
Personality, 168
Phenotype, 47
  Alzheimer's disease, 130–131,133
  behavior as, 165
  definition, 8,165
  mendelizing, 3–4,8
  reverse genetics and, 17
Phenylalanine, conversion, 193
Phenylalanine hydroxylase gene. *See*
    Phenylketonuria, phenylalanine
    hydroxylase gene
Phenylketonuria
  biochemical basis, 193
  carrier screening, 200
  clinical basis, 193
  intelligence quotient, 171–172
  phenylalanine hydroxylase gene, 13,193
    alleles, 196–198,199,200
    cDNA, 193–194,195
    chromosome 12 locus, 194
    deletion, 194
    molecular structure, 194–195
    mutant haplotypes, 196–200
    point mutation, 10
    restriction fragment length polymorphism,
      195,196,197
  prenatal diagnosis, 195–196
Phenylpyruvate, 193
Philadelphia (Ph') chromosome, 29
Pisum sativum, 47
Pleiotropy, 48,65–66
Polar body, 45
Polymorphism, 176,177
  definition, 56,57

  detection, 75
  of genetic markers, 156
  or red cell enzymes, 6–7
Polyneuropathy, amyloid, 6
Polyploidy, 26,30
Polysomy, 27
Population association study, 175
Porphobilinogen deaminase gene, 145–146
Porphyria, acute intermittent, 145
Positron emission tomography (PET),
  186,187–188
Prader-Willi syndrome, 31
Pre-pro-somatostatin gene, 94,95
Prophase, 43–45
Protein
  cytoskeletal, 123–125
  defect identification, 75
  as genetic marker, 156
Pseudohypoparathyroidism, 10
Pseudodominance, 55–56
Psychopathology
  heritability, 168–170
  major-gene linkages, 172–173
Psychosis
  chromosome 5 marker, 141
  steroid, 139
Putamen, in Huntington's disease, 186,187

Q

Quantitative genetics
  methods, 166–167
  multiple genes, 170–174
Quantitative trait loci, 175
Quinacrine, as chromosome banding stain, 23

R

Racial factors, in Huntington's disease, 182,
    184,187
Ragged-red fiber disease, 64,104–106,107,
    113,114
Random drift, 57
Rapid-eye-movement sleep induction, 155
Reading ability, 172
Recessiveness, 7–8
  autosomal, 54–57
  characteristics, 54
Recombinant inbred strain method, 171
Recombination, 40–41,48
  chromosomal crossing-over and, 42–43,44
  genetic marker alleles, 137–138
  genetic variance and, 41,42–43,44
Reproductive fitness, 50
Restriction fragment length polymorphism, 156
  availability, 143
  complete genome map, 161
  development, 11

Restriction fragment length polymorphism (*contd.*)
  major-depressive illness, 172
  phenylketonuria, 195,196,197
  schizophrenia, 137
  sickle cell anemia, 175
Retinitis pigmentosa, 104,107
Retinoblastoma, 31,61
rRibonucleic acid (rRNA)
  gene site, 21
  mtDNA-coding, 101
tRibonucleic acid (tRNA), mtDNA-coding, 101

S

Sanfilippo syndrome, 4,6
Scheie syndrome, 4,6
Schizoaffective disorder, chromosome 5 marker, 141
Schizophrenia
  adoption studies, 138,169
  chromosome 5 marker, 173
  familial factors, 173
  family studies, 138
  gene, 138–139
  HLA marker, 176
  linkage analysis, 137–152
    applications, 138
    candidate marker gene studies, 143–147
    chromosome 5 marker, 137,139–143
    gene mapping, 137
    genetic heterogeneity and, 138,141,142,143
    requirements, 142–143
  nongenetic factors, 170
  psychopathology, 168–170
  twin studies, 138,169,170
Scoliosis, 65–66
Segregation, 48. *See also* Mendel's laws
Segregation analysis, 1
  family studies, 12
  geriatric disease, 129–130
  schizophrenia, 144–146
Selection, 56,57
Serotonergic neurons, in Alzheimer's disease, 87
Serotonin theory, of alcoholism, 224–225
Sex chromosomes, 26. *See also* Chromosome X; Chromosome Y
  abnormalities, 27,30
Sex factors, in alcoholism, 219–220,224
Sexual reproduction, as genetic heterogeneity basis, 45–46
Shakespeare, William, 165
Sib pair method, 156,161
  affected, 173–174
Sickle cell, β-globin locus, 69
Sickle cell anemia, 8,10,49,175

Sickle cell disease, 56
Sickle cell trait, 53
Single-gene transmission, 170–171
Single major focus transmission model, 154
Sister chromatid, 21
  chiasma, 43,44
  isochromosome, 28
  meiosis, 42
  mitosis, 42
  synaptonemal complex, 44
Sleep, REM, 155
Somatization disorder, 169–170
Somatostatin, 94–95
Spatial ability, 172
Spectrin, 124
Spermatid, 45
Spermatocyte, 45
  continuous cycling, 51
  germ-line mosaicism, 52
  mutation, 51
Spermatogonium, 45
Spermatozoa, 40,45,46
Steinbeck, John, 220
Stillbirth, chromosomal abnormality-related, 30
Striatum, in Huntington's disease, 76,78, 184–187
Subcortical disorder, Huntington's disease as, 181,182,184–189,190
Synaptonemal complex, 44

T

Tay-Sachs disease, 11
Telomere, 21
Telophase, 44
Temporal gyrus, in Down's syndrome, 86
Testes-determining factor, 1,59
Tetrad, 42,43
Tetraploidy, 26
Thalamus, in Huntington's disease, 185
Thalassemia, 7,10
Thrombasthenia, Glanzmann, 11
Thyroglobulin gene, 13
Trait, 47
Translocation, chromosomal, 28–29
  Robertsonian, 29
Transthyretin gene, 6
Tricyclic antidepressants, as affective disorder treatment, 184
Triploidy, 26
Trisomy
  as abortion cause, 26,27,30
  frequency, 26,27,30
Trisomy 8, 26,27
Trisomy 9, 26,27
Trisomy 13, 26,27,29,30
Trisomy 14, 29

Trisomy 15, 29
Trisomy 16, 27,39
Trisomy 16 (mouse), 90–95,96
Trisomy 18, 26,27
Trisomy 19 (mouse), 91
Trisomy 21, 26–27,30,85
  Alzheimer's disease and, 129,133
  discovery, 1
  Down's syndrome severity and, 60
Trisomy 22, 29,30
Troyer syndrome, 55
Trypsin, as chromosome banding stain, 23
Tumor
  DNA, 18
  von Recklinghausen NF-I-related, 65
  Wilm's, 31
Turner's stigmata, 27,28
Turner's syndrome
  historical background, 1
  isochromosome, 28
  karyotype, 24–25
Twin study
  alcoholism, 169,206,222–223
  Alzheimer's disease, 129
  behavioral genetics, 167
  bipolar affective disorder, 153–154,169
  chronic obstructive pulmonary disease, 169
  cognitive function, 168
  diabetes mellitus, 169
  hypertension, 169
  intelligence quotient, 168
  ischemic heart disease, 169
  obesity, 205–209,211,215,217
  personality, 168
  schizophrenia, 138,169,170
Tyrosinase, gene loci, 15
Tyrosine, 155,193
Tyrosine hydroxylase, gene, 15,158

V
Variability, 48
  additive, 217
  anticipation and, 54
  causes, 66,67
  classification, 66
  definition, 66
  genetic influence and, 166
  intraspecific, 167
  meiosis and, 39–46
    chromosomal random distribution, 40
    chromosomal recombination, 40–41
    mitosis comparison, 42
    nondisjunction, 42
    prophase, 43–45
    sex differences, 45
    stages, 41
  nonadditive, 217
  quantitative analysis, 174
Vesalius, Andreas, 1–2
von Recklinghausen NF-I, 65–66

W
Wilm's tumor, 31
Wilson's disease, 187
Wolf-Hirschhorn syndrome, 28,76
Writers, alcoholics as, 220

X
X chromosome. *See* Chromosome X
X-linkage, 57–59
  bipolar affective disorder, 156,158–159, 161–162

Y
Y chromosome. *See* Chromosome Y
Y-linkage, 59

Z
Zygote, 40,45
Zygotene, 43,44